ERECTILE DYSFUNCTION

A MEDICAL DICTIONARY, BIBLIOGRAPHY, AND ANNOTATED RESEARCH GUIDE TO INTERNET REFERENCES

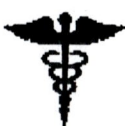

JAMES N. PARKER, M.D.
AND PHILIP M. PARKER, PH.D., EDITORS

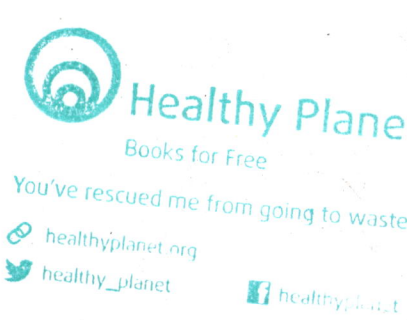

ICON Health Publications
ICON Group International, Inc.
4370 La Jolla Village Drive, 4th Floor
San Diego, CA 92122 USA

Printed in the United States of America.

Last digit indicates print number: 10 9 8 7 6 4 5 3 2 1

Publisher, Health Care: Philip Parker, Ph.D.
Editor(s): James Parker, M.D., Philip Parker, Ph.D.

Publisher's note: The ideas, procedures, and suggestions contained in this book are not intended for the diagnosis or treatment of a health problem. As new medical or scientific information becomes available from academic and clinical research, recommended treatments and drug therapies may undergo changes. The authors, editors, and publisher have attempted to make the information in this book up to date and accurate in accord with accepted standards at the time of publication. The authors, editors, and publisher are not responsible for errors or omissions or for consequences from application of the book, and make no warranty, expressed or implied, in regard to the contents of this book. Any practice described in this book should be applied by the reader in accordance with professional standards of care used in regard to the unique circumstances that may apply in each situation. The reader is advised to always check product information (package inserts) for changes and new information regarding dosage and contraindications before prescribing any drug or pharmacological product. Caution is especially urged when using new or infrequently ordered drugs, herbal remedies, vitamins and supplements, alternative therapies, complementary therapies and medicines, and integrative medical treatments.

Cataloging-in-Publication Data

Parker, James N., 1961-
Parker, Philip M., 1960-

Erectile Dysfunction: A Medical Dictionary, Bibliography, and Annotated Research Guide to Internet References / James N. Parker and Philip M. Parker, editors
                   p.   cm.
Includes bibliographical references, glossary, and index.
ISBN: 0-597-84210-8
1. Erectile Dysfunction-Popular works.   I. Title.

Disclaimer

This publication is not intended to be used for the diagnosis or treatment of a health problem. It is sold with the understanding that the publisher, editors, and authors are not engaging in the rendering of medical, psychological, financial, legal, or other professional services.

References to any entity, product, service, or source of information that may be contained in this publication should not be considered an endorsement, either direct or implied, by the publisher, editors, or authors. ICON Group International, Inc., the editors, and the authors are not responsible for the content of any Web pages or publications referenced in this publication.

Copyright Notice

Acknowledgements

The collective knowledge generated from academic and applied research summarized in various references has been critical in the creation of this book which is best viewed as a comprehensive compilation and collection of information prepared by various official agencies which produce publications on erectile dysfunction. Books in this series draw from various agencies and institutions associated with the United States Department of Health and Human Services, and in particular, the Office of the Secretary of Health and Human Services (OS), the Administration for Children and Families (ACF), the Administration on Aging (AOA), the Agency for Healthcare Research and Quality (AHRQ), the Agency for Toxic Substances and Disease Registry (ATSDR), the Centers for Disease Control and Prevention (CDC), the Food and Drug Administration (FDA), the Healthcare Financing Administration (HCFA), the Health Resources and Services Administration (HRSA), the Indian Health Service (IHS), the institutions of the National Institutes of Health (NIH), the Program Support Center (PSC), and the Substance Abuse and Mental Health Services Administration (SAMHSA). In addition to these sources, information gathered from the National Library of Medicine, the United States Patent Office, the European Union, and their related organizations has been invaluable in the creation of this book. Some of the work represented was financially supported by the Research and Development Committee at INSEAD. This support is gratefully acknowledged. Finally, special thanks are owed to Tiffany Freeman for her excellent editorial support.

About the Editors

James N. Parker, M.D.

Dr. James N. Parker received his Bachelor of Science degree in Psychobiology from the University of California, Riverside and his M.D. from the University of California, San Diego. In addition to authoring numerous research publications, he has lectured at various academic institutions. Dr. Parker is the medical editor for health books by ICON Health Publications.

Philip M. Parker, Ph.D.

Philip M. Parker is the Eli Lilly Chair Professor of Innovation, Business and Society at INSEAD (Fontainebleau, France and Singapore). Dr. Parker has also been Professor at the University of California, San Diego and has taught courses at Harvard University, the Hong Kong University of Science and Technology, the Massachusetts Institute of Technology, Stanford University, and UCLA. Dr. Parker is the associate editor for ICON Health Publications.

About ICON Health Publications

To discover more about ICON Health Publications, simply check with your preferred online booksellers, including Barnes&Noble.com and Amazon.com which currently carry all of our titles. Or, feel free to contact us directly for bulk purchases or institutional discounts:

ICON Group International, Inc.
4370 La Jolla Village Drive, Fourth Floor
San Diego, CA 92122 USA
Fax: 858-546-4341
Web site: **www.icongrouponline.com/health**

Table of Contents

FORWARD

In March 2001, the National Institutes of Health issued the following warning: "The number of Web sites offering health-related resources grows every day. Many sites provide valuable information, while others may have information that is unreliable or misleading."[1] Furthermore, because of the rapid increase in Internet-based information, many hours can be wasted searching, selecting, and printing. Since only the smallest fraction of information dealing with erectile dysfunction is indexed in search engines, such as **www.google.com** or others, a non-systematic approach to Internet research can be not only time consuming, but also incomplete. This book was created for medical professionals, students, and members of the general public who want to know as much as possible about erectile dysfunction, using the most advanced research tools available and spending the least amount of time doing so.

In addition to offering a structured and comprehensive bibliography, the pages that follow will tell you where and how to find reliable information covering virtually all topics related to erectile dysfunction, from the essentials to the most advanced areas of research. Public, academic, government, and peer-reviewed research studies are emphasized. Various abstracts are reproduced to give you some of the latest official information available to date on erectile dysfunction. Abundant guidance is given on how to obtain free-of-charge primary research results via the Internet. **While this book focuses on the field of medicine, when some sources provide access to non-medical information relating to erectile dysfunction, these are noted in the text.**

E-book and electronic versions of this book are fully interactive with each of the Internet sites mentioned (clicking on a hyperlink automatically opens your browser to the site indicated). If you are using the hard copy version of this book, you can access a cited Web site by typing the provided Web address directly into your Internet browser. You may find it useful to refer to synonyms or related terms when accessing these Internet databases. **NOTE:** At the time of publication, the Web addresses were functional. However, some links may fail due to URL address changes, which is a common occurrence on the Internet.

For readers unfamiliar with the Internet, detailed instructions are offered on how to access electronic resources. For readers unfamiliar with medical terminology, a comprehensive glossary is provided. For readers without access to Internet resources, a directory of medical libraries, that have or can locate references cited here, is given. We hope these resources will prove useful to the widest possible audience seeking information on erectile dysfunction.

The Editors

---

[1] From the NIH, National Cancer Institute (NCI): **http://www.cancer.gov/cancerinfo/ten-things-to-know**.

CHAPTER 1. STUDIES ON ERECTILE DYSFUNCTION

Overview

In this chapter, we will show you how to locate peer-reviewed references and studies on erectile dysfunction.

The Combined Health Information Database

The Combined Health Information Database summarizes studies across numerous federal agencies. To limit your investigation to research studies and erectile dysfunction, you will need to use the advanced search options. First, go to **http://chid.nih.gov/index.html**. From there, select the "Detailed Search" option (or go directly to that page with the following hyperlink: **http://chid.nih.gov/detail/detail.html**). The trick in extracting studies is found in the drop boxes at the bottom of the search page where "You may refine your search by." Select the dates and language you prefer, and the format option "Journal Article." At the top of the search form, select the number of records you would like to see (we recommend 100) and check the box to display "whole records." We recommend that you type "erectile dysfunction" (or synonyms) into the "For these words:" box. Consider using the option "anywhere in record" to make your search as broad as possible. If you want to limit the search to only a particular field, such as the title of the journal, then select this option in the "Search in these fields" drop box. The following is what you can expect from this type of search:

- **Gene Therapy: Future Therapy for Erectile Dysfunction**

  Source: Current Urology Reports. 2(6): 480-487. December 2001.

  Contact: Current Science, Inc. 400 Market Street, Suite 700, Philadelphia, PA 19106 (800) 427-1796. Fax (215) 574-2225. E-mail: info@current-reports.com. Website: http://www.current-reports.com.

  Summary: Advances in molecular biological techniques, completion of the Human Genome Project, and the ensuing age of molecular medicine, in conjunction with the sum of a decades-long accumulation of knowledge of the physiology of erection and the pathophysiology of erectile dysfunction (ED, formerly called impotence) have converged to make gene therapy for ED a distinct possibility. This report highlights the goals and strategies of gene therapy for erectile dysfunction and reviews the strategies that initially have been employed. Both the intrinsic complexities of mechanisms responsible for ensuring normal erection and the multifactorial nature of ED ensure that there is a relatively vast number of physiologically relevant molecular targets for gene therapy. The authors note that virtually every preclinical gene therapy strategy or target examined thus far has been largely successful in easing conditions associated with compromised erectile function in vivo or in vitro. While this preclinical data is quite preliminary in many regards, the results are nonetheless quite impressive and encouraging. If similar success is obtained in clinical trials, gene therapy for ED may provide the first concrete 'proof of concept' for using gene therapy in the treatment of human smooth muscle disorders. 3 figures. 2 tables. 25 references.

- **Smoking and Erectile Dysfunction: How Strong a Link?**

Source: Contemporary Urology. 15(3): 34, 36-38, 40. March 2003.

Contact: Available from Medical Economics Publishing Inc. Montvale, NJ 07645. (800) 432-4570.

Summary: Although the exact effect of smoking on penile function remains unclear, numerous studies suggest a correlation between smoking and erectile dysfunction (ED, formerly called impotence). This article examines what is currently known, and what remains to be discovered, about this link. ED is defined as the inability to achieve and maintain a penile erection sufficient for sexual intercourse. Topics include the physiology of erection, clinical evidence linking smoking and ED, the effect of smoking cessation, epidemiological evidence, and the interplay of smoking and oral pharmacotherapy (notably with sildenafil, Viagra). The authors conclude that more basic science and clinical investigation is necessary to ascertain the exact effects that smoking has on erectile function. 1 table. 28 references.

- **Erectile Dysfunction: The Role of Concomitant Diseases**

Source: Physician Assistant. 24(6 Supplement): 12-16. June 2000.

Contact: Available from Springhouse Corporation. Physician Assistant Journal, 1111 Bethlehem Pike, P.O. Box 908, Springhouse, PA 19477-0908. (215) 628-7758 or (800) 783-4903. Website: www.pajournal.com.

Summary: An estimated 20 to 30 million men and their partners are affected by erectile dysfunction (ED). However, patients and health care providers can often be uncomfortable discussing the subject. Understanding the causes of ED, which can range from alterations in the hemodynamics of penile blood flow to hormonal imbalances, can be helpful in dispelling the embarrassment and discomfort surrounding this disorder. Written for physician assistants, this article reviews the causes and concomitant diseases associated with ED, as well as the importance of early recognition and patient education. Hypertension (high blood pressure), arteriosclerosis (deposits of plaque in the arteries, causing 'hardening'), and lipid disorders are frequently associated with ED. Diabetes can affect the microvasculature (small blood vessels) of the nerves that regulate blood flow to and from the penis. Medications used to treat common diseases such as hypertension, cardiovascular disorders, and depression can precipitate ED, as can medications used for decongestion and appetite suppression. The causes of ED are categorized in three groups: organic, psychogenic, and mixed (organic and psychogenic). Psychogenic causes of ED include depression, anxiety, stress related disorders, religious orthodoxy, obsessive compulsive disorder, anhedonia, sexual phobias, and sexual deviance. The author stresses that if the clinician can identify an erectile problem early, psychosocial sequelae such as embarrassment, anxiety, self doubt, depression, withdrawal from relationships, divorce, or other problems may be averted. One table lists common drugs that can affect erectile function; another table reprints a five item sexual health inventory for men. 3 tables. 10 references.

- **Association of Type and Duration of Diabetes with Erectile Dysfunction in a Large Cohort of Men**

  Source: Diabetes Care. 25(8): 1458-1463. August 2002.

  Contact: Available from American Diabetes Association. 1701 North Beauregard Street, Alexandria, VA 22311. (800) 232-3472. Website: www.diabetes.org.

  Summary: Differences in risk of erectile dysfunction (ED, formerly called impotence) by characteristics of diabetes among older men are not well understood. This article reports on a large prospective cohort study that examined the association of type and duration of diabetes with erectile function in men older than 50 years of age. Subjects included 31,027 men aged 53 to 90 years who were in the Health Professionals Follow Up Study cohort. On a questionnaire mailed in 2000, participants rated their ability (without treatment) in the past 5 years to have and maintain an erection sufficient for intercourse. Men who reported poor or very poor function were considered to have ED. Diabetes information was ascertained via self-report and documented with supplementary medical data. Men with diabetes had an age-adjusted relative risk of 1.32 for having ED compared with men without diabetes. In analyses, men with type 1 and type 2 diabetes were at a significantly higher risk for ED than nondiabetic men. Men with type 2 diabetes had an increasingly greater risk of ED with increased duration since diagnosis. The authors conclude that, for men over age 50 years, increasing duration of diabetes was positively associated with increased risk of ED relative to men without diabetes. This association persisted despite the higher prevalence of other comorbid conditions. ED prevention and diabetes management efforts are likely to be appropriate together. 1 figure. 3 tables. 44 references.

- **Patient with Erectile Dysfunction: Psychological Issues**

  Source: Nurse Practitioner. 25(Supplement 6): 11-13. June 2000.

  Contact: Available from Nurse Practitioner. Circulation Department, P.O. Box 5053, Brentwood, TN 37024-5053. (800) 490-6580. Fax (615) 377-0525.

  Summary: Erectile dysfunction (ED) affects as many as 30 million men and their partners in the United States. Although clinicians now recognize that as many as 80 percent of ED cases have organic origins, psychological issues remain important. This article explores the psychological issues that may be involved. The author encourages health care providers to take the opportunity to begin discussions of ED with their patients. These discussions must be broader than simply focusing on the penis, but should take into account the entire range of interactions that affect sexual functions, including medical, psychological, and social conditions. Health care providers should be aware of the difficulties many patients have in discussing ED and endeavor to keep their own difficulties with sexual topics from affecting patient care. Treatment must be integrative, involving the partner as well. The article includes a five item sexual health inventory for men that can be a useful tool in initiating a conversation between health care provider and patient. 1 table. 9 references.

- **Sildenafil for Treatment of Erectile Dysfunction in Men with Diabetes: A Randomized Controlled Trial**

  Source: JAMA. Journal of the American Medical Association. 281(5): 421-426. February 3, 1999.

  Summary: Erectile dysfunction (ED) is common in men with diabetes. This article reports on a study undertaken to assess the efficacy and safety of oral sildenafil citrate (Viagra) in the treatment of erectile dysfunction in men with diabetes. The 1996 study involved 268 men (mean age, 57 years) with erectile dysfunction (mean duration, 5.6 years) and diabetes (mean duration, 12 years). Patients were randomized to receive sildenafil (n = 136) or placebo (n = 132) as needed, but not more than once daily, for 12 weeks. Patients took the study drug or placebo 1 hour before anticipated sexual activity. The starting dose of sildenafil citrate was 50 mg, with the option to adjust the dose to 100 mg or 25 mg based on efficacy and tolerability, to be taken as needed. The outcome measure was self reported ability to achieve and maintain an erection for sexual intercourse according to the International Index of Erectile Function and adverse events. Two hundred and fifty two patients (94 percent) completed the study (131 of 136 in the sildenafil group, 121 of 132 in the placebo group). At 12 weeks, 74 (56 percent) of 131 patients in the sildenafil group reported improved erections compared with 13 (10 percent) of 127 patients in the placebo group. The proportion of men with at least 1 successful attempt at sexual intercourse was 61 percent for the sildenafil groups versus 22 percent for the placebo group. Adverse events related to treatment were reported for 22 (16 percent) of the patients taking sildenafil and 1 (1 percent) of the patients receiving placebo. The most common adverse events were headache, dyspepsia, and respiratory tract disorder, predominantly sinus congestion or drainage. The authors conclude that oral sildenafil is an effective and well tolerated treatment for erectile dysfunction in men with diabetes. 2 figures. 4 tables. 24 references. (AA-M).

- **Status of Gene Therapy for Erectile Dysfunction**

  Source: Contemporary Urology. 14(10): 14, 16, 21-22, 25, 28, 30-31. October 2002.

  Contact: Available from Medical Economics Publishing Inc. Montvale, NJ 07645. (800) 432-4570.

  Summary: Erectile dysfunction (ED) is defined as the inability of a man to attain or maintain an erection long enough to complete sexual intercourse. Although medical therapy with sildenafil citrate (Viagra, Pfizer) acts by enhancing smooth muscle function, it is effective in only 50 to 65 percent of patients with ED. This article reviews the status of gene therapy for erectile dysfunction. The concept of up-regulating the function of erection-promoting enzymes is simply termed gene therapy. The authors review gene therapy for the treatment of ED, highlighting those genes that are involved in the normal process of cavernosal smooth muscle relaxation of the penis and, more specifically, those involved with the production of nitric oxide (NO), the chemical mediator of penile erections. Topics include penile structure and erectile physiology, how gene therapy works and why the penis is a likely target, current gene therapies in research or clinical application, and future directions. One sidebar offers an editorial comment on this subject. 1 figure. 1 table. 43 references.

- **Preliminary Observations of Sildenafil Treatment for Erectile Dysfunction in Dialysis Patients**

  Source: American Journal of Kidney Diseases. 37(1): 134-137. January 2001.

Contact: Available from W.B. Saunders Company. Periodicals Department, 6277 Sea Harbor Drive, Orlando, FL 32887-4800. (800) 654-2452 or (407) 345-4000.

Summary: Erectile dysfunction (ED, formerly called impotence) is common in dialysis patients. This article reports the authors' experience with sildenafil citrate (Viagra) in patients who are undergoing dialysis therapy. Male subjects attending the Outpatient Dialysis Unit at the University of Pennsylvania who were prescribed sildenafil by their primary physician or nephrologist were asked to complete the International Index of Erectile Function before their first dose of sildenafil and after at least 4 weeks of therapy. Subjects' mean age was 50.3 years (plus or minus 14.63 years). Ninety-three percent of the subjects were black. Based on a global efficacy question, 66.7 percent of the subjects believed that treatment had improved their erections. Subjects reported no increase sexual desire despite experiencing a significant increase in erectile function, orgasmic function, and satisfaction with intercourse. The authors summarize that sildenafil was well tolerated in a selected group of patients who reported improved sexual function with no major adverse effects. The authors stress that as advances are made to improve survival on hemodialysis therapy, improvement in quality of life should also be of utmost importance and should include an evaluation for ED. 1 table. 19 references.

- **Self-Esteem and Depression in Men Who Present with Erectile Dysfunction**

Source: Urologic Nursing. 18(3): 185-187, 208. September 1998.

Contact: Available from Society of Urologic Nurses and Associates, Inc. East Holly Avenue, Box 56, Pitman, NJ 08071-0056. (609) 256-2335. E-mail: suna@ajj.com.

Summary: Erectile dysfunction always has a psychologic component in addition to the underlying physical cause. This article reports on a study in which the extent of depression and reduced self esteem in patients who present with erectile dysfunction (ED) are investigated. Clinic patients diagnosed with ED during August and September of 1996 were asked to complete two test instruments; a total of 15 men agreed to participate anonymously. ED was defined as an inability to achieve an erection satisfactory for sexual intercourse due to organic factors as determined by two parameters: subjectively by a patient reported lack of morning erections on first waking; and objectively by low or negligible nocturnal erections as measured by Rigiscan. The results validate earlier work on the link between depression and ED with the subjects showing significant depression. In addition, the study demonstrates these men are lower in self esteem than the general population. The nurse should use this knowledge of depression and low self esteem as a guide when interviewing a patient with ED. Many treatment modalities for ED involve multiple office visits and continued erectile failure until a satisfactory response is achieved. Understanding the depth of depression on first presentation can often aid the nurse in preparing the patient for possible additional failure until the adoption of a successful treatment regimen. 9 references. (AA-M).

- **Health Outcomes Variables Important to Patients in the Treatment of Erectile Dysfunction**

Source: Journal of Urology. 159(5): 1541-1547. May 1998.

Summary: Erectile dysfunction is underreported and the rate of noncompliance with therapy is high. The National Institutes of Health Consensus Conference on Impotence endorsed the need for outcomes research of the various approaches to treatment. This article reports on an exploratory study undertaken to begin that process by identifying erectile dysfunction treatment outcome variables that are important to men. The study format consisted of focus group meetings. The goal of the discussions was to identify variables that are important to men when choosing among and judging the success of treatments for ED. After discussion, participants were asked individually to identify the 10 variables they considered important and to rank the 5 most important variables. An importance score reflecting group consensus was calculated for each variable. Success and negative outcomes were identified as the 2 most important outcome variables for all treatment modalities. Participants defined success in several ways. The most important measures were cure, pleasure, and partner satisfaction. Negative outcome was defined as negative consequences associated with treatment. The authors conclude that understanding the issues and outcomes important to ED patients is necessary to increase compliance with treatment and, thereby, increase the success of treatment for this widespread condition. Appendices list patient definitions and examples of success outcome measurements. 2 appendices. 6 tables. 8 references. (AA-M).

- **Oral Phentolamine as Treatment for Erectile Dysfunction**

  Source: Journal of Urology. 159(4): 1214-1216. April 1998.

  Contact: Available from Lippincott Williams and Wilkins. 12107 Insurance Way, Hagerstown, MD 21740. (800) 638-3030 or (301) 714-2334. Fax (301) 824-7290.

  Summary: For most patients with erectile dysfunction (impotence), oral agents are a preferred treatment option. Oral or buccal phentolamine has been shown to produce full erections in impotent subsets of study populations. This article reports on a study undertaken to evaluate the efficacy of oral phentolamine. After a comprehensive evaluation, 44 patients with recent onset (less than 3 years) of erectile dysfunction and a high likelihood of organogenic etiology underwent a prospective, double blind, placebo controlled trial with oral phentolamine after placebo. After placebo, 4 of 44 patients who reported full erections were excluded from study. Of the 40 patients in the double blind phase full erections were achieved by 2 of 10 with placebo, and 3 of 10 with 20 mg, 5 of 10 with 40 mg, and 4 of 10 with 60 mg phentolamine. There were no serious complications observed during the study, and only a single minor side effect occurred in 1 patient after 60 mg phentolamine. The authors conclude that oral phentolamine may be of benefit for the treatment of erectile dysfunction. 21 references.

- **Sildenafil Citrate for Treatment of Erectile Dysfunction in Men With Type 1 Diabetes**

  Source: Diabetes Care. 26(2): 279-284. February 2003.

  Contact: Available from American Diabetes Association. 1701 North Beauregard Street, Alexandria, VA 22311. (800) 232-3472. Website: www.diabetes.org.

  Summary: In 5 to 10 percent of men with type 1 diabetes, erectile dysfunction (ED) may be a particularly common and unwanted complication. This study focuses on the effects of sildenafil (Viagra) in men with type 1 diabetes and ED. A total of 188 patients were entered into a double-blind, placebo-controlled, parallel-group, flexible-dose study and were randomized to received sildenafil (n = 95) or placebo (n = 93) for 12 weeks. Efficacy was evaluated using questions three (Q3; achieving an erection) and four (Q4; maintaining an erection) from the International Index of Erectile Function (IIEF), a global efficacy question (GEQ) and a patient event log of sexual activity. Improvements in mean scores from baseline to end of treatment for IIEF Q3 (35.7 percent versus 19.9 percent) and Q4 (68.4 percent versus 26.5 percent) were significant in patients receiving sildenafil compared with those receiving placebo. Moreover, the percent of improved erections (GEQ, 66.6 versus 28.6 percent) and successful intercourse attempts (63 percent versus 33 percent) was significantly increased with sildenafil compared with placebo.

Improvements in sexual function were seen irrespective of the degree of ED severity. Adverse events were generally mild to moderate in severity, with headache (20 percent versus 8 percent), flushing (18 percent versus 3 percent), and dyspepsia (8 percent versus 1 percent) reported more often in the sildenafil than in placebo-treated patients. The authors conclude that treatment with sildenafil for ED was effective, resulting in an increased percentage of successful attempts at intercourse, and was well tolerated among men with type 1 diabetes. 2 figures. 2 tables. 32 references.

- **Viagra Revolution: Drug for Erectile Dysfunction is Redefining Our Ideas About Sexuality Among Older Couples (editorial)**

Source: Geriatrics. 53(10): 8-9. October 1998.

Contact: Available from Advanstar Communications. 131 West First Street, Duluth, MN 55802-2065. (888) 527-7008. Fax (218) 723-9437.

Summary: In this editorial, the author compares the impact of Viagra (sildenafil citrate) on older persons to the impact of the birth control pill on younger persons in the 1960's. The author considers how the popularity of Viagra may redefine general ideas about sexuality as an intimate expression in later life. The author notes that Viagra is neither an aphrodisiac nor a love potion for relationships in distress. It is a vehicle that can help couples enjoy the pleasures of sex and circumvent the disabling, demoralizing effects of erectile dysfunction. Physicians can advance the quality of life of older patients by appropriately prescribing Viagra after a careful medical history and physical examination. But they must also recommend psychological or marital counseling when the history reveals signs of emotional or interpersonal problems. The author reviews the administration and dosage, side effects, and economic considerations of Viagra. The author concludes that it is shortsighted of insurance or managed care companies to refuse to reimburse for Viagra. One additional dividend of Viagra is that it is motivating men in the 50-plus age group to seek medical treatment. This may allow earlier detection and control of chronic diseases, reducing morbidity and mortality and thereby resulting in cost savings.

- **Insights Into the Management of Erectile Dysfunction: Part I**

Source: Urologic Nursing. 19(4): 241-247. December 1999.

Contact: Available from Society of Urologic Nurses and Associates, Inc. East Holly Avenue, Box 56, Pitman, NJ 08071-0056. (609) 256-2335. E-mail: suna@ajj.com.

Summary: It is estimated that as many as 30 million men in the United States suffer from erectile dysfunction (ED). This article is the first in a series of 2 articles designed to help nurses and other health care professionals who care for and educate patients and health care workers regarding erectile dysfunction (impotence). Topics include the urologic condition of erectile dysfunction and appropriate patient care management for the client with erectile dysfunction, including interview, counseling, and monitoring of treatment. ED is defined as the consistent inability to achieve or sustain an erection satisfactory for sexual activity. More than 70 percent of cases of ED have a physiologic origin, including vascular, neurogenic, hormonal, mixed etiologies; or can be related to cavernosal abnormalities, cavernosal or local nerve damage, or drugs. The authors review the anatomy and physiology of a normal erection, then discuss assessment strategies for sexual health, including ED. Urologists and practitioners interested in treating men with ED and their partners can perform basic counseling regarding aging and environmental influences on sexual functioning. Part of the treatment process should include patient and partner education, including basic review of the anatomy and physiology of the sexual response, normal aging changes, overview of relevant etiology and associated risk factors, lifestyle factors (e.g., smoking), prescription drug effects, description of initial assessment and diagnostic testing results, and review of all treatment options, including potential risks and benefits. Most health care providers will suggest proceeding from the least invasive to the most invasive treatments if necessary. The treatment options are described in more detail in the second entry in the series (published in February 2000). Appended to the article is the posttest with which readers can obtain continuing education credits from the article. 1 figure. 2 tables. 10 references.

- **Psychological Impact of Erectile Dysfunction: Validation of a New Health Related Quality of Life Measure for Patients with Erectile Dysfunction**

Source: Journal of Urology. 168(5): 2086-2091. November 2002.

Contact: Available from Lippincott Williams and Wilkins. 12107 Insurance Way, Hagerstown, MD 21740. (800) 638-3030 or (301) 714-2334. Fax (301) 824-7290.

Summary: Male erectile dysfunction (ED, formerly called impotence) has a substantial impact on health related quality of life. This article reports on a study that examined the psychometric properties of two new scales created to measure the psychological impact of ED. Patients enrolled in a long-term study of men with ED completed clinical and health related quality of life (HRQOL) information at baseline and at three followup points. A total of 168 men completed the baseline quality of life questionnaire. The principal components analysis of the psychological impact of ED questions resulted in two new scales. Reliability was good with an internal consistency reliability of 0.91 for scale 1 and 0.72 for scale 2. Men reporting a greater psychological impact of ED also reported greater impairment in functional status, lower sexual self-efficacy, greater depression, and anxiety at the last intercourse. Each new scale significantly differentiated men with mild or moderate versus severe ED. The authors conclude that these new scales, named the Psychological Impact of Erectile Dysfunction instrument, comprehensively capture the psychological effect of ED on health related quality of life, which is not adequately assessed by existing patient-centered measures of erectile function. One appendix reprints the questionnaire instrument. 4 tables. 18 references.

- **Assessment of a Vacuum Constriction Device in Treating Erectile Dysfunction**

Source: Urologic Nursing. 18(1): 33-37. March 1998.

Contact: Available from Society of Urologic Nurses and Associates, Inc. East Holly Avenue, Box 56, Pitman, NJ 08071-0056. (609) 256-2335. E-mail: suna@ajj.com.

Summary: Male erectile dysfunction (ED, or impotence) is a common health concern, affecting an estimated 15 million men between the ages of 18 to 59. This article assesses the use of a vacuum constriction device in treating ED. A vacuum constriction device (VCD) is a mechanical apparatus that uses vacuum pressure to draw blood into the erectile tissue of the penis and a constriction ring worn at the base of the erect penis to maintain the erection during intercourse. The author reports on a study that included patients from a sexual dysfunction clinic; patients all had medical histories that provided ample evidence that their ED had an organic etiology (not a psychogenic etiology). After medical and psychosocial assessments that included interview, labs, and physical exam, a VCD was prescribed for each patient by the urologist. The author describes followup compliance and outcomes of the 110 patients who received VCDs in the clinic during 1995. Nine patients of the 110 who received VCDs and initial instruction sessions failed to keep their return appointments and, despite repeated attempts to contact them, they were not available for followup assessment. The overall assessment showed that 78 percent achieved and maintained an erection sufficient for sexual intercourse, indicating that the VCD method is a highly efficacious treatment. However, the treatment in the present study was inextricably combined with an evolved instructional protocol, with detailed followup, and with the outcome study itself. 1 figure. 1 table. 1 reference.

- **Erectile Dysfunction in the Ageing Man**

  Source: Current Opinion in Urology. 10(6): 625-628. November 2000.

  Contact: Available from Lippincott Williams and Wilkins. 241 Borough High Street, London, SE1 1GB, UK. +44 (0) 171940-7500. E-mail: sfrancis@lww.co.uk.

  Summary: Most studies have shown an increase in the prevalence of erectile dysfunction (ED, formerly called impotence) with aging. This article reviews the histologic and hemodynamic causes responsible for the erectile decline in the aging man. Penile erection is a vascular (blood system) phenomenon resulting from smooth muscle relaxation, arterial dilatation, and venous restriction. The atherosclerosis of the penis that occurs with aging causes a decrease in penile oxygen tension. This change in oxygen tension impacts directly upon both the physiologic function and the trabecular structure of the corpora cavernosa. Chronic ischemia (lack of blood flow) of the penis is associated with fibrosis of smooth muscle fibers and with endothelial and neuronal pathways. The effects of androgens (hormones) on libido and sexual behavior are well established, but their role in the erectile mechanism remains unclear. The author notes that a difficulty in assessing the pathophysiology of the decline of human erectile function with aging lies in the difficult discrimination between aging and concomitant diseases. The author concludes that, as the erectile dysfunction of aging appears to be a slowly progressive disorder, it appears wise for the patient to seek medical intervention earlier rather than later, and to find a new therapeutic approach to prevent the development of corporeal fibrosis. 23 references.

- **Erectile Dysfunction in Patients with Spina Bifida Is a Treatable Condition**

  Source: Journal of Urology. 164(3, Part 2): 958-961. September 2000.

  Contact: Available from Lippincott Williams and Wilkins. 12107 Insurance Way, Hagerstown, MD 21740. (800) 638-3030 or (301) 714-2334. Fax (301) 824-7290.

  Summary: Now that many individuals with spina bifida live well into adulthood, erectile dysfunction (ED) has become a recognized associated medical disorder. This article reports on a study undertaken to determine the ability to use sildenafil citrate (Viagra) to treat ED in men with spina bifida. ED was diagnosed in 15 men (19 to 35 years old) with spina bifida who were assigned to take 4 sets of tablets, 5 tablets per set, in a random order. All patients took 25 and 50 mg of sildenafil and 2 identical looking sets of corresponding placebos 1 hour before planned sexual activity. Improved erectile function was reported while on sildenafil by 12 (80 percent) men compared to baseline and placebos. There was a significant dose dependent improvement of erectile function with both 25 and 50 mg sildenafil compared to baseline, as mean erectile score increased by 50 percent and 88 percent, mean duration of erections increased by 192 percent and 266 percent, mean frequency of erections increased by 61 percent and 96 percent, and mean level of confidence increased by 33 percent and 63 percent, respectively. Furthermore, 50 mg sildenafil provided greater improvement in all 4 parameters compared to 25 mg. The placebo results were not significantly different compared to baseline for any of the parameters. The authors conclude that ED in patients with spina bifida is a medically treatable condition. Sildenafil is effective in this patient population and improves level of sexual confidence. 4 figures. 7 references.

- **Erectile Dysfunction: Workup and Management Tactics**

Source: Consultant. 41(12): 1573-1581. October 2001.

Contact: Available from Cliggott Publishing Company. 330 Boston Post Road, Darien, CT 06820-4027. (203) 661-0600.

Summary: Organic conditions are the most common cause of erectile dysfunction (ED, formerly called impotence), particularly in men older than 50 years. This article reviews the patient workup and management strategies for patients with ED. ED may signal an underlying treatable disorder, such as hypertension (high blood pressure), diabetes mellitus, hypercholesterolemia (high levels of cholesterol in the blood), heart disease, or peripheral vascular (blood vessel) disease. Other major risk factors are aging, obesity, cigarette smoking, medications (e.g., tranquilizers, antiulcer agents, antidepressants, antihistamines, and antihypertensives), and injury to the pelvic region. The absence of nocturnal (nighttime) erections or the lack of erections with masturbation or self-stimulation strongly suggests a physical cause of the patient's ED. Psychological factors play a role in a small percentage of long term cases. Physical examination of the patient should include an examination of the external genitalia for evidence of Peyronie disease, balanitis, and phimosis. Medical treatment options for ED include sildenafil (Viagra), testosterone therapy (for men with hypogonadism), vacuum erection devices, and prostaglandin therapy. Indications for referral to a urologist or psychiatrist include failure of medical therapy, Peyronie disease, severe vasculogenic ED, current nitroglycerin therapy that precludes the use of sildenafil, and severe depression or psychogenic ED. One sidebar reviews the mechanism of a normal erection. 2 tables. 14 references.

- **Penile Trauma: An Etiologic Factor in Peyronie's Disease and Erectile Dysfunction**

Source: Journal of Urology. 158(4): 1388-1390. October 1997.

Summary: Peyronie's disease is a common connective tissue disorder of the penis, presenting with painful erections, curvature, and palpable plaque. Most patients with Peyronie's disease have rigid erections but many develop difficulty with attaining or maintaining erections. Trauma to a penis that is either partially or fully erect may be a cause of Peyronie's disease. In addition, engaging in sexual relations with a partial erection due to mild impotence may also be a risk factor for the development of Peyronie's disease. This article reports on a study performed to determine whether patients with either Peyronie's disease or non-Peyronie's disease impotence had an increased rate of penile trauma compared with potent controls. The authors mailed surveys to 207 men who had been seen for management of Peyronie's disease, 250 impotent men without Peyronie's disease, and 275 age-matched urologic patients without a history of either impotence (erectile dysfunction) or Peyronie's disease. The survey inquired whether the individual had a history of penile trauma to the flaccid or erect phallus or injury during sexual intercourse. In addition, patients were questioned whether they had been engaging in sexual relations with a partial erection. The mean age of the impotent patients was slightly less than both the Peyronie's disease patients and controls. A similar response rate to the survey was found among the three groups. The mean duration of illness was 6 years for Peyronie's disease and 10 years for impotence. The frequency of penile trauma of any kind was significantly greater in both the Peyronie's disease (40 percent) and impotence (37 percent) patients than in the controls (11 percent). The Peyronie's disease patients had a lower frequency of attempting sexual relations with a partial erection than the other two groups. The authors conclude that these results demonstrate a significantly higher incidence of penile trauma in both patients with impotence and in patients with Peyronie's disease, compared to controls. The reduced incidence of engaging in sexual relations with a partial erection among the Peyronie's disease patients implies that partial impotence is not a predisposing factor for the disease. The survey instrument is provided as an appendix. 2 tables. 20 references. (AA-M).

- **Practical Approach to Erectile Dysfunction**

  Source: Hospital Medicine. 33(6): 41-44, 46, 49-50, 52. June 1997.

  Contact: Available from Hospital Medicine. 105 Raider Boulevard, Belle Mead, NJ 08502. (800) 783-4903 or (800) 976-4040.

  Summary: Probably no medical problem involves more diagnostic and therapeutic variety than erectile dysfunction. This article outlines a practical approach to erectile dysfunction that takes into consideration both cost and the patient's wishes. The authors describe a cost effective two-visit technique with which it is possible to evaluate most complaints of impotence and arrive at an individualized treatment plan. The authors first discuss the risk factors for impotence, including medication side effects. Antidepressants, including the tricyclics and the monoamine oxidase inhibitors, have been implicated in impotence, decreased libido, and impaired ejaculation. Most antihypertensives have been associated with some erectile impairment, but diuretics seem to have relatively little effect on erectile function. The calcium channel blockers and ACE inhibitors are associated with a low incidence of erectile dysfunction. The physical exam of a patient with impotence includes palpation of the neck for thyroidomegaly and alertness to any signs of excessive anxiety or hyperactivity that might suggest an adrenal or thyroid disorder. If a patient has normal-sized testes and intact libido, it is usually unnecessary to measure the serum testosterone level. Referral to a sex therapist is appropriate when the problem appears to be primarily psychogenic (e.g., premature ejaculation, abrupt onset associated with personal or occupational stress, partner-specific impotence). Treatment options outlined include testosterone supplementation, treating hyperprolactinemia, vacuum devices, and other nonsurgical options including self-injection and medical urethral system for erection (MUSE). 3 figures. 3 tables. 7 references. (AA-M).

- **Surgical Management of Erectile Dysfunction**

  Source: Diabetes Reviews. 6(1): 50-53. 1998.

  Contact: Available from American Diabetes Association. 1701 North Beauregard Street, Alexandria, VA 22311. (800) 232-3472.

  Summary: Revascularization of the corpus cavernosum of the penis has evolved into a well defined treatment choice in the management of traumatic arteriogenic erectile dysfunction (ED). This article describes the use of surgical management of ED as an approach for certain subpopulations, including men with diabetes. The author discusses patient evaluation and selection for penile revascularization, selection of the revascularization approach, complications, patient followup, penile venous ligation surgery, and the use of penile prostheses. The author emphasizes that penile revascularization by either an arterioarterial or arteriovenous approach is an effective longterm therapeutic option for arteriogenic erectile dysfunction in young men with pelvic, perineal, and penile trauma. This surgery can restore subjectively and objectively normal erectile function. However, its success depends on appropriate patient selection, careful diagnostic evaluation by specific erectile function studies, and an anatomically appropriate microsurgical approach. 11 references.

- **Erectile Dysfunction in Uremic Dialysis Patients: Diagnostic Evaluation in the Sildenafil Era**

Source: American Journal of Kidney Diseases. 38(4 Supplement 1): S115-S117. October 2001.

Contact: Available from W.B. Saunders Company. Periodicals Department, 6277 Sea Harbor Drive, Orlando, FL 32887-4800. (800) 654-2452 or (407) 345-4000.

Summary: Sexual dysfunction in men is a common and often distressing side effect of kidney (renal) failure. This article explores erectile dysfunction (ED, formerly called impotence) in dialysis patients with uremia, focusing on the diagnostic evaluation and the use of sildenafil (Viagra). The authors differentiate between ED and impotence, defining impotence as a general male sexual dysfunction that includes libidinal (sex drive), orgasmic, and ejaculatory dysfunction. ED is defined as the inability to achieve or maintain an erection sufficient to allow satisfactory sexual intercourse. Uremic men of different ages report a variety of sexual problems, including sexual hormonal pattern alterations, reduction in or loss of libido, infertility, and impotence, conditioning their well being status. In evaluating and treating sexual dysfunction, a nephrologist (kidney specialist) must consider factors involved in its pathogenesis (development), such as hypothalamic pituitary gonadal axis alterations, psychological problems related to chronic disease, secondary hyperparathyroidism, anemia, autonomic neuropathy, derangements in arterial supply or venous outflow, and the normal structure of cavernous body smooth muscle cells. The introduction of sildenafil to treat patients with impotence has completely changed the approach to evaluating these subjects (primarily because this drug is considered an effective, well tolerated treatment for men with ED). In the past, the authors proposed a complex algorithm to diagnose and treat ED. In this article, the authors propose a new algorithm to test the possibility of using sildenafil to obtain an erection, and to classify patients as responders or nonresponders to the sildenafil test. 1 figure. 11 references.

- **Oral Sildenafil in the Treatment of Erectile Dysfunction**

Source: New England Journal of Medicine. 338(20): 1397-1404. May 14, 1998.

Summary: Sildenafil is a potent inhibitor of cyclic guanosine monophosphate (GMP) in the corpus cavernosum and therefore increases the penile response to sexual stimulation. This article reports on a study that evaluated the efficacy and safety of sildenafil, administered as needed in two sequential double blind studies of men with erectile dysfunction of organic, psychogenic, or mixed causes. In a 24 week, dose response study, 532 men were treated with oral sildenafil (25, 50, or 100 mg) or placebo. In a 12 week, flexible dose escalation study, 329 different men were treated with sildenafil or placebo, with dose escalation to 100 mg based on efficacy and tolerance. After this dose escalation study, 225 of the 329 men entered a 32 week, open label extension study. The researchers assessed efficacy according to the International Index of Erectile Function, a patient log, and a global efficacy questionnaire. In the dose response study, increasing doses of sildenafil were associated with improved erectile function. In the last 4 weeks of treatment in the dose escalation study, 69 percent of all attempts at sexual intercourse were successful for the men receiving sildenafil, as compared with 22 percent for those receiving placebo. The mean numbers of successful attempts per month were 5.9 for the men receiving sildenafil and 1.5 for those receiving placebo. Headache, flushing, and dyspepsia (heartburn) were the most common adverse effects in the dose escalation study, occurring in 6 percent to 18 percent of the men. Ninety-two percent of the men completed the 32 week extension study. The researchers concluded that oral sildenafil is an effective, well tolerated treatment for men with erectile dysfunction. 2 figures. 3 tables. 14 references. (AA).

- **Diagnostic Steps in the Evaluation of Patients with Erectile Dysfunction**

Source: Journal of Urology. 168(8): 615-620. August 2002.

Contact: Available from Lippincott Williams and Wilkins. 12107 Insurance Way, Hagerstown, MD 21740. (800) 638-3030 or (301) 714-2334. Fax (301) 824-7290.

Summary: The need for a thorough diagnostic evaluation for erectile dysfunction (ED, formerly called impotence) has been questioned after the availability of effective oral therapies. This article reports on a study undertaken to determine the impact of the different diagnostic steps on the management strategy for ED. The study included all patients (n = 1,644) who presented at an andrology outpatient clinic during a 4 year period. Of these patients, 368 (22.4 percent) were excluded from the study due to severe psychiatric (5.2 percent) or cardiovascular (2.7 percent) disease, or to a history of ED less than 3 months in duration (14.5 percent). The remaining 1,276 patients were a mean age of 56 years (plus or minus 14 years) and had a mean duration of ED of 4.9 years (plus of minus 3.4 years). In these patients, medical history revealed ED-associated medical conditions in 57 percent, blood tests identified previously undiagnosed medical conditions in 6.2 percent, and physical examination and the intracavernous injection test were diagnostic in 13.9 percent and 2.6 percent, respectively. Initial screening was negative in 259 cases (20.3 percent), in which specific diagnostic procedures subsequently identified an underlying vascular (blood vessel) pathology in 165 men (12.9 percent) and unfavorable penile geometry in 16 men (1.3 percent). The remaining 78 men (6.1 percent) had no evidence of organic disease. The authors conclude that baseline diagnostic evaluation for ED can identify the underlying pathological condition or ED-associated risk factors in 80 percent of patients. Such screening may diagnose reversible causes of ED and also unmask medical conditions that manifest with ED as the first symptom. 4 figures. 3 tables. 28 references.

- **Diagnosis and Treatment of Erectile Dysfunction: The Process of Care Model**

Source: Nurse Practitioner. 25(Supplement 6): 4-10. June 2000.

Contact: Available from Nurse Practitioner. Circulation Department, P.O. Box 5053, Brentwood, TN 37024-5053. (800) 490-6580. Fax (615) 377-0525.

Summary: The new era of treating erectile dysfunction (ED), ushered in by the availability of an effective and safe oral medication (sildenafil, trade name Viagra), features the management of ED in the primary care setting. The Process of Care Model for the Evaluation and Treatment of Erectile Dysfunction was developed by the University of Medicine and Dentistry of New Jersey Robert Wood Johnson Medical School with input from multidisciplinary experts. This article discusses these guidelines. The key components of the model are a rational approach to diagnosis and treatment with emphasis on clinical history taking and a focused examination, specialized testing and referral in predefined situations, a stepwise management approach with ranking of treatment options, and incorporation of patient and partner needs and preferences in the decision making process when possible (a goal oriented approach). The essential first step in managing ED is taking a thorough sexual, medical, and psychosocial history. The history taking is also an opportunity for the health care provider to initiate patient and partner education and to facilitate communication. One sidebar reviews the anatomy and pathophysiology of ED. 1 figure. 1 table. 12 references.

- **Treating Erectile Dysfunction in Diabetes Patients**

  Source: Diabetes Educator. 23(1): 29-30, 32-33, 35-36, 38. January-February 1997.

  Summary: This article brings diabetes educators up to date on the treatment for erectile dysfunction (male impotence) in patients with diabetes. The authors stress that sensitive communication skills must be used to stimulate discussion with the patient and his significant other. This approach can help the patient understand the various treatment options that can be used to overcome erectile dysfunction. After a definition of erectile dysfunction (ED), the authors discuss the physiology of ED; the vascular, neurological, hormonal, psychological, and drug effect causes of impotence; treatment options, including vacuum constriction devices, penile prosthesis, vascular surgery, and drug therapy, notably self injection; priapism as a side effect of self injection; and patient evaluation techniques. The authors describe the three-drug combination of alprostadil, phentolamine, and papaverine as producing a better erection in ED of vascular origin (common in patients with diabetes). The authors also briefly discuss present research efforts, most notably those investigating new pharmaceutical agents. One full-page chart provides patient instructions for penile injection therapy. 2 figures. 4 tables. 40 references.

- **Erectile Dysfunction in Type 1 and Type 2 Diabetics in Italy**

  Source: International Journal of Epidemiology. 29(3): 524-531. June 2000.

  Contact: Available from Oxford University Press. Journals Subscription Department, Great Clarendon Street, Oxford OX2 6DP, UK. 44 (0)1865 267907. Fax 44 (0)1865 267485.

  Summary: This article describes a study that investigated the prevalence and determinants of self reported erectile dysfunction (ED) in men with type 1 and type 2 diabetes. Eligible for the study were men aged 20 to 69 years with a diagnosis of type 1 or type 2 diabetes who were observed on randomly selected days in 178 diabetes centers in Italy. ED was defined as a failure to achieve and maintain an erection sufficient for satisfactory sexual performance. The study population consisted of 1,383 men with type 1 diabetes and 8,373 men with type 2 diabetes. The prevalence of ED increased with age for both groups. After accounting for the effect of age, men who had type 2 diabetes tended to report ED less frequently (37 per 100) than men who had type 1 diabetes (51 per 100). A significant positive relationship was reported between ED and poor metabolic control. The odds ratio for ED were respectively for type 1 and type 2 1.5 and 1.7 in men with fair control and 1.8 and 2.3 in men with poor control. For both groups, history of diabetes related arterial, renal, or retinal diseases and neuropathy was associated with an increased risk of ED. Smoking was associated with an increased risk of ED in men with type 1 and type 2 diabetes, whereas high body mass index increased only the risk of ED in type 1 cases. Some medical conditions such as anxiety, depression, cardiopathy, hypercholesterolemia, and hypertension were associated with an increased risk of ED in both the type 1 and type 2 groups. ED was significantly more frequent in both groups taking certain medications, including tranquilizers, antihypertensives, cardiovascular medications, diuretics, and H2 antagonists. 1 appendix. 7 tables. 25 references.

- **What is Erectile Dysfunction?**

Source: Family Urology. p. 5-7. Fall 1997.

Contact: Available from American Foundation for Urologic Diseases, Inc. 300 West Pratt Street, Suite 401, Baltimore, MD 21201. (410) 727-2908.

Summary: This article discusses erectile dysfunction (impotence), defined as the inability to achieve or sustain an erection adequate for sexual intercourse. This article, written in a question and answer format, covers the causes of erectile dysfunction (ED), which doctors treat ED, age factors for treatment, the role of the partner in the patient's treatment, what to expect during the first visit to a health care provider for ED, how ED can affect a man psychologically, the impact of ED on the man's partner, the importance of adequate communication between partners, and treatment options. Physical causes of ED include blockage in the arteries, diabetes, neurological dsorders, disease of the erectile tissue of the penis, pelvic surgery or trauma, side effects of medications, chronic disease, hormonal abnormalities, alcoholism and drug abuse, heavy smoking, and Peyronie's disease. Psychological causes of impotence include stress and anxiety from work or home, worry about poor sexual performance, marital discord, unresolved sexual orientation, and depression. Treatment options outlined in the article include changing habits and medications, the use of hormone medications, professional counseling, vacuum devices, intraurethral therapy, injection therapy, penile prostheses, oral therapy, and surgical treatment. The author concludes that erectile dysfunction can usually be treated safely and effectively. The key to regaining long term sexual function is trust and open communication between the motivated man and his supportive partner. Success also requires a knowledgeable and caring health are provider who understands both the physical and psychological impact of the condition on both the patient and his partner. The article includes a brief glossary of terms and a list of resource organizations that can provide readers with additional information.

- **New Treatments for Erectile Dysfunction**

Source: Patient Care. 32(5): 30-32, 35, 39-40, 42, 45-46, 51-52. March 15, 1998.

Contact: Available from Medical Economics. 5 Paragon Drive, Montvale, NJ 07645. (800) 432-4570. Fax (201) 573-4956.

Summary: This article discusses the diagnosis and treatment of erectile dysfunction. This condition most often results from age-related diseases, medication side effects, or a condition such as diabetes mellitus. Diagnosing the problem involves starting a conversation with a patient about his sexual history, involving the partner, taking the medical and sexual history, performing a physical examination, conducting laboratory tests, and evaluating degrees of dysfunction. The article provides guidelines for treating underlying causes of erectile dysfunction, including age, medication side effects, smoking, alcohol consumption, chronic diseases, hormonal problems, vascular and neurologic problems, surgical procedures, anxiety, and depression. In addition, the article describes various options for treating erectile dysfunction that persists once any underlying causes are treated, including prescribing vacuum constriction devices, drug injection therapy, urethral suppositories, penile prosthetic implants and surgery, new oral therapies such as sildenafil, and marriage or sex therapy. Other topics include the problem of priapism, a painful condition in which an erection persists for more than 4 hours; the insurance aspects of erectile dysfunction treatment; discontinuation of treatment by the patient; and follow-up care. 1 figure. 8 references.

- **Erectile Dysfunction in Diabetes: Pills for Penile Failure**

Source: Clinical Diabetes. 16(3): 108-119. 1998.

Contact: Available from American Diabetes Association. 1701 North Beauregard Street, Alexandria, VA 22311. (800) 232-3472. Website: www.diabetes.org.

Summary: This article focuses on new oral therapies for erectile dysfunction (ED), particularly among men with diabetes. ED is the consistent inability to attain and maintain an erection adequate for sexual intercourse. Diabetes accounts for 30 percent of ED. The article explains the physiology of erection and the pathophysiology of ED in diabetes, describes the symptoms of ED, and discusses the evaluation and treatment of ED. Treatment is oriented toward removing the cause. There are three treatment options for men with diabetes and ED: no treatment, medical treatment, or surgery. The first choice involves having the patient withdraw from drugs likely to promote ED and participate in psychosexual counseling. The medical option involves administering androgens, bromergocriptine mesylate, or sildenafil; self-injecting drugs such as papaverine, phentolamine, and prostaglandin; and using the Medicated Urethral System for Erection (MUSE) or vacuum devices. The last option, surgery, involves either implanting semirigid, malleable, or inflatable prosthetic devices or undergoing revascularization procedures. The article also highlights future methods of reversing neuropathy, the major cause of ED in men with diabetes. 4 figures. 5 tables.

- **Psychological Aspects at the Interface of Diabetes and Erectile Dysfunction**

Source: Diabetes Reviews. 6(1): 41-49. 1998.

Contact: Available from American Diabetes Association. 1701 North Beauregard Street, Alexandria, VA 22311. (800) 232-3472. Website: www.diabetes.org.

Summary: This article focuses on the psychological issues affecting people with diabetes and erectile dysfunction. Diabetes-related erectile dysfunction is regarded as the typical model of organic impotence, with recognized organic pathogenesis and several effective treatments. Consideration has not always been given, however, to psychological factors that can affect the establishment, maintenance, and management of diabetes-induced impotence. The adoption of an either/or organic versus psychogenic paradigm fails to consider that psychology contributes to and can coexist with organicity. The article discusses several psychological issues affecting people with diabetes and erectile dysfunction. Diminished sexual desire often occurs in the impotent man and/or his partner. Partners may respond negatively, and sexual relationships tend to change as impotence develops. Performance anxiety or premature ejaculation may be secondary complications. The unwillingness of men to seek help for sexual difficulty and their poor compliance with prescribed treatments pose major obstacles to successful treatment. Continuing comprehensive care of men with diabetes aims to identify erectile dysfunction at its earliest manifestations. Effective intervention can then be instituted, and problems associated with chronic difficulties can be avoided. Optimal management of diabetes induced erectile dysfunction is best achieved by adopting an integrative treatment model that addresses the complex interplay of biological and psychological issues involved in sexual behavior. 66 references. (AA-M).

- **Evaluation, Treatment, and Management of Erectile Dysfunction: An Overview**

Source: Urologic Nursing. 18(2): 100-106. June 1998.

Contact: Available from Urologic Nursing. Mosby-Year Book, Inc. 11830 Westline Industrial Drive, St. Louis, MO 63146-3318. (314) 453-4351.

Summary: This article offers an overview of the evaluation, treatment, and management of erectile dysfunction (impotence). During the last decade there has been a significant change in the management of patients with sexual dysfunction, both because of improved understanding of erectile physiology and also because of the development of new and effective medical therapies. Erectile dysfunction is usually caused by an organic factor or disease, such as pelvic vascular disease, heart disease, hypertension and hypercholesteremia, diabetes mellitus, pelvic surgery and trauma, side effects of medications or neurodegenerative disorders, and the use of tobacco. Smoking doubles the probability of impotence with a given risk factor. Psychologic problems are also important contributing factors that can impair sexual performance, diminish self esteem, and disrupt personal relationships. A thorough medical, social, and sexual history, paired with a physical examination, is absolutely necessary in diagnosing the underlying problem. The author reviews specific diagnostic questions to ask the patient. Treatments are then reviewed, including vacuum devices, intracorporal injections, intraurethral applications, penile prostheses, and oral medications (such as sildenafil). The author concludes by emphasizing the importance of involving the man's partner (when possible) in any discussions of treatment options. 4 figures. 23 references.

- **Pelvic Floor Muscle Exercises and Manometric Biofeedback for Erectile Dysfunction and Postmicturition Dribble: Three Case Studies**

Source: Journal of WOCN. Wound, Ostomy, and Continence Nurses Society. 30(1): 44-52. January 2003.

Contact: Mosby, Inc. Periodicals Department, 6277 Sea Harbor Drive, Orlando, FL 32887-4800. (800) 654-2452.

Summary: This article presents three successful case studies of men receiving treatment for erectile dysfunction (ED, formerly called impotence) and postmicturition dribble (leakage of urine immediately after urination). The authors focus on the benefits of pelvic floor muscle exercises (PFME) for these men. Each of the three subjects reported normal erectile function following PFME and manometric biofeedback. Manometric biofeedback was chosen as a reliable method of monitoring anal pressure measurements. PFME, which included a 'squeeze out' pelvic floor muscle contraction after voiding urine, alleviated the small amount of postmicturition dribble experienced by two subjects. These case studies are reported to alert professionals to the possibility of the benefits of PFME for some men. A commentary is appended to the article. 2 figures. 3 tables. 20 references.

- **Treating Erectile Dysfunction in Diabetes Mellitus**

Source: Practical Diabetology. 16(2): 27-31, 34-35. June 1997.

Summary: This article provides information about treating erectile dysfunction in diabetes mellitus. The authors note that approximately 50 percent of men with diabetes in the United States complain of erectile dysfunction. Topics include how an erection occurs; diabetes and sexual dysfunction; evaluating erectile dysfunction; laboratory testing; studies; treatment; and future developments. Treatment categories include oral treatments; self-injection pharmacotherapy; vacuum constriction devices; sexual therapy; and penile prostheses. According to the article, impotence in men with diabetes may occur in three forms: as a first symptom of diabetes; as a secondary symptom after several years of diabetes; and as a temporary phenomenon associated with poor control of diabetes. Because impotence can be the presenting complaint in previously undiagnosed diabetes, it is important that all impotent men be screened for diabetes.

Health care professionals should be aware that since people with diabetes commonly use pharmacologic agents, drug use is one of the most frequent causes of sexual dysfunction. 4 figures. 7 references. (AA-M).

- **Epidemiology and Pathophysiology of Erectile Dysfunction**

Source: Journal of Urology. 161(1): 5-11. January 1999.

Summary: This article reports on a literature search of more than 400 studies on the epidemiology of erectile dysfunction and the physiology and pathophysiology of erectile function. The authors estimate that the prevalence of erectile dysfunction of all degrees is 52 percent in men 40 to 70 years old, with higher rates in those older than 70 years. Erectile dysfunction has a significant negative impact on quality of life. Risk factors for erectile dysfunction include aging, chronic illnesses, various medications, and cigarette smoking. A nitric oxide cyclic guanosine monophosphate mechanism has an important role in mediating the corporal smooth muscle relaxation necessary for erectile function. Other mechanisms involving neuropeptides, gap junctions, and ion channels also may modulate corporal smooth muscle tone. Erectile dysfunction can be due to vasculogenic, neurogenic, hormonal, or psychogenic factors as well as to alterations in the nitric oxide cyclic guanosine monophosphate pathway or other regulatory mechanisms, resulting in an imbalance in corporal smooth muscle contraction and relaxation. The authors conclude that erectile dysfunction is a common condition associated with aging, chronic illnesses, and various modifiable risk factors. Normal penile erection is a hemodynamic process that is dependent on corporal smooth muscle relaxation mediated by parasympathetic neurotransmission, nitric oxide, and possibly other regulatory factors and electrophysiological events. 2 figures. 78 references. (AA-M).

- **Treatment of Men With Erectile Dysfunction With Transurethral Alprostadil**

Source: New England Journal of Medicine. 336(1): 1-7. January 2, 1997.

Summary: This article reports on a study in which alprostadil (prostaglandin E1) is delivered transurethrally to treat erectile dysfunction in men. Alprostadil was delivered transurethrally in a double-blind, placebo-controlled study of 1,511 men, 27 to 88 years of age, who had chronic erectile dysfunction from various organic causes. The men were first tested in the clinic with up to four doses of the drug; those who had sufficient responses were randomly assigned to treatment with either the effective dose of alprostadil or placebo for three months at home. During in-clinic testing, 996 men (65.9 percent) had erections sufficient for intercourse. Of these men, 961 reported the results of at least one home treatment; 299 of the 461 treated with alprostadil (64.9 percent) had intercourse successfully at least once, as compared with 93 of the 500 who received placebo (18.6 percent). On average, 7 of 10 alprostadil administrations were followed by intercourse in men responsive to treatment. The efficacy of alprostadil was similar regardless of age or the cause of erectile dysfunction, including vascular disease, diabetes, surgery, and trauma. The most common side effect was mild penile pain, which occurred after 10.8 percent of alprostadil treatments, but the pain rarely resulted in refusal to continue in the study. Hypotension occurred in the clinic in 3.3 percent of men receiving alprostadil. Hypotension-related symptoms were uncommon at home. No men had priapism or penile fibrosis. 2 figures. 4 tables. 40 references. (AA-M).

- **Efficacy and Safety of Tadalafil for the Treatment of Erectile Dysfunction: Results of Integrated Analyses**

  Source: Journal of Urology. 168(4 Part 1): 1332-1336. October 2002.

  Contact: Available from Lippincott Williams and Wilkins. 12107 Insurance Way, Hagerstown, MD 21740. (800) 638-3030 or (301) 714-2334. Fax (301) 824-7290.

  Summary: This article reports on a study of the efficacy and safety of tadalafil, a potent selective phosphodiesterase 5 inhibitor, for the treatment of erectile dysfunction (ED, formerly called impotence). The study included a total of 1,112 men with a mean age of 59 years (range 22 to 82 years) and mild to severe ED of various etiologies (causes). Men were randomized to placebo or tadalafil, taken as needed without food or alcohol restrictions, at fixed daily doses in randomized, double-blind trials lasting 12 weeks. Compared with placebo, tadalafil significantly enhanced all efficacy outcomes. Patients receiving 20 milligrams of tadalafil experienced a significant mean improvement in an index of erectile function, 75 percent of intercourse attempts were successfully completed, and 81 percent reported improved erections at end point compared with 35 percent in the control group. Tadalafil was consistently effective across disease severities and etiologies, as well as in patients of all ages. Tadalafil was well tolerated, with headache and dyspepsia (indigestion) as the most frequent adverse events. 4 tables. 14 references.

- **Effect of Erectile Dysfunction on Quality of Life: Psychometric Testing of a New Quality of Life Measure for Patients with Erectile Dysfunction**

  Source: Journal of Urology. 167(1): 212-217. January 2002.

  Contact: Available from Lippincott Williams and Wilkins. 12107 Insurance Way, Hagerstown, MD 21740. (800) 638-3030 or (301) 714-2334. Fax (301) 824-7290.

  Summary: This article reports on a study that assessed the psychometric properties of the newly developed Erectile Dysfunction Effect on Quality of Life (ED EQoL) instrument for quantifying the effect of erectile dysfunction (ED, formerly called impotence) on quality of life. The questionnaire was assessed in a cohort of 283 men recruited from 11 centers in the United Kingdom. Internal consistency, test-retest reliability, construct validity, and responsiveness were evaluated. The results showed the ED-EQoL was simple to complete and captured wide variation in quality of life. The test demonstrated good internal consistency and reliability, and generally correlated in an expected manner with other quality of life measures. Correlation with initial erectile function was relatively low, but the change in function after treatment was reflected by the change in quality of life. The authors conclude that when assessing ED in clinical practice or research, it is important to consider the effect on quality of life in addition to function. Combined with a measure of erectile function, the ED-EQoL is recommended for use in routine clinical practice and research to provide a holistic approach to the assessment of ED and its treatment. The appendix of the article reprints the instrument. 5 tables. 11 references.

- **Efficacy of Oral Sildenafil in Hemodialysis Patients with Erectile Dysfunction**

  Source: JASN. Journal of the American Society of Nephrology. 13 (11): 2770-2775. November 2002.

  Contact: Available from Lippincott Williams and Wilkins. 12107 Insurance Way, Hagerstown, MD 21740. (800) 638-6423.

Summary: This article reports on a study undertaken to evaluate the efficacy and safety of oral sildenafil (Viagra) to treat erectile dysfunction (ED) in chronic renal (kidney) failure in patients on hemodialysis (HD). The double-blind, randomized, placebo-controlled study included oral sildenafil (50 milligrams) administered as required in HD patients; 21 patients received placebo and 20 received sildenafil. Baseline clinical and demographic parameters were similar in both groups. Sildenafil was associated with improvement in the score of all questions and domains of the IIEF (International Index of Erectile Function), except those related to sexual desire. Using the erectile function domain to evaluate primary efficacy, improvement was observed in 85 percent of the sildenafil patients, compared with 9.5 percent of placebo patients. Sildenafil use resulted in normal EF scores in 35 percent of sildenafil patients. Sildenafil was well tolerated. Headache and flushing occurred in both groups. Dyspepsia was reported by two patients in the sildenafil group. The authors conclude that oral sildenafil seems to be an effective and safe treatment for ED in selected patients with chronic renal (kidney) failure on hemodialysis. 4 tables. 20 references.

- **First-line Therapies for Erectile Dysfunction**

Source: JAAPA. Journal of the American Academy of Physician Assistants. 14(10): 17-20. October 2001.

Contact: Available from Medical Economics. 5 Paragon Drive, Montvale, NJ 07645. (800) 432-4570. Fax (201) 573-4956.

Summary: This article reviews the first line therapies that are now recommended for erectile dysfunction (ED, formerly called impotence). The article, designed as a continuing education lesson for physician assistants, reviews the definition of ED, the major etiologic (causative) factors for ED, and how to know when a diagnostic workup for ED is warranted. The author notes that the introduction of an oral medication (sildenafil, Viagra) to treat ED generated widespread publicity and brought many men to their health care providers. As awareness and patients' willingness to discuss ED have grown, so too has the role of primary care as an appropriate setting for the workup and initial treatment of ED. The author reviews the options for treatment, including sildenafil, testosterone replacement, and vacuum constriction devices.1 table. 8 references.

- **Novel Strategy for Individualizing Erectile Dysfunction Treatment**

Source: Patient Care. 34(2): 91-94, 99. January 30, 2000.

Contact: Available from Medical Economics. 5 Paragon Drive, Montvale, NJ 07645. (800) 432-4570. Fax (201) 573-4956.

Summary: This article reviews the increasing selection of drugs for the treatment of patients with erectile dysfunction (ED), focusing on individualizing treatment. The authors describe a matrix classification system that physicians can use to support this decision making process. The classification system divides drugs according to their anatomic and physiologic actions. The authors stress that ED is a quality of life impairment, so the opinions of the patient and the patient's partner are especially important. In the absence of a logical, validated diagnostic schedule, classification of ED can be made by response to treatment. Drugs for treating ED can be classified as initiators of an erection or conditioners (drugs that help maintain an erection). Drugs for ED act on either the central nervous system (CNS) or on the peripheral end organ (the penis). By classifying the drugs used for ED, physicians can understand the differences and similarities among these drugs. For example, a patient who responds to drugs from one class, such as the CNS initiators, is likely to respond to other drugs from the same class. One case study is offered to illustrate this patient care strategy. 1 figure. 11 references.

- **Men's Health. Erectile Dysfunction: Outta Here**

Source: PA Today. 6(22): 19-23. October 26, 1998.

Contact: Available from Great Valley Publishing Company, Inc. 1288 Valley Forge Road, P.O. Box 2224, Valley Forge, PA 19482-2224. (610) 917-9300. Website: www.gvpub.com.

Summary: This article, from a journal for physician assistants, is the first of two articles on erectile dysfunction (impotence). Erectile dysfunction (ED) is commonly defined as the consistent inability to maintain or achieve an erection that permits satisfactory intercourse or other sexual activity. The article reviews the typical etiology and epidemiology of ED, focusing on the common risk factors including vascular, other systemic diseases (including kidney failure and diabetes), neurogenic, endocrine, penile, psychiatric or social, hematologic, infectious, chemical, and other factors such as pain, fatigue, and poor nutrition. The author then reviews the components of assessment for ED, including medical history, sexual history, psychosocial history, physical examination, neurological function assessment, and laboratory evaluation. The author describes the changes in sexual response that normally accompany aging (ED is not one of those changes) and emphasizes the importance of patient education in preventing psychogenic ED. The author also focuses on the need to include the patient's partner in the assessment and treatment process. The author concludes that the majority of men with ED can be treated successfully by physician assistants in an office practice. Treatment is individualized and begins with the correction of any primary medical conditions (the second article in the series addresses treatment options).

- **Erectile Dysfunction in Older Men**

Source: Topics in Geriatric Rehabilitation. 12(4): 40-52. 1997.

Summary: This journal article discusses erectile dysfunction in older men including possible causes, diagnosis, and treatment. Erectile dysfunction may result from neurogenic causes such as Alzheimer's disease (AD), Parkinson's disease, and stroke. The article reviews the physiology of an erection, possible organic disease causes, and steps involved in the diagnostic process. Some of the treatments for erectile dysfunction include nonspecific therapies which may be appropriate for men with AD and other irreversible causes of the dysfunction. 53 references.

- **Management of Erectile Dysfunction by the Geriatrician**

Source: Journal of the American Geriatrics Society. 45(10): 1240-1246. October 1997.

Contact: Available from Williams and Wilkins. 351 West Camden Street, Baltimore, MD 21201-2436. (800) 638-6423. Fax (410) 528-8596.

Summary: This review article covers the management of erectile dysfunction (ED or impotence). The authors first provide information on the pathophysiology, evaluation, and treatment of ED. The authors note that ED is the most common health disorder to afflict elderly men. Although 67 percent of men aged 70 years have ED, and their interest in sexual intercourse remains high, less than 5 percent receive adequate treatment. The authors encourage geriatricians and other primary care providers to treat men with ED, noting that only in rare cases does a patient with ED need to be referred to a specialist. The article outlines the neural and vascular components of erection; the pathophysiology of libido, vascular disease, neurological disease, medication-induced ED, and orgasmic dysfunction. The authors discuss diagnostic issues and describe different nonsurgical treatment options, including sex therapy, medication adjustment, vacuum devices, intracavernosal injection therapy, and some unproven therapies including yohimbine, trazodone, and vitamin E. 5 figures. 67 references. (AA-M).

- **Erectile Dysfunction in Diabetes**

Source: Practical Diabetology. 19(2): 16, 18-23. June 2000.

Contact: Available from R.A. Rapaport Publishing, Inc. 150 West 22nd Street, New York, NY 10011. (800) 234-0923.

Summary: This review article discusses the etiology, pathology, diagnosis, and management of erectile dysfunction (ED) in men who have diabetes. The causes of ED generally fall within the categories of organic or psychogenic. Organic causes include the categories of vascular, traumatic or postsurgical, neurologic, endocrinologic, and drug induced. Psychogenic causes include mood and anxiety disorders and relationship difficulties. Among men who have diabetes, risk factors for developing ED include age, poor glycemic control, hypertension, smoking, excessive alcohol intake, the presence of claudication, and neuropathy. The natural history of ED in men who have diabetes usually progresses gradually. Autonomic neuropathy appears to be a major contributor to the development of ED in men who have diabetes. Diagnosis of ED is based on the medical history, physical examination, and several simple diagnostic tests. The management of ED usually involves the use of oral agents such as sildenafil, yohimbine, apomorphine, and phentolamine. In men who are not candidates for oral therapy, intracavernosal injection with alprostadil can be an acceptable alternative. Other agents that have been used in injection therapy include papaverine, phentolamine, and moxisylyte hydrochloride. Mechanical treatments are also available for patients who are not candidates for drug therapy. These treatment options include external vacuum devices and constriction rings. Surgical therapy may also be considered when other forms of therapy have not been successful. The most utilized surgical procedure has been prosthetic penile implantation. Penile revascularization is another surgical option. Several preventive measures can help minimize the risk of developing ED, including improving glycemic control, quitting smoking, reducing excessive alcohol intake, and controlling hypertension. 1 figure. 3 tables. 23 references.

- **It Takes Two: Coping with Erectile Dysfunction**

Source: Harvard Women's Health Watch. 7(7): 2-3. March 2000.

Contact: Available from Harvard Women's Health Watch. P.O. Box 420068, Palm Coast, FL 32142-0068. (800) 829-5921 or (904) 445-4662.

Summary: This women's health newsletter article offers information about coping with erectile dysfunction (impotence). The author notes that women can play an important role in helping their partners seek treatment and turn this often difficult experience into an opportunity to learn new ways to enjoy each other sexually. The article defines erectile dysfunction as an inability to attain and maintain an erection sufficient for intercourse at least 25 percent of the time. The author then explains the various causes of erectile dysfunction, including nervous system problems, cardiovascular disease, the interplay and normal function of the nerves and blood vessels, spinal cord injury, drug effects, diabetes, and psychological problems. The author stresses that a common pattern can develop among couples dealing with erectile dysfunction that features a series of unsuccessful tries at sexual intercourse, then emotional withdrawal, lack of initiation of sex (for fear of failure), and finally more emotional and physical separation between the couple. The author explains how communication is the best way to combat these isolating behaviors. The author encourages patients to consult a physician, and the article briefly lists the possible treatment options available for erectile dysfunction. The article concludes with a discussion of strategies for coping with erectile dysfunction issues, emphasizing the incorporation of sensuality and sexuality into a regular, loving, and playful interchange between the partners. A brief list of resources is also provided.

- **Oral Medications for Erectile Dysfunction**

Source: Family Urology. 5(2): 19-20. 2000.

Contact: Available from American Foundation for Urologic Disease. 1126 North Charles Street, Baltimore, MD 21201. (800) 242-2383 or (410) 468-1800. Fax (410) 468-1808. Website: www.afud.org.

Summary: Today there are effective, safe, and easy to use oral medications for erectile dysfunction (ED, formerly called impotence). This article summarizes key information for three oral treatments for ED: sildenafil (Viagra), yohimbine (Yocon), and apomorphine SL (Uprima). For each drug, the author reviews efficacy, time to effect, side effects and contraindications, and interactions with other drugs. Sildenafil relaxes smooth muscle cells and allows increased blood flow into the erectile tissue, thus enhancing erection in the presence of sexual stimulation. It is indicated for the treatment of ED or organic, psychological, or combined causes. Sildenafil is effective for about 70 to 80 percent of men with ED; the drug is effective approximately an hour after oral ingestion. Yohimbine is a medicinal herb whose primary action is to increase blood flow to erectile tissue. Its effectiveness is relatively low, but it also has a low incidence of side effects. Beneficial effects are achieved after two to three weeks of taking yohimbine. Taken sublingually (under the tongue), Apomorphine SL is a centrally acting drug the stimulates erection through the brain and nervous system. The drug takes effect in 10 to 25 minutes and is effective in approximately half the men who use it; the drug has proven to be reliable and consistent in patients who have taken it for a year or more.

- **Newer Pharmacologic Alternatives for Erectile Dysfunction**

Source: American Family Physician. 60(4): 1159-1166. September 15, 1999.

Contact: Available from American Academy of Family Physicians. 11400 Tomahawk Creek Parkway, Leawood, KS 66211-2672. (800) 274-2237. Website: www.aafp.org.

Summary: With the introduction of effective pharmacologic therapies for erectile dysfunction (ED, previously called impotence), more men are seeking treatment. This article reviews the newer pharmacologic alternatives for ED. The underlying cause of ED is usually a chronic medical illness or a side effect of certain drugs. Less commonly, the problem is psychogenic. Even after optimal treatment of common medical disorders such as diabetes mellitus and hypertension, ED may persist. The authors note that drug therapy, such as the intracavernosal (injected into the cavernosa of the penis) or transurethral administration of alprostadil (Caverject or MUSE) or the use of the new oral medication sildenafil (Viagra), may offer patients substantial benefit. However, before any of these drugs are prescribed, consideration should be given to existing medical illnesses and medications, partner satisfaction, comfort with the method of administration, and the side effect profile. The authors note that the development of sildenafil has prompted an unprecedented number of men to seek treatment. Even for those patients for whom sildenafil is not appropriate, other therapeutic options may be of benefit. A thoughtful evaluation of the patient may reveal treatable causes and provide family physicians with an opportunity to become involved in the comprehensive health care of men who otherwise would not have sought medical attention. Accompanying the article is a fact sheet for patients on drug treatments for ED. 5 tables. 23 references.

Federally Funded Research on Erectile Dysfunction

The U.S. Government supports a variety of research studies relating to erectile dysfunction. These studies are tracked by the Office of Extramural Research at the National Institutes of Health.[2] CRISP (Computerized Retrieval of Information on Scientific Projects) is a searchable database of federally funded biomedical research projects conducted at universities, hospitals, and other institutions.

Search the CRISP Web site at **http://crisp.cit.nih.gov/crisp/crisp_query.generate_screen**. You will have the option to perform targeted searches by various criteria, including geography, date, and topics related to erectile dysfunction.

For most of the studies, the agencies reporting into CRISP provide summaries or abstracts. As opposed to clinical trial research using patients, many federally funded studies use animals or simulated models to explore erectile dysfunction. The following is typical of the type of information found when searching the CRISP database for erectile dysfunction:

- **Project Title: CLINICAL TRIAL DEVELOPMENT IN CHRONIC PELVIC PAIN SYNDR***

  Principal Investigator & Institution: Shoskes, Daniel A.; Professor; Cleveland Clinic Foundation 9500 Euclid Ave Cleveland, Oh 44195

  Timing: Fiscal Year 2003; Project Start 05-SEP-2003; Project End 28-FEB-2008

  Summary: (provided by applicant): Chronic Pelvic Pain Syndrome (CPPS) is a prevalent multifactorial disorder with variable and often disappointing response to therapy. There is evidence for infection, inflammation and neuromuscular spasm as the underlying cause in different patients despite identical clinical presentation. Large multicenter clinical trials are required to help delineate effective therapies and to identify which patients have the highest chance of success for a particular intervention. The Chronic Prostatitis Clinic at the Cleveland Clinic Florida has a high volume of patients, both newly diagnosed and longstanding. We have done numerous clinical trials in chronic prostatitis with rapid enrolment, 100% accrual of set targets and high rates of retention. We have a team of clinical specialists in allied fields important to the understanding of this condition, including experts in **erectile dysfunction,** rectal dysfunction, chronic pain management, complementary therapies (acupuncture, phytotherapy) and neuropsychology. We also maintain a basic science laboratory which would be equipped to perform any necessary molecular or biochemical ancillary studies such as real time PCR, oxidative stress markers, cytokines and genetic polymorphisms. Through our participation in the CPCRN and first NIH chronic prostatitis randomized clinical trial, we have demonstrated the ability to work collaboratively and to participate in

---

[2] Healthcare projects are funded by the National Institutes of Health (NIH), Substance Abuse and Mental Health Services (SAMHSA), Health Resources and Services Administration (HRSA), Food and Drug Administration (FDA), Centers for Disease Control and Prevention (CDCP), Agency for Healthcare Research and Quality (AHRQ), and Office of Assistant Secretary of Health (OASH).

study design and execution. As an example of a potential clinical trial, a study of water induced thermotherapy is outlined.

Website: http://crisp.cit.nih.gov/crisp/Crisp_Query.Generate_Screen

- **Project Title: CRYSTAL STRUCT. OF CYCLIC NUCLEOTIDE PHOSPHODIESTERASE**

Principal Investigator & Institution: Ke, Hengming; Associate Professor; Biochemistry and Biophysics; University of North Carolina Chapel Hill Office of Sponsored Research Chapel Hill, Nc 27599

Timing: Fiscal Year 2001; Project Start 01-APR-2000; Project End 31-MAR-2004

Summary: (Verbatim from the Applicant's Abstract) Cyclic nucleotide phosphodiesterase (PDE) catalyzes the hydrolysis of adenosine 3',5'-cyclic monophosphate (cAMP) and guanosine 3',5'-cyclic monophosphate (cGMP) to produce, respectively, 5'-AMP and 5'-GMP. PDE is a key enzyme to control cellular concentrations of cAMP that is known as "second messenger" and mediates the response of cells to a wide variety of hormones and neurotransmitters. Ten families and twenty two subtypes of human PDE have been identified. The mRNAs of the 22 subtype PDEs are further spliced to generate over 60 isoforms of PDE. The distinct isoforms of PDE are located in different cellular compartments and possess different specificity of substrate. These two features of PDE have attracted great attention from pharmaceutical companies in the past decade. Many selective PDE inhibitors have been studied as therapeutic agents such as cardiotonic agents, vasodilators, antiasthma, atithrombic compounds, smooth muscle relaxants and antidepressants. For example, VIAGRA, an inhibitor of PDE5, is a prescription drug for **erectile dysfunction** of male patients. This proposal aims at characterization of substrate specificity and inhibitor selectivity by the approach of crystallography. The specific aims are to determine crystal structures of PDEs and their complexes with inhibitors including (1) the catalytic domain of PDE4B, (2) the catalytic domain of PDE4B complexed with the inhibitors rolipram and iodonated cAMP, (3) full length PDE4D and its complexes with the inhibitors rolipram and denbufylline and (4) the catalytic domain of PDE3 and its complex with cilostamide. The structures in this proposal will reveal the details of inhibitor binding at the active site and provide insight into catalytic mechanism. Docking cGMP into the active site of PDE4B, together with the structure of PDE4B-cAMP analog, will shed light on the substrate specificity. Comparison of the structures of PDE-inhibited complexes will shed light on the selectivity of inhibition of different families of PDE, and thus provide a structural basis for design of selective drugs. The structures will be determined by multiple isomorphous replacement, multiwavelength anomalous diffraction, or molecular replacement. The structural models will be built with the program O and refined by the program CNS.

Website: http://crisp.cit.nih.gov/crisp/Crisp_Query.Generate_Screen

- **Project Title: DIABETES AND UROGENITAL SMOOTH MUSCLE FUNCTION IN VIVO**

Principal Investigator & Institution: Melman, Arnold; Professor & Chairman; Albert Einstein College of Medicine

Timing: Fiscal Year 2003; Project Start 01-DEC-2002; Project End 30-NOV-2007

Summary: Neuronal alterations, as a consequence of diabetes mellitus, aging, or other diseases, can cause organ dysfunciton ranging from mild to severe in scope. Urinary incontinence and **erectile dysfunction** are two such aspects of the human condition that may be caused by neuronal dysfunction. Each condition can have a severely adverse effect on the quality of life at great monetary expense and emotional distress to the individual. In addition to diabetes and the aging process (which affects the entire population) the neuropathies caused by stroke, Parkinson's disease, and multiple sclerosis, are examples of common illnesses that millions of people with potential bladder and penile dysfunction. We will employ the Streptozotocin (STZ) and BBAN rat diabetic models in vivo, to study the effects of diabetic neuropathy on bladder and erectile function. The effects of 1-8 months of diabetic neurepathy on bladder and erectile function be studied on consecutive days in THE SAME MALE RAT in vivo. The working hypothesis is that bladder and erectile tissue are imbued w{th significnat plasticity and that the neuronal loss, in each organ, induces a series of compensatory and/or adaptive tissue, cellular and subcellular changes. The Project, which is designed to measure the physiological effects of diabetic neuropathy, is divided into three Specific Aims. In Specific Aim #1 we will study IN THE SAME RAT ON CONSECUTIVE DAYS, the effects of diabetic neuropathy on bladder (cystometry) and erectile (cavernosometry) function, in vivo. In Specific Aim #2 we will use immunohistochemistry to study the extent of the structural changes in neural status in bladder and erectile tissue from the SAME RAT used in Aim #1; thus permitting us to directly evaluate the effects of neuronal changes on organ function in the SAME RAT. In Specific Aim #3, we will utilize microarray gene chip technologies to study diabetes-related changes in gene expression in bladder and erectile tissue obtained from animals whom have already been evaluated in Aim #1; again, permitting us to evaluate the relationship between diabetic neuropathy, organ function and gene expression.

Website: http://crisp.cit.nih.gov/crisp/Crisp_Query.Generate_Screen

- **Project Title: DYADIC SOCIAL SUPPORT FOR MEN WITH PROSTATE CANCER**

Principal Investigator & Institution: Weber, Bryan A.; Adult and Elderly Nursing; University of Florida Gainesville, Fl 32611

Timing: Fiscal Year 2001; Project Start 01-SEP-2001; Project End 31-AUG-2003

Summary: (Applicant's Description) This 2 year study, "Dyadic Social Support For Men with Prostate Cancer," will investigate the effects of dyadic social support on self-efficacy, social support, and depression for men with prostate cancer, which is the leading form of cancer for American men. Improvements in screening and medical management of prostate cancer have prolonged life expectancy for the 180,000 men to be diagnosed this year. The diagnosis and treatment side effects, particularly urinary and **erectile dysfunction** from radical prostatectomy, are known to lead to depression. Although support groups have been found to reduce depression for cancer patients, few men participate in such groups. One-to-one support with another man as in the proposed dyadic intervention may be more acceptable than support groups to these men. The purpose of the study is to test the effects of a dyadic intervention based on Bandura's Self-Efficacy Theory (vicarious experience, performance and attribute similarity) that links men who are newly diagnosed with prostate cancer with those who are long-term survivors (> 5 years). One hundred men (50 years and older) with prostate cancer and having a radical prostatectomy will be recruited within 100 days of the diagnosis. Excluded will be those with prior history of cancer and death of a loved one within 1 year. Subjects will be randomized to control or experimental groups. Experimental subjects will be matched according to race with a long-term survivor volunteer who had a prostatectomy for prostate cancer. After training in the study protocol, long-term survivors will meet with subjects 8 times during a 60-day period to discuss feelings, thoughts, and concerns associated with prostate cancer. The investigator will monitor the intervention through weekly telephone calls and weekly logs recorded by the long-term survivors that will be used to assess the quality of the interaction, the number and duration of sessions, and topics discussed. Baseline and post-test measures of self-efficacy (Stanford Inventory of Cancer Patient Adjustment), social support (Modified Inventory of Socially Supportive Behaviors), and depression (Geriatric Depression Scale) will be used to determine if the dyadic intervention decreases depression and increases self-efficacy and social support. Comorbidity (Charlson Index), and urinary and sexual dysfunction (UCLA Prostate Cancer Index) are expected to influence depression, hence data will be collected and these factors will be controlled. If dyadic interventions are shown to enhance survival and/or reduce depression among this group, results may be extended to others with cancer. Hence, this may be integrated in the treatment of cancer survivors in the future.

Website: http://crisp.cit.nih.gov/crisp/Crisp_Query.Generate_Screen

- **Project Title: ENGINEERING MANGANESE METALLOENZYMES**

Principal Investigator & Institution: Christianson, David W.; Professor; Chemistry; University of Pennsylvania 3451 Walnut Street Philadelphia, Pa 19104

Timing: Fiscal Year 2002; Project Start 01-MAY-1994; Project End 31-JAN-2006

Summary: (provided by applicant): In order to establish a base of structural knowledge concerning structure, function, and regulation in the enigmatic family of manganese metalloenzymes, we have selected the metallohydrolase rat liver arginase as the paradigm for protein engineering and rational ligand design experiments. This enzyme is extraordinary in that it contains a binuclear, spin-coupled manganese cluster in its active site that is implicated in the chemistry of ariginine hydrolysis. In addition to yielding the first structure of a mammalian urea cycle enzyme (where cytosolic arginase catalyzes the hydrolysis of arginine into omithine plus urea), our structural studies of arginase complement studies of its role in nitric oxide (NO) biology. The activities of nitric oxide synthase and arginase in various tissues are reciprocally coordinated in order to modulate NO-dependent processes. In this role, we have implicated arginase as a potential target for therapeutic intervention in the treatment of **erectile dysfunction.** We have achieved key goals outlined in the original grant proposal, and we now request continued support for X-ray crystallographic studies of arginase, its site-specific variants, and its inhibitor complexes. Additionally, building on our successful design and evaluation of potent boromc acid-based arginase inhibitors in the current funding period, we request support for exploring the development of new inhibitors in a structure-based design approach. New inhibitor designs may exhibit enhanced properties such as affinity and membrane permeability, which may facilitate physiological studies of arginase inhibition in the laboratories of our collaborators.

Website: http://crisp.cit.nih.gov/crisp/Crisp_Query.Generate_Screen

- **Project Title: ERECTILE DYSFUNCTION AND NITRIC OXIDE SYNTHASE IN AGING**

Principal Investigator & Institution: Gonzalez-Cadavid, Nestor F.; Harbor-Ucla Research & Educ Inst 1124 W Carson St Torrance, Ca 90502

Timing: Fiscal Year 2001; Project Start 01-MAY-1999; Project End 30-APR-2003

Summary: Erectile dysfunction, the inability of the penis to [attain or maintain] a rigid erection, is associated with aging. In the aging rat model, a defective relaxation of the penile corpora cavernosal smooth muscle results from a loss of tissue compliance, [and/or, possibly excessive sympathetic tone,] and/or, 61 reduced synthesis of nitric oxide (NO), the main mediator of penile erection. Our laboratory found and cloned PnNOS, a novel variant of neuronal nitric oxide synthase (nNOS), and showed it is the only nNOS expressed in the rat penis [both as full- length and shorter protein variants. A putative endothelial NOS (eNOS) variant was also detected. We have also shown that a protein Inhibitor of NOS activity (PIN), is expressed in the rat and human penis.] We also found that the aging-associated **erectile dysfunction** in the rat can be ameliorated by gene therapy with cDNA constructs of penile inducible NOS (iNOS). The aims of this project are first to determine whether aging affects the expression pattern of PnNOS and NOS (eNOS) variants in the penis by western and northern blots, RT/PCR, immunocytochemistry and in situ hybridization, and whether the reduction in penile NOS enzyme activity in very old animals is caused by NOS binding to inhibitors or by NOS glycation. Gene therapy of the corpora cavernosa in aged rats with PnNOS Will then be investigated, using several regimes and cDNA constructs in conjunction with L-arginine, to stimulate NOS activity. The ability to increase the erectile response of aged rats to electrical field stimulation (EFS) of the cavernosal nerve, and penile reflexes, will be determined. [Finally, the effects of aging on the levels of PIN binding to PnNOS variants will be determined in the rat penis with immunodetection techniques. An anti-PIN gene therapy with the cDNA for the truncated PnNOS unable to bind PIN (PnNOSbeta) will be tested to stimulate PIN-independent NOS activity. Alternatively, the cDNA for the nNOS protein domain that binds PIN will be given to quench PIN effects, and antisense PIN oligonucleotides will be investigated for a possible down-regulation of PIN translation. Other putative protein modulators of PnNOS activity will be searched for using the random display peptide library]. The long-term goal is to validate pre-clinically the use of these agents for medical treatment of **erectile dysfunction** associated with aging.

Website: http://crisp.cit.nih.gov/crisp/Crisp_Query.Generate_Screen

- **Project Title: ERECTILE FUNCTION AND THE INFLUENCE OF RHO-KINASE**

Principal Investigator & Institution: Wingard, Christopher J.; Assistant Professor; Phys Med and Rehabilitation; Medical College of Georgia 1120 15Th St Augusta, Ga 30912

Timing: Fiscal Year 2001; Project Start 21-SEP-2001; Project End 31-AUG-2005

Summary: (Adapted from the Applicant's Abstract): An estimated 30 million American men are reported to have some form of **erectile dysfunction** with close to 75 percent having an organic origin. The erectile response in the penis is dependent on the reactive state of the smooth muscle of the cavernosal sinuses and of the arteries supplying blood to those sinuses. A variety of pathways can sensitize the cavernosal vasculature and suppress the normal erectile response. Our preliminary studies, using an in vivo model of erectile function have demonstrated both ET-1 and pheneylphrine can suppress the erectile response and that an inhibitor of Rho-kinase is capable of reversing this sensitization. We hypothesize that an active RhoA/Rho-kinase signal transduction pathway exerts a potent vasoconstrictive action on the cavernosal smooth muscle thus maintaining the penis in a flaccid state. Activation of the RhoA pathway results in increased activity of Rho-associated kinase (ROK or Rho-kinase) which enhances contractile sensitivity. The goal of this proposal is to understand the role of the RhoA/Rho-kinase signaling vasoactive pathways and mechanisms by which Rho-kinase modulates cavernosal smooth muscle contractile activity. Specific aim 1 is to demonstrate the functional role of the RhoA/Rho-kinase signal transduction pathway in normal erectile response. Specific aim 2 is to elucidate how Rho-kinase activated cavernosal smooth muscle contraction influences he erectile response mediated by neural stimulation or pharmacological intervention. Specific aim 3 is to determine if the

RhoA/Rho-kinase pathway contributes to the diminished erectile response in an animal model of **erectile dysfunction.** With use of both in vivo and in vitro approaches, this proposal will generate new information relevant to the regulation of cavernosal circulation and its role in **erectile dysfunction.** If our hypothesis is correct, future studies may examine other modulators of this novel regulatory pathway and how potential alterations of this pathway may aid in treatment of **erectile dysfunction.**

Website: http://crisp.cit.nih.gov/crisp/Crisp_Query.Generate_Screen

- **Project Title: EXPANDIBILITY AS A MEASURE OF FIBROSIS INDUCED IMPOTENCE**

  Principal Investigator & Institution: Udelson, Daniel G.; Aerospace and Mechanical Engineering; Boston University Charles River Campus 881 Commonwealth Avenue Boston, Ma 02215

  Timing: Fiscal Year 2003; Project Start 15-SEP-2003; Project End 31-AUG-2006

  Summary: (provided by applicant): **Erectile dysfunction** is common, developing in 52% of men aged 40-70 years, and the host significant physiological correlate is increasing age. Independent of vascular disease, erectile tissue undergoes progressive loss of corporal trabacular smooth muscle and increase of corporal connective tissue. If clinicians were able to accurately measure in a non-invasive manner the degree of corporal fibrosis, they would be in a position to develop management strategies to prevent or delay the onset of **erectile dysfunction.** The clinical utility of an assessment of corpus cavernosum fibrosis is primarily early detection of initial structural disease, a critical component of **erectile dysfunction** prophylaxis. The broad, long-term objective of this engineering-based medical research is the development of a clinically-applicable method to assess corpus cavernosum fibrosis. The specific aims to achieve this goal will be to: (i) develop a refined engineering model that illustrates the relationship between cavernosal percent smooth muscle and cavernosal "expandibility". (2) demonstrate, in a group of patients, correlation between cavernosal "expandibility" (obtained during pre-operative dynamic infusion pharmacocavernosometry) and cavernosal percent smooth muscle (obtained by histomorphometric analysis of the cavernosal tissue harvested during penile implant surgery). This would verify that the correlation between these two parameters, which was shown to exist in a previous animal study, also exists in humans; and (3) clinically test a circular strain gauge device that automatically measures penile geometry versus intracavernosal pressure which is necessary for the calculation of cavernosal "expandibility". It is anticipated that this project will contribute substantially to a new clinical assessment of the structural effects of aging on **erectile dysfunction** which is necessary to develop rational effective clinical strategies to offset the age-related decline in erectile function.

  Website: http://crisp.cit.nih.gov/crisp/Crisp_Query.Generate_Screen

- **Project Title: GENE THERAPY OF DIABETIC PENILE ENDOTHELIAL DYSFUNCTION**

  Principal Investigator & Institution: Wessells, Hunter; Associate Professor; Urology; University of Washington Seattle, Wa 98195

  Timing: Fiscal Year 2001; Project Start 15-SEP-2000; Project End 30-JUN-2005

  Summary: Gene therapy of diabetic penile endothelial dysfunction. Half of the 7.5 million diabetic men in the US will develop **erectile dysfunction** (ED). Despite advances in our understanding of erectile physiology, treatments for diabetic impotence remains limited, and phosphodiesterase-specific therapy (Viagra) fails in the majority of diabetics with ED. It is known that endothelium- dependent smooth muscle relaxation is impaired in vascular and penile tissue from diabetics. Nitric oxide generated in the endothelium is involved in vasorelaxation and is an important supporter of cardiovascular homeostasis. But the role of the endothelial cell during flaccidity and erection is not understood. We hypothesize that the endothelial cell is critical to the homeostasis of the corpus cavernosum and that iNOS gene therapy of the penile endothelium can mitigate the development of **erectile dysfunction.** The goals of this project are 1) to demonstrate that diabetes impairs endothelium-dependent erectile responses through changes in eNOS homeostasis and endothelial cytoskeletal organization and 2) to repair the penile endothelium with iNOS gene therapy. Specific Aim 1 will characterize the time course and severity of endothelium dependent erection in the normal and streptozotocin- induced diabetic rat. Specific Aims 2 and 3 will examine the effects of hyperglycemia on corporal endothelial structure and function in vitro and in vivo. Cultured corporal endothelial cells and a detailed analysis of rat and human diabetic corpora will provide different methodological approaches to characterize eNOS expression and activity, cytoskeletal integrity, and disturbances in the cell cycle. Specific Aim 4 will determine whether transplantation of iNOS-transduced endothelial cells will generate high levels of nitric oxide, repair the corporal endothelium, and augment erectile responses in diabetic rats. By providing a more detailed understanding of the corporal endothelium, and the alterations induced by diabetes, we can develop a novel therapeutic strategy targeted to the endothelial cell and endothelium-dependent mechanisms of **erectile dysfunction.** Such a strategy may ultimately be beneficial to men with ED due to diabetes as well as smoking, hypercholesterolemia, and aging.

Website: http://crisp.cit.nih.gov/crisp/Crisp_Query.Generate_Screen

- **Project Title: HORMONES AND ERECTILE DYSFUNCTION IN AGING MEN**

Principal Investigator & Institution: Mckinlay, John B.; Senior Vice President and Director; New England Research Institutes, Inc. 9 Galen St Watertown, Ma 02472

Timing: Fiscal Year 2001; Project Start 19-MAY-1995; Project End 31-AUG-2005

Summary: (provided by applicant): The Massachusetts Male Aging Study (MMAS) is considered a landmark research effort in the fields of aging, urology, and endocrinology. It employs a random sample of community-dwelling men (not a convenience sample of patient volunteers). Its size permits estimation of even relatively rare phenomena (e.g., hypogonadism). It is longitudinal (intra-subject variation) not cross-sectional (inter-subject variation) and has successfully followed a cohort from 987-89 (T1) through 1995-97 (T2). Worldwide, it remains the largest male endocrine database. It is the first and still the only major longitudinal study of ED. It is multidisciplinary. The MMAS team has been extraordinarily productive. Emphasis has been given to the practical clinical applications of scientific findings. The proposed project ("EPIDEMIOLOGY OF HORMONES AND **ERECTILE DYSFUNCTION** IN AGING MEN") is designed to extend the highly productive MMAS by following a projected 800 already participating subjects through a third wave (T3). Building directly on earlier work we will: continue investigation of life-span changes in 14 carefully selected hormones in the same subjects; precisely delineate any hypogonadal syndrome and its major correlates; continue pioneering work on **erectile dysfunction** (ED) and its various predictors; precisely measure the hypothesized relation between ED (sentinel event) and subsequent CVD; extend knowledge concerning ED-related utilization behavior and quality of life in older men; and assess the validity of the single question measure of ED against a clinical urologic examination by a nationally-respected urologist blinded to subjects' self-reported ED status. Methods of data collection will be identical to those used previously for the MMAS. The proposed research will continue to provide the most comprehensive and reliable information available on ED, life-span hormonal changes and their physiological, psychosocial, anthropometric, and behavioral predictors in normally aging men. Prior to the MMAS there was: (a) no well-designed prospective study describing life span changes in endocrine functioning (hormones) in normally aging men; and (b) no definitive population-based study of ED and its biobehavioral correlates.

Website: http://crisp.cit.nih.gov/crisp/Crisp_Query.Generate_Screen

- **Project Title: MOLECULAR MECHANISM FOR ERECTILE FUNCTION & DYSFUNCTION**

Principal Investigator & Institution: Disanto, Michael E.; Assistant Professor; Surgery; University of Pennsylvania 3451 Walnut Street Philadelphia, Pa 19104

Timing: Fiscal Year 2001; Project Start 29-SEP-1998; Project End 30-JUN-2003

Summary: Erection(tumescence) is a complex neurophysiologic event that leads to relaxation of the smooth muscle cells in the corpus cavernosum penis which allows filling of blood into the cavernous spaces causing an increase in the size and rigidity of the penis. Flaccidity (detumescence) is initiated and maintained by contraction of the corpus cavernosum smooth muscle (CCSM) cells. The CCSM is unique since it remains in the contracted state most of the time. It is not know whether the Ca2+-calmodulin-MLCK pathway or other then filament- mediated regulation (via the actin-binding protein caldesmon) plays a role in keeping these cells in the contracted state, for the penis to remain flaccid. A third possibility is that the myosin isoforms in CCSM play a role in determining the velocity of force generation and the tonicity. A recent study conducted by this investigator showed that the aortic smooth muscle, which is considered tonic, contains one type of myosin isoform whereas the smooth muscle cells in small muscular arteries contain a different myosin isoform. The latter isoform is encoded by a myosin heavy chain mRNA that is alternatively spliced to insert a 21-nucleotide sequence that encodes a region near the ATP-binding site on the myosin head. This insert encodes a 7-amino acid peptide, and the resulting myosin isoform has a two-fold increase in the actin-activated myosin ATPase activity and an associated increase in shortening velocity (Vmax). Similar studies conducted on CCSM in our lab show that the CCSM contains both inserted (as in small muscular arteries and all visceral smooth muscles which show phasic characteristics) and non-inserted (as in aortic smooth muscle which is tonic) myosin heavy chain isoforms. Specially, using CCSM from normal rabbits, normal humans, and patients with erectile dysfunctions, we will address the following questions: (1) Are the differences in the contractile characteristics of CCSM compared to smooth muscle from other sources due to a difference in the composition of smooth muscle myosin isoforms that are produced by alternative splicing of the myosin pre-mRNA at the 3' end (resulting in SM1 and SM2) or the 5' end (resulting in inserted myosin)? (2) What role does myosin light chain phosphorylation play in erectile function and do CCSM cells have higher kinase or lower phosphatase activity compared to other smooth muscle cells (e.g. bladder smooth muscle)? (3) What is the level of expression of myosin light chain kinase and caldesmon in the CCSM and is it altered in patients with erectile dysfunction? Thus, the results from experiments proposed in this application will provide the molecular mechanisms for the regulation of CCSM contraction and delineate specific steps in the pathways for cross-bridge cycling and contractility of smooth muscle cells in the normal corporus cavernosum penis. It will also provide and explanation for changes in contractility of smooth muscle cells seen in patients with **erectile dysfunction.**

Website: http://crisp.cit.nih.gov/crisp/Crisp_Query.Generate_Screen

- **Project Title: MOLECULAR MECHANISMS OF PDE5 REGULATION**

Principal Investigator & Institution: Corbin, Jackie D.; Molecular Physiol & Biophysics; Vanderbilt University 3319 West End Ave. Nashville, Tn 372036917

Timing: Fiscal Year 2001; Project Start 01-MAY-2001; Project End 30-APR-2006

Summary: (Applicant's abstract): Interest in mammalian cGMP cascades has recently been intense. Much research in this area has centered on the signal receptors and guanylyl cyclases that modulate cGMP formation, as well as on cellular actions of cGMP. Natural signals (natriuretic peptides, guanylins and nitric oxide), in addition to many medications, stimulate cGMP cascades by activating these cyclases. Cyclic nucleotide phosphodiesterases (PDEs), which are also highly modulated enzymes, participate in regulating cellular cAMP and cGMP levels by catalyzing breakdown of cAMP and cGMP. The subject of this application is the cGMP-binding cGMP-specific PDE (PDE5), which is specific for cGMP over cAMP at its allosteric cGMP-binding sites and at its catalytic site. The long-term goal is to determine the mechanism of action and cellular regulation of PDE5, a major determinant of cGMP level in many tissues. Classical effects of cGMP include relaxation of smooth muscle, inhibition of platelet activation, neutrophil degranulation, and mediation of vision. New discoveries have expanded this list to include regulation of gene expression, chloride transport in intestine and kidney, watertransport, bone resorption, melanogenesis in skin, long-term nerve depression, and opioid effects. Therapeutic agents that elevate cGMP include PDE inhibitors (e.g., caffeine, papaverine, and sildenafil) and nitrovasodilators (e.g., nitroglycerin). Certain enterotoxins cause secretory diarrhea by elevating cGMP. Dr. Corbin recently demonstrated that in some instances cGMP acts by "crossactivating" cAMP receptors. However, PDE5 is a specific intracellular receptor for cGMP. The present proposal represents a thorough biochemical and physiological investigation of PDE5 regulation. This enzyme is the specific target of sildenafil (Viagra.), which is used in treatment of male **erectile dysfunction** associated with diabetes, aging, spinal cord injuries and other pathologies. Effects of phosphorylation of PDE5 by cyclic nucleotide-dependent protein kinases on catalysis and allosteric cGMP binding will be explored, and effects of mutating the phosphorylation site, Ser- 102 (human), to Ala, Glu, and Asp will be examined. The principal investigator will study the PDE5 regulatory domain structure and function by expressing truncation mutants that include various combinations of the two allosteric cUMP-binding sites and the phosphorylation site of the enzyme but exclude the catalytic domain. Small angle x-ray scattering and Fourier transformed infra-red spectroscopy will be used to study effects of cGMP and phosphorylation on conformation of these domains. Crystallography of certain truncated regulatory domains will be attempted. The specificity and efficacy with which phosphoprotein phosphatases of vascular smooth muscle extracts catalyze dephosphorylation of Ser-102 will be investigated. Short-term regulation of PDE5 in intact vascular smooth muscle by cGMP analogs, phosphoprotein phosphatase inhibitors, and agents that elevate cGMP will be studied. The possibility that hese agents could alter enzyme activity, subcellular localization, or cGMP levels (feedback mechanism) will be examined. Potential non-covalent modulators of PDE5 other than cGMP will be sought. The possibility that PDE5 allosteric sites represent a sequestration site for cGMP in cells will be explored. Results of these studies will provide a basis for understanding fundamental questions relating to cGMP signaling in many tissues.

Website: http://crisp.cit.nih.gov/crisp/Crisp_Query.Generate_Screen

- **Project Title: MOLECULAR STUDIES OF EXPERIMENTAL DIABETIC NEUROPATHY**

Principal Investigator & Institution: Christ, George J.; Professor; Urology; Yeshiva University 500 W 185Th St New York, Ny 10033

Timing: Fiscal Year 2001; Project Start 01-MAR-2001; Project End 31-DEC-2003

Summary: (Adapted from the Applicant's Abstract): More than 50 percent of patients with diabetes have **erectile dysfunction,** with autonomic neuropathy playing a proximal role. However, the precise contribution of autonomic neuropathy to diabetic **erectile dysfunction** remains undefined. Part of the difficulty in establishing the etiologic role of the autonomic nervous system in diabetic **erectile dysfunction** is related to the fact that the penis is endowed with multiple mechanisms for preserving syncytial tissue function. In particular, the interaction among: 1. neuronal innervation, 2. cell-to-cell communication, and 3. myogenic intracellular signal transduction processes, are critical to guarantee erectile function over a wide range of physiological conditions. Such plasticity is expected of an organ critical to the survival of the species and the physiological well being of men and their sexual partners. The explicit aim of these studies is to utilize an established rat model of experimental diabetic neuropathy to evaluate the effects of diabetes on autonomic innervation in the penis, and any correlative changes that occur in intercellular communication and myogenic responsivity. In particular, we will test the hypothesis that autonomic neuropathy is associated with global alterations in tissue function, that result, at least in part, from alterations in ion flow through potassium (K) and gap junction channels. Specifically, we shall induce a 1-6 month period of streptozotocin (STZ)-diabetes in Fischer-344 (F-344) rats, and: 1. Evaluate the functional correlates of molecular changes in K channels and gap junctions that are associated with experimental diabetic neuropathy/hyperglycemia, and 2. To evaluate the functional correlates of the molecular changes in K channels and gap junctions that are produced by a novel gene therapy approach for the amelioration of **erectile dysfunction.** To this end, we will utilize techniques ranging from in vivo animal studies, through in vitro studies at the tissue, cellular, subcellular and molecular/genetic levels. By bringing to bear such a diverse array of techniques on this important medical problem we hope to gain the greatest insight possible into the functional correlates in vivo of well quantified molecular alterations.

Website: http://crisp.cit.nih.gov/crisp/Crisp_Query.Generate_Screen

- **Project Title: MYOSIN LIGHT CHAIN KINASE FUNCTION IN SMOOTH MUSCLE**

Principal Investigator & Institution: Stull, James T.; Professor and Chair; Physiology; University of Texas Sw Med Ctr/Dallas Dallas, Tx 753909105

Timing: Fiscal Year 2001; Project Start 01-APR-1995; Project End 31-MAR-2004

Summary: The overall objectives of the research projects described in this proposal are to provide insights into how myosin light chain kinase (MLCK) is regulated by Ca^{2+} / calmodulin in vivo and in vitro and to establish the importance of kinase binding to actin-containing filaments in smooth muscle. Specific aim I will test the hypothesis that Ca^{2+} / calmodulin activation of MLCK involves sequential binding steps between the two domains of calmodulin with the calmodulin-binding sequence and catalytic core. Low-angle X-ray and neutron-scattering studies will be combined with protein fragment complementation and protein cross-linking to identify sites of interactions between the catalytic core, the regulatory segment, and calmodulin. Specific aim II will determine the temporal and spatial distributions of calmodulin binding to MLCK in vivo with a biosensor MLCK containing fluorescent indicator proteins. The relationship between calmodulin-bound kinase and the extent of myosin regulatory light chain phosphorylation will be established. A biosensor MLCK will be expressed in transgenic mice with a smooth muscle-specific promoter for physiological studies on aortic and bladder tissues. Specific aim III will determine the biochemical mechanism for MLCK binding to actin-containing filaments. We will test the hypothesis that all three motifs cooperatively confer high-affinity binding and that spacing between the motifs is important. Specific aim IV will investigate the importance of MLCK binding to actin-containing filaments in vivo. We will test the hypothesis that the bound kinase is not translocated from F-actin filaments to the cytosol with increases in [Ca2+] in smooth muscle cells in culture and in tissues. Smooth muscle tissues play important roles in many body functions and are crucial for maintaining the homeostatic environment. The investigations proposed in this application address fundamental mechanisms involved in contractile regulation of smooth muscle. Investigations dealing with the primary biochemical pathway controlling smooth muscle contractility are essential for understanding derangements in smooth muscle-based diseases such as asthma, hypertension, **erectile dysfunction** and irritable bowl syndrome.

Website: http://crisp.cit.nih.gov/crisp/Crisp_Query.Generate_Screen

- **Project Title: N O S AND NEUROPATHIC AND ENDOTHELIAL INDUCED ED**

Principal Investigator & Institution: Mcvary, Kevin T.; Associate Professor; Urology; Northwestern University Office of Sponsored Programs Chicago, Il 60611

Timing: Fiscal Year 2001; Project Start 30-SEP-1998; Project End 31-AUG-2003

Summary: (adapted from the application) **Erectile dysfunction** (ED) is a devastating pathologic development affecting 10-30 million American men and costing in excess of $150 million for inpatient urologic care alone (1985 dollars). Diabetes mellitus (DM) is a common risk factor for ED as it effects 15 million Americans and contributes to ED in 50% of affected males. The pathogenesis of this ED is controversial because of the mixed angiopathy and neuropathy found in human DM. Recently, we reported an animal model of DM with evidence supporting neuropathy alone as a cause for ED. We found, using the Bio- breeding Wistar (BBWOR) diabetic rat model, diffuse neuropathic changes resulting in ED without a confounding vasculopathy. We have identified profound deficits in the sexual behavior of diabetics as well as deficits in sexual reflexes and physiologic erections suggesting a CNS dysfunction and a concurrent diffuse peripheral neuropathic process(es) resulting in ED. We have recent evidence that nitric oxide (NO), a central and peripheral autonomic neurotransmitter and regulatory of penile erection, is decreased in diabetic rats. Our goal is to characterize DM's impact on autonomic regulation of penile smooth muscle (SM) relaxation. We postulate that ED in our model is due to a central and peripheral change in neural NO content and subsequent impaired transmission. This change in NO level is secondary to down regulated NOS expression in neural and corporal SM tissues. The following four specific aims are proposed: 1) test the hypothesis that multiple nitric oxide synthase (NOS) subtypes are present in the penile SM and spinal cord of control and diabetic rats using Western immunoblot and immunohistochemistry, 2) test the hypothesis that the content and expression of NOS subtypes are down regulated at spinal cord and penile level in diabetics, 3) test the hypothesis that diabetics have decreased NOS enzymatic activity and altered levels of secondary messengers (cGMP) in the penile SM, and 4) test they hypothesis that NOS deficits in the CNS and the PNS/penis are responsible are the differences seen in diabetic rats by the use of NOS antagonists to induce diabetic- like sexual dysfunction in control rats. Results of this research will aid in the understanding of how diabetic neuropathy contributes to sexual dysfunction in control rats. Results of this research will aid in the understanding of how diabetic neuropathy contributes to sexual dysfunction and elucidate possible mechanisms to prevent them.

Website: http://crisp.cit.nih.gov/crisp/Crisp_Query.Generate_Screen

- **Project Title: NITRIC OXIDE INHIBITS RHOA/RHO-KINASE IN PENILE ERECTION**

Principal Investigator & Institution: Webb, R Clinton.; Chairperson; Phys Med and Rehabilitation; Medical College of Georgia 1120 15Th St Augusta, Ga 30912

Timing: Fiscal Year 2003; Project Start 04-APR-2003; Project End 31-MAR-2007

Summary: (provided by applicant): Over 30 million men suffer from **erectile dysfunction** in the United States. Constriction and dilation of the cavernosal vasculature determines penile erection. In the absence of arousal stimuli, Ca2+-sensitizing RhoA/Rho-kinase signaling maintains vasoconstriction, keeping the penis non-erect. Upon arousal, nitric oxide (NO), released from nerves and endothelial cells, induces dilation and erection. Although NO stimulates erection, the cellular mechanism of NO is unknown. NO binds soluble guanylate cyclase to stimulate an increase in cyclic GMP (cGMP) and the subsequent activation of cGMP-dependent protein kinase (cGK). In the penis, cGK has been proposed to induce dilation through activation of membrane K+ channels to cause hyperpolarization, inhibition of membrane Ca2+ channels to decrease activator Ca+, and stimulation of sarcoplasmic reticular Ca2+ uptake to sequester the cation. However, recent work suggests that high levels of activator Ca2+ are not maintained during constriction and it is the Ca2+-sensitizing effect of RhoAJRho-kinase that must be overcome to cause dilation. We hypothesize that cGK inhibits RhoA translocation to the membrane leading to a reduction in Rho-kinase activity and removal of its inhibitory action on myosin light chain (MLC) phosphatase. This dis-inhibition leads to reduced MLC phosphorylation, smooth muscle relaxation and erection. We further hypothesize that the long-term expression of components of the RhoA/Rho-kinase signaling pathway are inversely related to NO bioavailability. These hypotheses will be tested by 3 specific aims: 1) to determine if NO/cGMP/cGK signaling antagonizes RhoA activation to evoke dilation and penile erection; 2) to determine if gene transfer of endothelial nitric oxide synthase (eNOS) to the penis will down-regulate RhoA/Rho-kinase signaling to augment erection; and 3) to determine if reduced NO bioavailability (pharmacological blockade and denervation) leads to up-regulation of the RhoA/Rho-kinase pathway and **erectile dysfunction.** The approach will utilize rat and mouse models of erection. The experiments will determine the effect of NO/cGMP/cGK on biochemical, pharmacological and physiological measures of the RhoA/Rho-kinase pathway in the intact penis and in isolated cavernosal strips. Gene transfer of dominant-negative RhoA and endothelial NOS to the penis will provide a powerful tool to manipulate the activity of the RhoA/Rho-kinase pathway. Contractile force measurements in isolated cavernosal strips (intact and permeablizied) will provide evidence for Ca2+ sensitization and its regulation by cGMP/cGK. These studies will define the molecular basis for NO-mediated cavernosal vasodilation in the normal state and how long-term changes in the Ca 2+ sensitizing mechanism contribute to **erectile dysfunction.**

Website: http://crisp.cit.nih.gov/crisp/Crisp_Query.Generate_Screen

- **Project Title: NITRIC OXIDE REGULATORY SYSTEM IN THE PENIS**

Principal Investigator & Institution: Burnett, Arthur L.; Associate Professor; Urology; Johns Hopkins University 3400 N Charles St Baltimore, Md 21218

Timing: Fiscal Year 2001; Project Start 16-APR-1998; Project End 31-MAR-2003

Summary: (adapted from the application) It is currently accepted that the mechanism of vascular and trabecular smooth muscle relaxation in the penis required for penile erection depends upon nitric oxide. This novel biochemical mediator is well understood to be synthesized and released from nerve terminals within the erectile tissue of the penis. Some evidence also exists for its release from the endothelial component of the erectile tissue. As nitric oxide exerts such a significant role in the physiology of the penis, it would be pertinent to also understand the control mechanisms effecting its release and action in this organ. It is entirely conceivable that nitric oxide operates much like other mediators which are neither released constantly or unchangeably but are precisely regulated by modulatory substances. Regulation of the nitric oxide signal transduction pathway in the penis may significantly affect erectile tissue function and dysfunction. An improved understanding of the regulatory basis for nitric oxide effects in the penis would be expected to advance the biochemical and pharmacological approaches to promote erectile tissue function and dysfunction. An improved understanding of the regulatory basis for nitric oxide effects in the penis would be expected to advance the biochemical and pharmacologic approaches to promote erectile integrity and to minimize structural and functional damage involving the erectile tissue of the penis. Such an advance is welcomed in view of the established 10-20 percent rate of **erectile dysfunction** present in the American male population. This research proposal centers on two primary objectives, the regulatory basis for nitric oxide in the physiology of the penis and that possibly influencing penile pathophysiology. Specific aims are: (1) to examine the effects of selective an combined nitric oxide synthase isoform deletions on penile erections in genetically altered mutant mice and determine whether compensatory mechanisms develop which preserve erectile function in these mice; (2) to investigate the effects of stimulation and inhibition of neural and humoral factors commonly associated with erectile function and dysfunction on the maintenance of penile erections in mutant mice with selecting and combined deletions of nitric oxide synthase isoforms; and (3) to evaluate neurotrophic mechanisms that may result in physiologic upregulation of nitric oxide synthase in the penis applying neurotrophin delivery to experiments paradigms of **erectile dysfunction.** The experimental strategies employed by this proposal prominently feature a mutant mouse paradigm in which nitric oxide synthase genes are genetically disrupted. Consequences of this model on erectile function at baseline and following perturbations such as androgen withdrawal, neurotransmitter stimulation, neurotrophin exposure, and diabetogenesis will be studied using immunoblot analysis to confirm nitric oxide synthase expressions, immunohistochemistry to confirm nitric oxide synthase localizations, nitric oxide synthase assay to confirm nitric oxide synthase activity, and both physiologic erection and isometric tension studies of isolated erectile tissue to determine the effects of erectile function.

Website: http://crisp.cit.nih.gov/crisp/Crisp_Query.Generate_Screen

- **Project Title: PILOT--CHEMICAL PROFILING OF ORPHAN NUCLEAR RECEPTORS**

Principal Investigator & Institution: Downes, Michael; Baylor College of Medicine 1 Baylor Plaza Houston, Tx 77030

Timing: Fiscal Year 2002; Project Start 15-AUG-2002; Project End 31-JUL-2007

Summary: A solid clinical rationale exists for the discovery of novel orphan nuclear receptor (ONR) therapeutic ligands. The intimate associate, for example, between PPARgamma and carbohydrate and lipid metabolism, for example, finds clear expression in a variety of metabolic and aging disorders from atherosclerosis and lipid metabolism, for example, finds clear expression in a variety of metabolic and aging disorders, from atherosclerosis and diabetes, to Alzheimer's disease, decreased skin elasticity, male **erectile dysfunction,** pulmonary fibrosis, and atherosclerosis, and ocular diseases such as diabetic retinopathy, glaucoma, cataract formation, and age-related macular degeneration (AMD). This proposal will focus on the discovery of novel chemical tools for the purpose of advancing ONR research. A technology platform will be assembled that will facilitate the screening of chemical compound libraries for molecules able to modulate ONR-mediated transcription. Chemical screens that will be established to achieve this objective will consist of both in vivo and in vitro bas assays developed specifically for a high throughput (HTS) 384 well format. The assays developed exploit the agonist induced association of receptor ligand binding domains (LBDs) with nuclear receptor co-regulators and their derivative peptides. Currently we have diverse 18000 chemical compound library of mostly synthetic compounds that we have demonstrated to be viable for screening against ONRs. A pilot a screen of these compounds against FXR and identified novel compounds that robustly activate transcription of this ONR. The major goal of this project is to identify potent, specific compounds and make them freely available to the academic community to contribute high quality and unrestricted research on ONR function.

Website: http://crisp.cit.nih.gov/crisp/Crisp_Query.Generate_Screen

- **Project Title: QUALITATIVE STUDY OF PROSTATE CANCER SYMPTOM MANAGEMENT**

Principal Investigator & Institution: Latini, David M.; Urology; University of California San Francisco 500 Parnassus Ave San Francisco, Ca 94122

Timing: Fiscal Year 2003; Project Start 30-SEP-2003; Project End 31-MAR-2005

Summary: (provided by applicant.) Prostate cancer is the second-most common cancer among American men Various options for treatment exist, with approximately equal effectiveness However, the choice of treatment can result in different side effects that severely impact quality of life These side-effects include medical problems, such as **erectile dysfunction** and urinary and bowel incontinence The experience of those side-effects can cause a number of emotional and psychological concerns, including changes in self-concept, difficulties in a man's primary relationship, and social isolation to avoid the embarrassment of incontinence in a social setting Numerous interventions have been developed for patients with other types of cancers, but few interventions have been developed for men with localized prostate cancer None of the existing prostate cancer interventions focus on symptom management, an important part of the prostate cancer survivor's quality of life Moreover, interventions that target more general cancer symptoms (e g, pain or nausea) have less relevance for the unique needs of men with localized prostate cancer Our study proposes to use the Critical Incident Technique to collect data on how patients with treatment-related side-effects are able to successfully manage the physical and psychosocial impact of their symptoms The critical incident reports will be organized into a taxonomy of effective and ineffective symptom management practices. As part of the proposed study, the investigator will accomplish the following aims: 1. Collect qualitative data describing effective and ineffective symptom management knowledge, skills, and behaviors in men treated for localized prostate cancer from prostate cancer patients, their partners, and health care providers.

2. Analyze the critical incidents to develop a hierarchical classification or taxonomy of critical symptom management competencies. 3. Using the taxonomy of symptom management competencies from Specific Aim 2, develop the instructional objectives for a tailored intervention that will help men treated for prostate cancer manage their treatment-related side-effects and related psychosocial concerns more effectively.

Website: http://crisp.cit.nih.gov/crisp/Crisp_Query.Generate_Screen

- **Project Title: REGULATION OF PDE 5 IN HUMAN PENILE SMOOTH MUSCLE CELLS**

Principal Investigator & Institution: Kim, Noel N.; Urology; Boston University Medical Campus 715 Albany St, 560 Boston, Ma 02118

Timing: Fiscal Year 2001; Project Start 01-SEP-1999; Project End 31-JUL-2003

Summary: The nitric oxide/cGMP signalling pathway is a major regulator of penile vascular smooth muscle tone and plays a critical role in erection. Phosphodiesterases, enzymes which hydrolyze cyclic nucleotides, are an integral part of this signalling pathway. Phosphodiesterase type 5 (PDE 5) is one of the main phosphodiesterases expressed in penile corpus cavernosum smooth muscle. Sildenafil, a reversible PDE 5 selective inhibitor, has been successfully utilized in the clinical treatment of **erectile dysfunction.** The efficacy of this inhibitor in ameliorating erectile function in men with impotence, resulting from a broad range of etiologies, emphasizes the crucial aspect which PDE5 plays in regulating penile smooth muscle tone. Yet the regulation of PDE 5 expression or activity is not well understood and the consequences of prolonged inhibition of this enzyme are unknown. Fundamental knowledge of the cellular and molecular mechanisms which regulate PDE 5 expression and/or activity is important to the understanding of erectile function. The novel perspective that intracellular cGMP levels are actively regulated by PDE 5 broadens our understanding of the cGMP signalling pathway and the integrated mechanisms which control penile trabecular smooth muscle tone. Thus, in this study we will investigate potential regulatory mechanisms which may alter the expression and/or activity of PDE 5 in human penile corpus cavernosum smooth muscle. We will utilize primary cultures of human penile trabecular smooth muscle cells to study and characterize mechanisms of PDE 5 regulation without disrupting the intracellular regulatory pathways which are under investigation. Using cyclic nucleotide radioimmunoassays, Northern and Western blot analyses, and enzyme activity assays, we will investigate: 1) the effects of nitric oxide and cGMP on PDE 5 expression and/or activity; 2) the effects of cAMP and agonists which stimulate adenylate cyclase on PDE 5 expression and/or activity; 3) the effects of cAMP and agonists which stimulate adenylate cyclase on PDE 5 expression and/or activity; 4) cross-talk regulation between cyclic nucleotides and their respective protein kinases, and estrogen and testosterone signalling pathways. This investigation of multiple signalling systems and their influence on PDE 5 will increase our current understanding of the extensive nature by which distinct signalling pathways can interact and provide integrated regulation of smooth muscle tone. This work will provide new and useful information on regulation of PDE5 which will improve treatment strategies for management o **erectile dysfunction.**

Website: http://crisp.cit.nih.gov/crisp/Crisp_Query.Generate_Screen

- **Project Title: REGULATION OF SOLUBLE GUANYLYL CYCLASE, THE NO-RECEPTOR**

Principal Investigator & Institution: Beuve, Annie V.; Pharmacology and Physiology; Univ of Med/Dent Nj Newark Newark, Nj 07103

Timing: Fiscal Year 2003; Project Start 15-APR-2003; Project End 31-MAR-2008

Summary: (provided by applicant): The cellular processes that are regulated by nitric oxide (NO) are central to many aspects of biology and disease, particularly in the cardiovascular system and the central and peripheral nervous systems. Despite the widely recognized importance of NO, little is known about the mechanism of regulation of the NO receptor, the soluble guanylyl cyclase (sGC). sGC is a heme-containing heterodimer that catalyzes the formation of cGMP from the substrate GTP. Upon binding of NO to the heme, the sGC is activated several hundred-fold and it is thought that the NO-cGMP signaling cascade is a key player in regulation of blood pressure, synaptic plasticity and inhibition of platelet aggregation. The proposed studies seek to understand the structural basis of mechanisms of regulation of the sGC and to identify modulators of its activity: 1) Our recent work suggests that sGC contains an allosteric regulatory site. We seek to identify residues that dictate the structure and nature of the proposed allosteric site. Guided by homology with adenylyl cyclases, we conducted a mutational analysis that identifies specific regions of interactions between the two subunits that seem to mediate allosteric activation. We shall characterize these mutants by biochemical studies integrated with molecular modeling. 2) Recent work from our laboratory and others, suggests that there is an endogenous regulator for the sGC. We have discovered but not yet identified a novel endogenous activator. We will identify this activator and screen for others. 3) The wild-type and mutant sGC will be used to test a newly generated chemical library derived from a synthetic activator, YC-1. Active compounds and sGC will be used as templates for molecular modeling. This modeling combined with structure-activity relationship studies will be used to generate detailed and testable hypotheses regarding the physiological modulation of the NO-cGMP signaling pathway. Understanding the mechanisms of regulation of sGC and identifying regulatory molecules will be key to uncovering the molecular basis of some types of hypertension, atherosclerosis and **erectile dysfunction.**

Website: http://crisp.cit.nih.gov/crisp/Crisp_Query.Generate_Screen

- **Project Title: SHH, A POTENTIAL REGULATOR OF PENILE DEVELOPMENT**

Principal Investigator & Institution: Podlasek, Carol A.; Assistant Professor; Urology; Northwestern University Office of Sponsored Programs Chicago, Il 60611

Timing: Fiscal Year 2003; Project Start 23-DEC-2002; Project End 30-NOV-2004

Summary: (provided by applicant): The proposed research will examine the significance of Sonic hedgehog (Shh) signaling during postnatal development of the penis and will examine the potential regulation of Shh by testosterone. Shh is a secreted glycopeptide that is critically important to mesenchymal-epithelial interactions between tissue layers during embryogenesis. A significant function for Shh in postnatal development has only recently been identified in an organ that undergoes considerable postnatal morphogenesis, the prostate (Podlasek et al., 1999a). Thus Shh function is not restricted to the embryonic period and in organs that undergo extensive postnatal differentiation, Shh activity may be substantial. Like the prostate, development in the penis is primarily a postnatal event, with extensive development taking place after birth. We will present preliminary evidence in the adult that establishes Shh to be absolutely essential for maintaining penile homeostasis. This is significant since diabetic rats exhibit profoundly altered Shh signaling. This same rat model (BB/WOR) has a high incidence of **erectile dysfunction** (McVary et al., 1997). Thus there is evidence to suggest a potential link between disrupted Shh signaling and the physiological abnormality of **erectile dysfunction.** Diabetic impotence is a devastating pathologic development that affects 10-30 million American men, and costs in excess of $150 million for inpatient urologic care alone (1985 dollars). As individuals live longer there is a greater concern for quality of life and treatment options for individuals with **erectile dysfunction** are only partially effective (Vale et al., 2000). A better understanding of how penile morphology is established and maintained in the juvenile would significantly enhance the potential for improved treatment. The proposed experiments are ideally suited to satisfy the goals of this RFA since innovative technology is used to identify novel signaling molecules involved in urologic tissue development and altered regulation of this molecule is prominent in urologic complications of diabetes. The power of this proposal is its potential to provide novel and critically important insight into the mechanism of diabetes induced **erectile dysfunction.**

Website: http://crisp.cit.nih.gov/crisp/Crisp_Query.Generate_Screen

- **Project Title: SPORE IN PROSTATE CANCER**

Principal Investigator & Institution: Lee, Chung; Professor; Urology; Northwestern University Office of Sponsored Programs Chicago, Il 60611

Timing: Fiscal Year 2001; Project Start 01-JUN-2001; Project End 30-APR-2006

Summary: provided by applicant) This SPORE application submitted in response to the RFA from the National Cancer Institute, will take advantage of the strengths in prostate cancer research and treatment that exist at the Robert H. Lurie Comprehensive Cancer Center. The SPORE will provide the infrastructure to bring together basic scientists and clinicians to rapidly test new approaches in the prevention, early detection, diagnosis and treatment of human prostate cancer. The specific themes of the SPORE are: 1. Cell and molecular biology of prostate cancer 2. Prevention and risk factors in prostate cancer development 3. Prostate cancer innovative therapeutics and rehabilitation 4. Quality of life and outcomes research in prostate cancer The SPORE application consists of six principal research projects, three career development projects, five pilot projects and four Core facilities to support the research. The principal research projects are: 1) Clusterin and resistance to apoptosis (Lee), 2) Suppressive role of calreticulin in prostate cancer (Wang), 3) Prostate cancer dependent generation of angiostatin 4.5 (Soff), 4) Molecular mechanisms of **erectile dysfunction** (McVary), 5) Effects of lycopene on prostatic tissue (Gann), 6) Quality of life item banking in prostate cancer (Cella). The Core facilities include: Administration, Tissue Resource, Clinical and Biostatistical Cores. The investigators selected to be part of the SPORE Program come from a variety of disciplines ranging from Clinical Programs to Chemical Engineering, Pathology and Chemistry. To maintain meaningful communication between investigators, we will have monthly meetings of SPORE investigators, an annual retreat and monthly meetings of the Executive Committee. Based on the infrastructure described, our large patient population and our track record of productivity, we believe that the Robert H. Lurie Comprehensive Cancer Center is well suited for the SPORE program.

Website: http://crisp.cit.nih.gov/crisp/Crisp_Query.Generate_Screen

- **Project Title: STRUCTURAL AND MECHANISTIC ANALYSIS OF LIVER ARGINASE**

Principal Investigator & Institution: Ash, David E.; Professor; Biochemistry; Temple University 406 Usb, 083-45 Philadelphia, Pa 19122

Timing: Fiscal Year 2002; Project Start 01-DEC-1993; Project End 30-JUN-2006

Summary: (provided by applicant): Arginase catalyzes the Mn(II)-dependent hydrolysis of L-arginine to produce L-ornithine and urea. In liver, this reaction is catalyzed by type I arginase and constitutes the final step of the urea cycle. Type II arginase is mitochondnal and found in tissues such as kidney, mammary gland and macrophages, where it provides a source of L-ornithine for the biosynthesis of proline and polyamines. Recent studies in this laboratory and the laboratories of our collaborators have provided compelling evidence that both type I and type II arginases are involved in regulating the production of nitric oxide. A major goal of these studies is to dissect structure-function and structure-activity relationships for the arginase family of enzymes. We have recently determined high-resolution structures for product complexes and for complexes of the enzyme with potent boronic acid-based inhibitors. These structures are consistent with our proposed mechanism for arginase, which involves attack of a metal-bridging hydroxide on the guanidinium carbon.An expression system for the production of type I and type II arginases in E. coli has been developed for site directed mutagenesis of critical amino acids identified in the crystal structure. The origin of the exceptional substrate specificity of the enzyme will be explored through mutagenesis of residues implicated in substrate binding. The role of H141 as a proton shuttle will be evaluated through mutagenesis, chemical quench and structure determinations. Novel inhibitors of arginase will be developed and screened for potency and isozyme selectivity. Such inhibitors have therapeutic potential in the treatment of smooth muscle disorders such as **erectile dysfunction.** Mutagenesis studies will identify critical amino acid residues in type II arginase, and we will vigorously pursue efforts to determine the three-dimensional structure of this poorly characterized isozyme. Arginase will serve as a paradigm in structure-function analyses of the enigmatic class of Mn-metalloenzymes, including the Mn-catalases.

Website: http://crisp.cit.nih.gov/crisp/Crisp_Query.Generate_Screen

- **Project Title: THE ROLE OF OXYTOCIN IN MALE SEXUAL FUNCTION**

Principal Investigator & Institution: Mckenna, Kevin E.; Professor; Physiology; Northwestern University Office of Sponsored Programs Chicago, Il 60611

Timing: Fiscal Year 2001; Project Start 11-JAN-2000; Project End 31-DEC-2002

Summary: (applicant's abstract): **Erectile dysfunction** is a common and personally devastating disease. Effective therapies are dependent on knowledge of the fundamental mechanisms underlying normal function. Recently, there has been considerable progress in understanding of the peripheral mechanisms of penile erections. Unfortunately, CNS mechanisms have lagged far behind. The pathways by which the hypothalamus excites the spinal erectile and ejaculatory centers remain undefined. Our laboratories have joined together to make a concerted effort at one important aspect of this CNS control. We have identified a direct hypothalamic pathway from the paraventricular nucleus to lumbosacral spinal cord as a potent facilitator of penile erection and ejaculation. The neurotransmitter for this excitation is the peptide oxytocin. We propose a broad comprehensive plan to examine the mechanism of the role of oxytocin in male sexual function. Electrophysiological studies in anesthetized rats will examine the excitation of erection and ejaculation by PVN stimulation. These will be combined with neuroanatomical staining for oxytocin and pharmacological blockade of oxytocin to verify that the effects of PVN stimulation are mediated by oxytocin. Several spinal sexual reflexes will be tested to see if they are facilitated by PVN stimulation and intrathecal administration of oxytocin. An extensive anatomical study is proposed looking at the relationship between oxytocin fibers in the lumbosacral cord and identified pelvic efferents and intereurons. Interneurons will be identified by transneuronal viral tracing, Fos staining and neurochemical identification. Our preliminary studies demonstrate that oxytocin exerts its facilitatory effects on male sexual function via a spinal nitric oxide pathway. We propose a series of pharmacological studies to examine the mechanisms of the oxytocin-nitric oxide interaction. We further propose that our results of this interdisciplinary program be validated using behavioral and pharmacological testing in unanesthetized animals.

Website: http://crisp.cit.nih.gov/crisp/Crisp_Query.Generate_Screen

- **Project Title: TOLERABILITY/PHARMACOLOGY OF PNU-83757 IN PATIENTS WITH ERECTILE DYSFUNCTION**

Principal Investigator & Institution: Carson, Culley C.; University of North Carolina Chapel Hill Office of Sponsored Research Chapel Hill, Nc 27599

Timing: Fiscal Year 2001

Summary: This abstract is not available.

Website: http://crisp.cit.nih.gov/crisp/Crisp_Query.Generate_Screen

- **Project Title: TREATMENT OF ED IN PATIENTS TREATED FOR PROSTATE CANCER**

Principal Investigator & Institution: Bruner, Deborah W.; American College of Radiology 1101 Market St, 14Th Fl Philadelphia, Pa 19107

Timing: Fiscal Year 2001; Project Start 30-SEP-2001; Project End 31-AUG-2004

Summary: (provided by applicant): Antiandrogens are often combined with radiation therapy (RT) or surgery as neoadjuvant, adjuvant or concurrent therapy in an attempt to decrease disease relapse and improve survival. However, the optimal combination and timing of antiandrogen therapy remains controversial. The Radiation Therapy Oncology Group (RTOG) recently activated a Phase III clinical trial, RTOG 99-10, to study the optimal duration of neoadjuvant total androgen suppression (TAS) and RT in stage II-III prostate cancer. However, it is possible that diminished QGL, particularly related to sexual function, will accompany the improved clinical outcomes associated with TAS. Specifically, TAS and RT have a significant impact on erectile function. If interventions are available to treat **erectile dysfunction** (ED) after prostate cancer therapy, QOL impairments may be minimized. Sildenafil (Viagra TM, Pfizer) is a FDA approved drug for the treatment of ED. Small, nonrandomized; single institution studies have shown significant improvements in ED in men treated with sildenafil after RT. However, the effectiveness of sildenafil for ED as a consequence of combined treatment with RT with TAS has not been adequately described. Conventional wisdom held that after RT plus neoadjuvant or concurrent TAS, erectile function would be equivalent to that after RT alone (once the TAS are discontinued). However, we observed a higher ED rate with the combination of RT and TAS (even after the antiandrogens were discontinued) compared with RT alone in our preliminary work. Antiandrogens affect erectile function through a different mechanism than the etiologies previously studied. If sildenafil is efficacious in this setting, it may assist in both patient decision-making regarding choice of therapy and in clinical management of post-therapy ED. Since most men with prostate cancer have partners, a critical part of the sexual experience, currently lacking in the literature, is an assessment of relationship factors that may interact with ED therapy to predict or modify response to treatment. This knowledge would allow for more effective treatment approaches based on a clinical strategy that provides instruction both on the technical use of the medication as well as on the importance of creating an appropriate psychosexual environment. This study targets men (N=332) recruited for participation from RTOG 99-10, treated with either 8 or 28 weeks of neoadjuvant TAS and RT with concurrent (8 week duration) TAS. The primary aim of this study is to determine, in a randomized, double-blind crossover study, if there is a significant difference in erectile function between men treated with sildenafil versus placebo after RT plus neoadjuvant TAS for prostate cancer. The secondary aim is to determine if there is a significant difference in overall sexual function and satisfaction between men treated with sildenafil versus placebo, and the third and fourth aims are to assess differences in partner sexual satisfaction and dyad marital adjustment between the sildenafil versus placebo arms of this study. Lastly, this study will assess factors associated with response to ED therapy such as age, pre-treatment sexual functions, and tobacco use among others.

Website: http://crisp.cit.nih.gov/crisp/Crisp_Query.Generate_Screen

- **Project Title: ULTRASOUND IMAGING AND THERAPY FOR PROSTATE CANCER**

  Principal Investigator & Institution: Sanghvi, Narendra T.; President; Focus Surgery, Inc. 3940 Pendleton Way Indianapolis, in 46226

  Timing: Fiscal Year 2003; Project Start 15-SEP-2000; Project End 31-MAY-2005

  Summary: (provided by applicant): Prostate cancer is the second leading cause of cancer death among American men, after lung cancer. Since early 1990s, Focus Surgery, Inc. (FSI) has developed and commercialized the Sonablate TM system, which makes use of a novel technology based on high intensity focused ultrasound (HIFU) for the minimally invasive treatment of prostate diseases. The latest version of the device, the Sonablate TM 500, has been specifically developed and clinically used for minimally invasive image-guided HIFU treatment of localized and recurrent prostate cancer. Following the successful accomplishments of the Phase I study, in this Phase II proposal we plan to refine and enhance the ultrasound imaging, treatment planning, and treatment execution aspects of the current Sonablate TM 500 system for a safe, effective, and minimally invasive prostate cancer treatment. The proposed R & D efforts will minimize side effects such as **erectile dysfunction** and impotency related to prostate cancer treatment. This goal will be accomplished by the stated specific aims: (1) add Doppler imaging support to aid in the detection of treatment exclusion zones such as neuro-vascular bundles, enhance 2D multi-slice and 3D ultrasound imaging and visualization (2) develop innovative computer-assisted 3D shape models from patient-specific 3D ultrasound data for on-line treatment planning and visualization, (3) develop a full 3D treatment planning tool geared toward both whole and partial (selective) prostate ablation, (4) integrate the new hardware and software enhancements into the Sonablate TM 500 device in preparation for clinical evaluation, and (5) complete an in vivo canine prostate study (both non-cancerous and cancerous prostate models) to evaluate and test the new features. Successful completion of this project, together with currently undergoing prostate cancer clinical trials, will bring the Sonablate TM 500 device to a status ready for widespread clinical use for the safe and minimal side effect treatment of early detected localized (T1 and T2) and recurrent prostate cancer.

  Website: http://crisp.cit.nih.gov/crisp/Crisp_Query.Generate_Screen

- **Project Title: UROLOGICAL DYSFUNCTION AND NO CONTROL IN DIABETES**

  Principal Investigator & Institution: Bauer, John A.; Associate Professor; None; Ohio State University 1960 Kenny Road Columbus, Oh 43210

  Timing: Fiscal Year 2001; Project Start 30-SEP-1998; Project End 31-JAN-2002

  Summary: (adapted from the application) **Erectile dysfunction** and bladder dysfunction are prevalent problems associated with diabetes. These debilitating problems often progress throughout a patient's life span and are irreversible. Despite their common occurrence, the mechanisms by which the diabetes related urological problems develop are not well studied or understood. The focus of our application is to investigate the mechanisms of erectile and bladder dysfunction during diabetes progression, an to devise rational and innovative therapeutic strategies to intervene. A key mediator of both vascular and genitourinary smooth muscle function is nitric oxide (NO). Under normal physiological conditions, NO acts as a critical signal transduction agent in these tissues, serving as the primary controller of local erectile responses and urinary sphincter control. Recent studies have shown that superoxide anion destroys NO, reduces its efficacy as a signal transduction agent, and promotes the formation of peroxynitrite, a highly reactive intermediate known to cause nitration of protein associated tyrosine residues and cellular oxidative damage. Thus, loss of NO control may impair signal transduction pathways, cause enzyme inactivation, and induce cellular apoptosis and/or necrosis. Since diabetes is associated with elevated oxidant conditions in both blood and tissues, dysregulation of NO (particularly a shift from "good effects" to toxicological consequences) may be an important mechanisms for the developing urological dysfunction. Here biochemical and molecular measures of NO production and destruction pathways will be related to erectile and bladder dysfunction and apoptosis during experimental diabetes progression. Our aims are: 1) test the hypothesis that NO dysregulation participates in **erectile dysfunction** during experimental diabetes; 2) test the hypothesis that diabetes induced bladder dysfunction is related to modulation of NO production and/or destruction within bladder and/or urethral sphincter smooth muscle; 3) test the hypothesis that cellular apoptosis is a contributor to diabetes induced urological dysfunction; and (4) rationally design and test experimental therapeutic strategies for the prevention or reversal of diabetes induced urological complications, including small molecules and gene therapy. These collaborative investigations will provide important new insights regarding the mechanisms of and treatment options for an emerging health problem. These studies will also contribute valuable basic understanding of erectile and bladder physiology and pharmacology, and the participation of NO in disease.

Website: http://crisp.cit.nih.gov/crisp/Crisp_Query.Generate_Screen

E-Journals: PubMed Central[3]

PubMed Central (PMC) is a digital archive of life sciences journal literature developed and managed by the National Center for Biotechnology Information (NCBI) at the U.S. National Library of Medicine (NLM).[4] Access to this growing archive of e-journals is free and unrestricted.[5] To search, go to **http://www.ncbi.nlm.nih.gov/entrez/query.fcgi?db=Pmc**, and type "erectile dysfunction" (or synonyms) into the search box. This search gives you access to full-text articles. The following is a sample of items found for erectile dysfunction in the PubMed Central database:

---

[3] Adapted from the National Library of Medicine: **http://www.pubmedcentral.nih.gov/about/intro.html**.

[4] With PubMed Central, NCBI is taking the lead in preservation and maintenance of open access to electronic literature, just as NLM has done for decades with printed biomedical literature. PubMed Central aims to become a world-class library of the digital age.

[5] The value of PubMed Central, in addition to its role as an archive, lies in the availability of data from diverse sources stored in a common format in a single repository. Many journals already have online publishing operations, and there is a growing tendency to publish material online only, to the exclusion of print.

- **Coronary artery flow reserve in diabetics with erectile dysfunction using sildenafil.** by Dietz U, Tries HP, Merkle W, Jaursch-Hancke C, Lambertz H.; 2003;
  http://www.pubmedcentral.gov/articlerender.fcgi?tool=pmcentrez&artid=194431

- **Erectile dysfunction in cyclic GMP-dependent kinase I-deficient mice.** by Hedlund P, Aszodi A, Pfeifer A, Alm P, Hofmann F, Ahmad M, Fassler R, Andersson KE.; 2000 Feb 29;
  http://www.pubmedcentral.gov/articlerender.fcgi?tool=pmcentrez&artid=15804

- **Incidence of erectile dysfunction and characteristics of patients before and after the introduction of sildenafil in the United Kingdom: cross sectional study with comparison patients.** by Kaye JA, Jick H.; 2003 Feb 22;
  http://www.pubmedcentral.gov/articlerender.fcgi?tool=pmcentrez&artid=149443

- **Oral sildenafil (Viagra[TM]) in male erectile dysfunction: use, efficacy and safety profile in an unselected cohort presenting to a British district general hospital.** by Sairam K, Kulinskaya E, Hanbury D, Boustead G, McNicholas T.; 2002;
  http://www.pubmedcentral.gov/articlerender.fcgi?tool=pmcentrez&artid=111060

- **Sildenafil (Viagra) for male erectile dysfunction: a meta-analysis of clinical trial reports.** by Moore RA, Edwards JE, McQuay HJ.; 2002;
  http://www.pubmedcentral.gov/articlerender.fcgi?tool=pmcentrez&artid=115867

The National Library of Medicine: PubMed

One of the quickest and most comprehensive ways to find academic studies in both English and other languages is to use PubMed, maintained by the National Library of Medicine.[6] The advantage of PubMed over previously mentioned sources is that it covers a greater number of domestic and foreign references. It is also free to use. If the publisher has a Web site that offers full text of its journals, PubMed will provide links to that site, as well as to sites offering other related data. User registration, a subscription fee, or some other type of fee may be required to access the full text of articles in some journals.

To generate your own bibliography of studies dealing with erectile dysfunction, simply go to the PubMed Web site at **http://www.ncbi.nlm.nih.gov/pubmed**. Type "erectile dysfunction" (or synonyms) into the search box, and click "Go." The following is the type of output you can expect from PubMed for erectile dysfunction (hyperlinks lead to article summaries):

- **A comparison of the International Index of Erectile Function and erectile dysfunction studies.**
  Author(s): Cappelleri JC, Rosen RC.
  Source: Bju International. 2003 October; 92(6): 654.
  http://www.ncbi.nlm.nih.gov:80/entrez/query.fcgi?cmd=Retrieve&db=PubMed&list_uids=14511061&dopt=Abstract

---

[6] PubMed was developed by the National Center for Biotechnology Information (NCBI) at the National Library of Medicine (NLM) at the National Institutes of Health (NIH). The PubMed database was developed in conjunction with publishers of biomedical literature as a search tool for accessing literature citations and linking to full-text journal articles at Web sites of participating publishers. Publishers that participate in PubMed supply NLM with their citations electronically prior to or at the time of publication.

- **A comparison of the International Index of Erectile Function and erectile dysfunction studies.**
  Author(s): Kassouf W, Carrier S.
  Source: Bju International. 2003 May; 91(7): 667-9.
  http://www.ncbi.nlm.nih.gov:80/entrez/query.fcgi?cmd=Retrieve&db=PubMed&list_uids=12699481&dopt=Abstract

- **A double-blind crossover study evaluating the efficacy of korean red ginseng in patients with erectile dysfunction: a preliminary report.**
  Author(s): Hong B, Ji YH, Hong JH, Nam KY, Ahn TY.
  Source: The Journal of Urology. 2002 November; 168(5): 2070-3.
  http://www.ncbi.nlm.nih.gov:80/entrez/query.fcgi?cmd=Retrieve&db=PubMed&list_uids=12394711&dopt=Abstract

- **A historical review of erectile dysfunction.**
  Author(s): Valiquette L.
  Source: Can J Urol. 2003 February; 10 Suppl 1: 7-11.
  http://www.ncbi.nlm.nih.gov:80/entrez/query.fcgi?cmd=Retrieve&db=PubMed&list_uids=12625844&dopt=Abstract

- **A Rho-kinase inhibitor, soluble guanylate cyclase activator and nitric oxide-releasing PDE5 inhibitor: novel approaches to erectile dysfunction.**
  Author(s): Cellek S, Rees RW, Kalsi J.
  Source: Expert Opinion on Investigational Drugs. 2002 November; 11(11): 1563-73. Review.
  http://www.ncbi.nlm.nih.gov:80/entrez/query.fcgi?cmd=Retrieve&db=PubMed&list_uids=12437503&dopt=Abstract

- **A shared care approach to the management of erectile dysfunction in the community.**
  Author(s): Wagner G, Claes H, Costa P, Cricelli C, De Boer J, Debruyne FM, Dean J, Dinsmore WW, Fitzpatrick JM, Ralph DJ, Hackett GI, Heaton JP, Hatzichristou DG, Mendive J, Meuleman EJ, Mirone V, Montorsi F, Raineri F, Schulman CC, Stief CG, Von Keitz AT, Wright PJ; Lygon Arms Group.
  Source: International Journal of Impotence Research : Official Journal of the International Society for Impotence Research. 2002 June; 14(3): 189-94. Review.
  http://www.ncbi.nlm.nih.gov:80/entrez/query.fcgi?cmd=Retrieve&db=PubMed&list_uids=12058246&dopt=Abstract

- **A systematic approach to erectile dysfunction in the cardiovascular patient: a Consensus Statement--update 2002.**
  Author(s): Jackson G, Betteridge J, Dean J, Eardley I, Hall R, Holdright D, Holmes S, Kirby M, Riley A, Sever P.
  Source: Int J Clin Pract. 2002 November; 56(9): 663-71. Review.
  http://www.ncbi.nlm.nih.gov:80/entrez/query.fcgi?cmd=Retrieve&db=PubMed&list_uids=12469980&dopt=Abstract

- **ACE gene I/D and NOS3 G894T polymorphisms and response to sildenafil in men with erectile dysfunction.**
  Author(s): Eisenhardt A, Sperling H, Hauck E, Porst H, Stief C, Rubben H, Muller N, Siffert W.
  Source: Urology. 2003 July; 62(1): 152-7.
  http://www.ncbi.nlm.nih.gov:80/entrez/query.fcgi?cmd=Retrieve&db=PubMed&list_uids=12837457&dopt=Abstract

- **Achieving treatment optimization with sildenafil citrate (Viagra) in patients with erectile dysfunction.**
  Author(s): McCullough AR, Barada JH, Fawzy A, Guay AT, Hatzichristou D.
  Source: Urology. 2002 September; 60(2 Suppl 2): 28-38.
  http://www.ncbi.nlm.nih.gov:80/entrez/query.fcgi?cmd=Retrieve&db=PubMed&list_uids=12414331&dopt=Abstract

- **Activators of soluble guanylate cyclase for the treatment of male erectile dysfunction.**
  Author(s): Brioni JD, Nakane M, Hsieh GC, Moreland RB, Kolasa T, Sullivan JP.
  Source: International Journal of Impotence Research : Official Journal of the International Society for Impotence Research. 2002 February; 14(1): 8-14. Review.
  http://www.ncbi.nlm.nih.gov:80/entrez/query.fcgi?cmd=Retrieve&db=PubMed&list_uids=11896472&dopt=Abstract

- **Age dependent secretion of LH and ACTH in healthy men and patients with erectile dysfunction.**
  Author(s): Derouet H, Lehmann J, Stamm B, Luhl C, Romer D, Georg T, Isenberg E, Gebhardt T, Stoeckle M.
  Source: European Urology. 2002 February; 41(2): 144-53; Discussion 153-4.
  http://www.ncbi.nlm.nih.gov:80/entrez/query.fcgi?cmd=Retrieve&db=PubMed&list_uids=12074401&dopt=Abstract

- **An ethical dilemma: erectile dysfunction in the HIV-positive patient: to treat or not to treat.**
  Author(s): Kell P, Sadeghi-Nejad H, Price D.
  Source: International Journal of Std & Aids. 2002 June; 13(6): 355-7. Review.
  http://www.ncbi.nlm.nih.gov:80/entrez/query.fcgi?cmd=Retrieve&db=PubMed&list_uids=12015005&dopt=Abstract

- **An investigation into the relationship between prostate size, peak urinary flow rate and male erectile dysfunction.**
  Author(s): Green JS, Holden ST, Bose P, George DP, Bowsher WG.
  Source: International Journal of Impotence Research : Official Journal of the International Society for Impotence Research. 2001 December; 13(6): 322-5.
  http://www.ncbi.nlm.nih.gov:80/entrez/query.fcgi?cmd=Retrieve&db=PubMed&list_uids=11918247&dopt=Abstract

- **Anagrelide-induced erectile dysfunction.**
  Author(s): Braester A, Laver B.
  Source: The Annals of Pharmacotherapy. 2002 July-August; 36(7-8): 1291.
  http://www.ncbi.nlm.nih.gov:80/entrez/query.fcgi?cmd=Retrieve&db=PubMed&list_uids=12086566&dopt=Abstract

- **Androgens improve cavernous vasodilation and response to sildenafil in patients with erectile dysfunction.**
  Author(s): Aversa A, Isidori AM, Spera G, Lenzi A, Fabbri A.
  Source: Clinical Endocrinology. 2003 May; 58(5): 632-8.
  http://www.ncbi.nlm.nih.gov:80/entrez/query.fcgi?cmd=Retrieve&db=PubMed&list_
  uids=12699447&dopt=Abstract

- **Apomorphine-induced brain modulation during sexual stimulation: a new look at central phenomena related to erectile dysfunction.**
  Author(s): Montorsi F, Perani D, Anchisi D, Salonia A, Scifo P, Rigiroli P, Zanoni M, Heaton JP, Rigatti P, Fazio F.
  Source: International Journal of Impotence Research : Official Journal of the International Society for Impotence Research. 2003 June; 15(3): 203-9.
  http://www.ncbi.nlm.nih.gov:80/entrez/query.fcgi?cmd=Retrieve&db=PubMed&list_
  uids=12904807&dopt=Abstract

- **Are patients and the general public like-minded about the effect of erectile dysfunction on quality of life?**
  Author(s): Stolk EA, Busschbach JJ.
  Source: Urology. 2003 April; 61(4): 810-5.
  http://www.ncbi.nlm.nih.gov:80/entrez/query.fcgi?cmd=Retrieve&db=PubMed&list_
  uids=12670570&dopt=Abstract

- **Arteriosclerosis of penile arteries: histological findings and their significance in the treatment of erectile dysfunction.**
  Author(s): Grein U, Schubert GE.
  Source: Urologia Internationalis. 2002; 68(4): 261-4.
  http://www.ncbi.nlm.nih.gov:80/entrez/query.fcgi?cmd=Retrieve&db=PubMed&list_
  uids=12053029&dopt=Abstract

- **Assessing patients with actual or potential erectile dysfunction.**
  Author(s): Steggall MJ, Gann SY.
  Source: Prof Nurse. 2002 November; 18(3): 155-9. Review.
  http://www.ncbi.nlm.nih.gov:80/entrez/query.fcgi?cmd=Retrieve&db=PubMed&list_
  uids=12465540&dopt=Abstract

- **Assessment of andropause awareness and erectile dysfunction among married men in Ile-Ife, Nigeria.**
  Author(s): Fatusi AO, Ijadunola KT, Ojofeitimi EO, Adeyemi MO, Omideyi AK, Akinyemi A, Adewuyi AA.
  Source: The Aging Male : the Official Journal of the International Society for the Study of the Aging Male. 2003 June; 6(2): 79-85.
  http://www.ncbi.nlm.nih.gov:80/entrez/query.fcgi?cmd=Retrieve&db=PubMed&list_
  uids=12898791&dopt=Abstract

- **Barriers to recognition of erectile dysfunction among diabetic Mexican-American men.**
  Author(s): Zweifler J, Padilla A, Schafer S.
  Source: The Journal of the American Board of Family Practice / American Board of Family Practice. 1998 July-August; 11(4): 259-63.
  http://www.ncbi.nlm.nih.gov:80/entrez/query.fcgi?cmd=Retrieve&db=PubMed&list_uids=9719347&dopt=Abstract

- **Benign prostatic hyperplasia and erectile dysfunction: a review.**
  Author(s): Altwein JE, Keuler FU.
  Source: Urologia Internationalis. 1992; 48(1): 53-7. Review.
  http://www.ncbi.nlm.nih.gov:80/entrez/query.fcgi?cmd=Retrieve&db=PubMed&list_uids=1376011&dopt=Abstract

- **Benign prostatic hyperplasia and erectile dysfunction--is there a link?**
  Author(s): Vale J.
  Source: Current Medical Research and Opinion. 2000; 16 Suppl 1: S63-7. Review.
  http://www.ncbi.nlm.nih.gov:80/entrez/query.fcgi?cmd=Retrieve&db=PubMed&list_uids=11329825&dopt=Abstract

- **Beyond Viagra. Psychological issues in the assessment and treatment of erectile dysfunction.**
  Author(s): McDowell AJ, Snellgrove CA, Bond MJ.
  Source: Aust Fam Physician. 2001 September; 30(9): 867-73.
  http://www.ncbi.nlm.nih.gov:80/entrez/query.fcgi?cmd=Retrieve&db=PubMed&list_uids=11676316&dopt=Abstract

- **Biochemical screening in the assessment of erectile dysfunction: what tests decide future therapy?**
  Author(s): Earle CM, Stuckey BG.
  Source: Urology. 2003 October; 62(4): 727-31.
  http://www.ncbi.nlm.nih.gov:80/entrez/query.fcgi?cmd=Retrieve&db=PubMed&list_uids=14550452&dopt=Abstract

- **Biofeedback and facilitation of erection in men with erectile dysfunction.**
  Author(s): Reynolds BS.
  Source: Archives of Sexual Behavior. 1980 April; 9(2): 101-13.
  http://www.ncbi.nlm.nih.gov:80/entrez/query.fcgi?cmd=Retrieve&db=PubMed&list_uids=6156665&dopt=Abstract

- **Biweekly intracavernous administration of papaverine for erectile dysfunction.**
  Author(s): Mooradian AD, Morley JE, Kaiser FE, Davis SS, Viosca SP, Korenman SC.
  Source: The Western Journal of Medicine. 1989 November; 151(5): 515-7.
  http://www.ncbi.nlm.nih.gov:80/entrez/query.fcgi?cmd=Retrieve&db=PubMed&list_uids=2603417&dopt=Abstract

- **Bladder and erectile dysfunction before and after rectal surgery for cancer.**
  Author(s): Leveckis J, Boucher NR, Parys BT, Reed MW, Shorthouse AJ, Anderson JB.
  Source: British Journal of Urology. 1995 December; 76(6): 752-6.
  http://www.ncbi.nlm.nih.gov:80/entrez/query.fcgi?cmd=Retrieve&db=PubMed&list_uids=8535720&dopt=Abstract

- **Blood gas changes in the corpora cavernosa: metabolic and histomorphometric implications in the patient with erectile dysfunction.**
  Author(s): Sasso F, Falabella R, Gentile G, Servello C, Gulino G.
  Source: The Journal of Urology. 2003 June; 169(6): 2270-4.
  http://www.ncbi.nlm.nih.gov:80/entrez/query.fcgi?cmd=Retrieve&db=PubMed&list_uids=12771768&dopt=Abstract

- **Blunt trauma: the pathophysiology of hemodynamic injury leading to erectile dysfunction.**
  Author(s): Munarriz RM, Yan QR, ZNehra A, Udelson D, Goldstein I.
  Source: The Journal of Urology. 1995 June; 153(6): 1831-40.
  http://www.ncbi.nlm.nih.gov:80/entrez/query.fcgi?cmd=Retrieve&db=PubMed&list_uids=7752329&dopt=Abstract

- **Bulbocavernosus reflex studies and autonomic testing in the diagnosis of erectile dysfunction.**
  Author(s): Bird SJ, Hanno PM.
  Source: Journal of the Neurological Sciences. 1998 January 21; 154(1): 8-13.
  http://www.ncbi.nlm.nih.gov:80/entrez/query.fcgi?cmd=Retrieve&db=PubMed&list_uids=9543316&dopt=Abstract

- **Bulbocavernosus reflex testing in 100 consecutive cases of erectile dysfunction.**
  Author(s): Wabrek AJ.
  Source: Urology. 1985 May; 25(5): 495-8.
  http://www.ncbi.nlm.nih.gov:80/entrez/query.fcgi?cmd=Retrieve&db=PubMed&list_uids=3992774&dopt=Abstract

- **Bupropion and sexual function: a placebo-controlled prospective study on diabetic men with erectile dysfunction.**
  Author(s): Rowland DL, Myers L, Culver A, Davidson JM.
  Source: Journal of Clinical Psychopharmacology. 1997 October; 17(5): 350-7.
  http://www.ncbi.nlm.nih.gov:80/entrez/query.fcgi?cmd=Retrieve&db=PubMed&list_uids=9315985&dopt=Abstract

- **Central nervous system agents in the treatment of erectile dysfunction: how do they work?**
  Author(s): Allard J, Giuliano F.
  Source: Curr Urol Rep. 2001 December; 2(6): 488-94. Review.
  http://www.ncbi.nlm.nih.gov:80/entrez/query.fcgi?cmd=Retrieve&db=PubMed&list_uids=12084236&dopt=Abstract

- **Central oxytocinergic neurotransmission: a drug target for the therapy of psychogenic erectile dysfunction.**
  Author(s): Melis MR, Argiolas A.
  Source: Current Drug Targets. 2003 January; 4(1): 55-66. Review.
  http://www.ncbi.nlm.nih.gov:80/entrez/query.fcgi?cmd=Retrieve&db=PubMed&list_uids=12528990&dopt=Abstract

- **Challenges in oral therapy for erectile dysfunction.**
  Author(s): Seftel AD.
  Source: Journal of Andrology. 2002 November-December; 23(6): 729-36. Review.
  http://www.ncbi.nlm.nih.gov:80/entrez/query.fcgi?cmd=Retrieve&db=PubMed&list_uids=12399513&dopt=Abstract

- **Changing practice patterns in erectile dysfunction: a diagnostic algorithm for the new millennium.**
  Author(s): Broderick GA.
  Source: Adv Ren Replace Ther. 1999 October; 6(4): 314-26. Review.
  http://www.ncbi.nlm.nih.gov:80/entrez/query.fcgi?cmd=Retrieve&db=PubMed&list_uids=10543711&dopt=Abstract

- **Chronic illness and the psychology of erectile dysfunction.**
  Author(s): Sank LI.
  Source: Adv Ren Replace Ther. 1999 October; 6(4): 310-3. Review.
  http://www.ncbi.nlm.nih.gov:80/entrez/query.fcgi?cmd=Retrieve&db=PubMed&list_uids=10543710&dopt=Abstract

- **Cigarette smoking as risk factor for erectile dysfunction: results from an Italian epidemiological study.**
  Author(s): Mirone V, Imbimbo C, Bortolotti A, Di Cintio E, Colli E, Landoni M, Lavezzari M, Parazzini F.
  Source: European Urology. 2002 March; 41(3): 294-7.
  http://www.ncbi.nlm.nih.gov:80/entrez/query.fcgi?cmd=Retrieve&db=PubMed&list_uids=12180231&dopt=Abstract

- **Clinical safety profile of sildenafil in Singaporean men with erectile dysfunction: pre-marketing experience (ASSESS-I evaluation).**
  Author(s): Lim PH, Ng FC, Cheng CW, Wong MY, Chee CT, Moorthy P, Vasan SS.
  Source: J Int Med Res. 2002 March-April; 30(2): 137-43.
  http://www.ncbi.nlm.nih.gov:80/entrez/query.fcgi?cmd=Retrieve&db=PubMed&list_uids=12025521&dopt=Abstract

- **Clomiphene increases free testosterone levels in men with both secondary hypogonadism and erectile dysfunction: who does and does not benefit?**
  Author(s): Guay AT, Jacobson J, Perez JB, Hodge MB, Velasquez E.
  Source: International Journal of Impotence Research : Official Journal of the International Society for Impotence Research. 2003 June; 15(3): 156-65.
  http://www.ncbi.nlm.nih.gov:80/entrez/query.fcgi?cmd=Retrieve&db=PubMed&list_uids=12904801&dopt=Abstract

- **Color Doppler imaging of erectile dysfunction: a new place in strategy?**
  Author(s): Grenier N.
  Source: European Radiology. 2002 September; 12(9): 2133-5.
  http://www.ncbi.nlm.nih.gov:80/entrez/query.fcgi?cmd=Retrieve&db=PubMed&list_
  uids=12353494&dopt=Abstract

- **Colour duplex Doppler ultrasonography evaluation of non-vasculogenic male erectile dysfunction: An Indian perspective.**
  Author(s): Bhargava R, Srivastava DN, Thulkar S, Berry M, Gupta NP.
  Source: Australasian Radiology. 2002 June; 46(2): 170-3.
  http://www.ncbi.nlm.nih.gov:80/entrez/query.fcgi?cmd=Retrieve&db=PubMed&list_
  uids=12060156&dopt=Abstract

- **Combination therapy for erectile dysfunction: where we are and what's in the future.**
  Author(s): Nehra A, Kulaksizoglu H.
  Source: Curr Urol Rep. 2002 December; 3(6): 467-70. Review.
  http://www.ncbi.nlm.nih.gov:80/entrez/query.fcgi?cmd=Retrieve&db=PubMed&list_
  uids=12425869&dopt=Abstract

- **Common conditions of the aging male: erectile dysfunction, benign prostatic hyperplasia, cardiovascular disease and depression.**
  Author(s): Zakaria L, Anastasiadis AG, Shabsigh R.
  Source: International Urology and Nephrology. 2001; 33(2): 283-92. Review.
  http://www.ncbi.nlm.nih.gov:80/entrez/query.fcgi?cmd=Retrieve&db=PubMed&list_
  uids=12092641&dopt=Abstract

- **Comparison of a needle-free high-pressure injection system with needle-tipped injection of intracavernosal alprostadil for erectile dysfunction.**
  Author(s): Harding LM, Adeniyi A, Everson R, Barker S, Ralph DJ, Baranowski AP.
  Source: International Journal of Impotence Research : Official Journal of the International Society for Impotence Research. 2002 December; 14(6): 498-501.
  http://www.ncbi.nlm.nih.gov:80/entrez/query.fcgi?cmd=Retrieve&db=PubMed&list_
  uids=12494285&dopt=Abstract

- **Comparison of finasteride and alpha-blockers as independent risk factors for erectile dysfunction.**
  Author(s): Sadeghi-Nejad H, Sherman N, Lue J.
  Source: Int J Clin Pract. 2003 July-August; 57(6): 484-7.
  http://www.ncbi.nlm.nih.gov:80/entrez/query.fcgi?cmd=Retrieve&db=PubMed&list_
  uids=12918887&dopt=Abstract

- **Comparison of nocturnal penile tumescence monitoring and cavernosal smooth muscle content in patients with erectile dysfunction.**
  Author(s): Yilmaz E, Yaman O, Bozlu M, Inal T, Tokatli Z, Anafarta K.
  Source: International Urology and Nephrology. 2002; 34(1): 117-20.
  http://www.ncbi.nlm.nih.gov:80/entrez/query.fcgi?cmd=Retrieve&db=PubMed&list_
  uids=12549653&dopt=Abstract

- **Comparison of satisfaction rates and erectile function in patients treated with sildenafil, intracavernous prostaglandin E1 and penile implant surgery for erectile dysfunction in urology practice.**
  Author(s): Rajpurkar A, Dhabuwala CB.
  Source: The Journal of Urology. 2003 July; 170(1): 159-63.
  http://www.ncbi.nlm.nih.gov:80/entrez/query.fcgi?cmd=Retrieve&db=PubMed&list_uids=12796670&dopt=Abstract

- **Counseling the patient with erectile dysfunction: a primary care physician perspective.**
  Author(s): Kuritzky L.
  Source: J Am Osteopath Assoc. 2002 December; 102(12 Suppl 4): S7-11.
  http://www.ncbi.nlm.nih.gov:80/entrez/query.fcgi?cmd=Retrieve&db=PubMed&list_uids=12572635&dopt=Abstract

- **Current drug use as risk factor for erectile dysfunction: results from an Italian epidemiological study.**
  Author(s): Ricci E, Parazzini F, Mirone V, Imbimbo C, Palmieri A, Bortolotti A, Di Cintio E, Landoni M, Lavezzari M.
  Source: International Journal of Impotence Research : Official Journal of the International Society for Impotence Research. 2003 June; 15(3): 221-4.
  http://www.ncbi.nlm.nih.gov:80/entrez/query.fcgi?cmd=Retrieve&db=PubMed&list_uids=12904809&dopt=Abstract

- **Current oral treatments for erectile dysfunction.**
  Author(s): Kalsi JS, Cellek S, Muneer A, Kell PD, Ralph DJ, Minhas S.
  Source: Expert Opinion on Pharmacotherapy. 2002 November; 3(11): 1613-29. Review.
  http://www.ncbi.nlm.nih.gov:80/entrez/query.fcgi?cmd=Retrieve&db=PubMed&list_uids=12437495&dopt=Abstract

- **Current status of standardized questionnaires in the measurement of erectile dysfunction.**
  Author(s): Beasley KA, De Young LX, Brock GB.
  Source: Curr Urol Rep. 2000 December; 1(4): 285-90.
  http://www.ncbi.nlm.nih.gov:80/entrez/query.fcgi?cmd=Retrieve&db=PubMed&list_uids=12084305&dopt=Abstract

- **Deciphering erectile dysfunction drug trials.**
  Author(s): Mulhall JP.
  Source: The Journal of Urology. 2003 August; 170(2 Pt 1): 353-8. Review.
  http://www.ncbi.nlm.nih.gov:80/entrez/query.fcgi?cmd=Retrieve&db=PubMed&list_uids=12853774&dopt=Abstract

- **Deep venous thrombosis and venous thrombophlebitis associated with alprostadil treatment for erectile dysfunction.**
  Author(s): Barthelmes L, Chezhian C, Aihaku EK.
  Source: International Journal of Impotence Research : Official Journal of the International Society for Impotence Research. 2002 June; 14(3): 199-200. Review.
  http://www.ncbi.nlm.nih.gov:80/entrez/query.fcgi?cmd=Retrieve&db=PubMed&list_uids=12058249&dopt=Abstract

- **Dehydroepiandrosterone in the treatment of erectile dysfunction in patients with different organic etiologies.**
  Author(s): Reiter WJ, Schatzl G, Mark I, Zeiner A, Pycha A, Marberger M.
  Source: Urological Research. 2001 August; 29(4): 278-81.
  http://www.ncbi.nlm.nih.gov:80/entrez/query.fcgi?cmd=Retrieve&db=PubMed&list_uids=11585284&dopt=Abstract

- **Depression, antidepressant therapies, and erectile dysfunction: clinical trials of sildenafil citrate (Viagra) in treated and untreated patients with depression.**
  Author(s): Nurnberg HG, Seidman SN, Gelenberg AJ, Fava M, Rosen R, Shabsigh R.
  Source: Urology. 2002 September; 60(2 Suppl 2): 58-66. Review.
  http://www.ncbi.nlm.nih.gov:80/entrez/query.fcgi?cmd=Retrieve&db=PubMed&list_uids=12414334&dopt=Abstract

- **Determination of human angiotensin converting enzyme (ACE) gene polymorphisms in erectile dysfunction: frequency differences of ACE gene polymorphisms according to the method of analysis.**
  Author(s): Kim DS, Choi SI, Lee HS, Park JK, Yi HK.
  Source: Clinical Chemistry and Laboratory Medicine : Cclm / Fescc. 2001 January; 39(1): 11-4.
  http://www.ncbi.nlm.nih.gov:80/entrez/query.fcgi?cmd=Retrieve&db=PubMed&list_uids=11256792&dopt=Abstract

- **Determination of nitric oxide metabolites by means of the Griess assay and gas chromatography-mass spectrometry in the cavernous and systemic blood of healthy males and patients with erectile dysfunction during different functional conditions of the penis.**
  Author(s): Becker AJ, Uckert S, Tsikas D, Noack H, Stief CG, Frolich JC, Wolf G, Jonas U.
  Source: Urological Research. 2000 December; 28(6): 364-9.
  http://www.ncbi.nlm.nih.gov:80/entrez/query.fcgi?cmd=Retrieve&db=PubMed&list_uids=11221914&dopt=Abstract

- **Development of surgical procedures in the treatment of erectile dysfunction. A historical overview.**
  Author(s): Hauri D.
  Source: Urologia Internationalis. 2003; 70(2): 124-31.
  http://www.ncbi.nlm.nih.gov:80/entrez/query.fcgi?cmd=Retrieve&db=PubMed&list_uids=12592041&dopt=Abstract

- **Diabetes, hypertension and erectile dysfunction.**
  Author(s): Ledda A.
  Source: Current Medical Research and Opinion. 2000; 16 Suppl 1: S17-20. Review.
  http://www.ncbi.nlm.nih.gov:80/entrez/query.fcgi?cmd=Retrieve&db=PubMed&list_uids=11329816&dopt=Abstract

- **Diagnosis and management of endocrine disorders of erectile dysfunction.**
  Author(s): Zonszein J.
  Source: The Urologic Clinics of North America. 1995 November; 22(4): 789-802. Review.
  http://www.ncbi.nlm.nih.gov:80/entrez/query.fcgi?cmd=Retrieve&db=PubMed&list_uids=7483129&dopt=Abstract

- **Diagnosis and treatment of erectile dysfunction.**
  Author(s): Levine LA.
  Source: The American Journal of Medicine. 2000 December 18; 109 Suppl 9A: 3S-12S; Discussion 29S-30S. Review.
  http://www.ncbi.nlm.nih.gov:80/entrez/query.fcgi?cmd=Retrieve&db=PubMed&list_uids=11137497&dopt=Abstract

- **Diagnostic steps in the evaluation of patients with erectile dysfunction.**
  Author(s): Hatzichristou D, Hatzimouratidis K, Bekas M, Apostolidis A, Tzortzis V, Yannakoyorgos K.
  Source: The Journal of Urology. 2002 August; 168(2): 615-20.
  http://www.ncbi.nlm.nih.gov:80/entrez/query.fcgi?cmd=Retrieve&db=PubMed&list_uids=12131320&dopt=Abstract

- **Did men with erectile dysfunction discuss their condition with partner and physicians? A survey of men attending a free call information service.**
  Author(s): Mirone V, Gentile V, Zizzo G, Terry M, Longo N, Fusco F, Parazzini F.
  Source: International Journal of Impotence Research : Official Journal of the International Society for Impotence Research. 2002 August; 14(4): 256-8.
  http://www.ncbi.nlm.nih.gov:80/entrez/query.fcgi?cmd=Retrieve&db=PubMed&list_uids=12152114&dopt=Abstract

- **Dietary supplements and other alternative medicines for erectile dysfunction. What do I tell my patients?**
  Author(s): Moyad MA.
  Source: The Urologic Clinics of North America. 2002 February; 29(1): 11-22, Vii.
  http://www.ncbi.nlm.nih.gov:80/entrez/query.fcgi?cmd=Retrieve&db=PubMed&list_uids=12109338&dopt=Abstract

- **Do impotent men with diabetes have more severe erectile dysfunction and worse quality of life than the general population of impotent patients? Results from the Exploratory Comprehensive Evaluation of Erectile Dysfunction (ExCEED) database.**
  Author(s): Penson DF, Latini DM, Lubeck DP, Wallace KL, Henning JM, Lue TF; Comprehensive Evaluation of Erectile Dysfunction (ExCEED) database.
  Source: Diabetes Care. 2003 April; 26(4): 1093-9.
  http://www.ncbi.nlm.nih.gov:80/entrez/query.fcgi?cmd=Retrieve&db=PubMed&list_uids=12663579&dopt=Abstract

- **Do lipid-lowering drugs cause erectile dysfunction? A systematic review.**
  Author(s): Rizvi K, Hampson JP, Harvey JN.
  Source: Family Practice. 2002 February; 19(1): 95-8. Review.
  http://www.ncbi.nlm.nih.gov:80/entrez/query.fcgi?cmd=Retrieve&db=PubMed&list_uids=11818357&dopt=Abstract

- **Does bicycling contribute to the risk of erectile dysfunction? Results from the Massachusetts Male Aging Study (MMAS).**
  Author(s): Marceau L, Kleinman K, Goldstein I, McKinlay J.
  Source: International Journal of Impotence Research : Official Journal of the International Society for Impotence Research. 2001 October; 13(5): 298-302.
  http://www.ncbi.nlm.nih.gov:80/entrez/query.fcgi?cmd=Retrieve&db=PubMed&list_uids=11890518&dopt=Abstract

- **Doppler US evaluation of erectile dysfunction.**
  Author(s): Kim SH.
  Source: Abdominal Imaging. 2002 September-October; 27(5): 578-87.
  http://www.ncbi.nlm.nih.gov:80/entrez/query.fcgi?cmd=Retrieve&db=PubMed&list_uids=12173002&dopt=Abstract

- **Double-blind, crossover comparison of 3 mg apomorphine SL with placebo and with 4 mg apomorphine SL in male erectile dysfunction.**
  Author(s): Dula E, Bukofzer S, Perdok R, George M; Apomorphine SL Study Group.
  Source: European Urology. 2001 May; 39(5): 558-3; Discussion 564.
  http://www.ncbi.nlm.nih.gov:80/entrez/query.fcgi?cmd=Retrieve&db=PubMed&list_uids=11464037&dopt=Abstract

- **Drug combinations in the therapy of low response to phosphodiesterase 5 inhibitors in patients with erectile dysfunction.**
  Author(s): Dunzendorfer U, Behm A, Dunzendorfer E, Dunzendorfer A.
  Source: In Vivo. 2002 September-October; 16(5): 345-8.
  http://www.ncbi.nlm.nih.gov:80/entrez/query.fcgi?cmd=Retrieve&db=PubMed&list_uids=12494876&dopt=Abstract

- **Drug therapy and prevalence of erectile dysfunction in the Massachusetts Male Aging Study cohort.**
  Author(s): Derby CA, Barbour MM, Hume AL, McKinlay JB.
  Source: Pharmacotherapy. 2001 June; 21(6): 676-83.
  http://www.ncbi.nlm.nih.gov:80/entrez/query.fcgi?cmd=Retrieve&db=PubMed&list_uids=11401181&dopt=Abstract

- **Effects of moxonidine and metoprolol in penile circulation in hypertensive men with erectile dysfunction: results of a pilot study.**
  Author(s): Piha J, Kaaja R.
  Source: International Journal of Impotence Research : Official Journal of the International Society for Impotence Research. 2003 August; 15(4): 287-9.
  http://www.ncbi.nlm.nih.gov:80/entrez/query.fcgi?cmd=Retrieve&db=PubMed&list_uids=12934058&dopt=Abstract

- **Efficacy and tolerability of vardenafil for treatment of erectile dysfunction in patient subgroups.**
  Author(s): Porst H, Young JM, Schmidt AC, Buvat J; International Vardenafil Study Group.
  Source: Urology. 2003 September; 62(3): 519-23; Discussion 523-4.
  http://www.ncbi.nlm.nih.gov:80/entrez/query.fcgi?cmd=Retrieve&db=PubMed&list_uids=12946758&dopt=Abstract

- **Efficacy of shunt surgery for refractory low flow priapism: a report on the incidence of failed detumescence and erectile dysfunction.**
  Author(s): Nixon RG, O'Connor JL, Milam DF.
  Source: The Journal of Urology. 2003 September; 170(3): 883-6.
  http://www.ncbi.nlm.nih.gov:80/entrez/query.fcgi?cmd=Retrieve&db=PubMed&list_uids=12913722&dopt=Abstract

- **Efficacy of sildenafil in an open-label study as a continuation of a double-blind study in the treatment of erectile dysfunction after radiotherapy for prostate cancer.**
  Author(s): Incrocci L, Hop WC, Slob AK.
  Source: Urology. 2003 July; 62(1): 116-20.
  http://www.ncbi.nlm.nih.gov:80/entrez/query.fcgi?cmd=Retrieve&db=PubMed&list_uids=12837434&dopt=Abstract

- **Efficacy of tadalafil for the treatment of erectile dysfunction at 24 and 36 hours after dosing: a randomized controlled trial.**
  Author(s): Porst H, Padma-Nathan H, Giuliano F, Anglin G, Varanese L, Rosen R.
  Source: Urology. 2003 July; 62(1): 121-5; Discussion 125-6.
  http://www.ncbi.nlm.nih.gov:80/entrez/query.fcgi?cmd=Retrieve&db=PubMed&list_uids=12837435&dopt=Abstract

- **Erectile dysfunction after radical prostatectomy treatment and challenge.**
  Author(s): Lin JS.
  Source: J Chin Med Assoc. 2003 January; 66(1): 2-3. No Abstract Available.
  http://www.ncbi.nlm.nih.gov:80/entrez/query.fcgi?cmd=Retrieve&db=PubMed&list_uids=12728967&dopt=Abstract

- **Erectile dysfunction and culture in South Africa.**
  Author(s): Levinson B.
  Source: Journal of Sex & Marital Therapy. 1999 October-December; 25(4): 267-70.
  http://www.ncbi.nlm.nih.gov:80/entrez/query.fcgi?cmd=Retrieve&db=PubMed&list_uids=10546164&dopt=Abstract

- **Erectile dysfunction in Singapore: prevalence and its associated factors--a population-based study.**
  Author(s): Tan JK, Hong CY, Png DJ, Liew LC, Wong ML.
  Source: Singapore Med J. 2003 January; 44(1): 20-6.
  http://www.ncbi.nlm.nih.gov:80/entrez/query.fcgi?cmd=Retrieve&db=PubMed&list_uids=12762559&dopt=Abstract

- **Erectile dysfunction in the Australian community.**
  Author(s): Lowy MP.
  Source: The Medical Journal of Australia. 1999 October 4; 171(7): 342-3.
  http://www.ncbi.nlm.nih.gov:80/entrez/query.fcgi?cmd=Retrieve&db=PubMed&list_uids=10590719&dopt=Abstract

- **Erectile dysfunction in the cardiac patient: how common and should we treat?**
  Author(s): Kloner RA, Mullin SH, Shook T, Matthews R, Mayeda G, Burstein S, Peled H, Pollick C, Choudhary R, Rosen R, Padma-Nathan H.
  Source: The Journal of Urology. 2003 August; 170(2 Pt 2): S46-50; Discussion S50. Review.
  http://www.ncbi.nlm.nih.gov:80/entrez/query.fcgi?cmd=Retrieve&db=PubMed&list_uids=12853773&dopt=Abstract

- **Erectile dysfunction in the community: a prevalence study.**
  Author(s): Pinnock CB, Stapleton AM, Marshall VR.
  Source: The Medical Journal of Australia. 1999 October 4; 171(7): 353-7.
  http://www.ncbi.nlm.nih.gov:80/entrez/query.fcgi?cmd=Retrieve&db=PubMed&list_uids=10590723&dopt=Abstract

- **Erectile dysfunction in the elderly: epidemiology, etiology and approaches to treatment.**
  Author(s): Seftel AD.
  Source: The Journal of Urology. 2003 June; 169(6): 1999-2007. Review.
  http://www.ncbi.nlm.nih.gov:80/entrez/query.fcgi?cmd=Retrieve&db=PubMed&list_uids=12771705&dopt=Abstract

- **Erectile dysfunction.**
  Author(s): Ferri RS.
  Source: Nurs Spectr (Wash D C). 1998 March 23; 8(6): 15. No Abstract Available.
  http://www.ncbi.nlm.nih.gov:80/entrez/query.fcgi?cmd=Retrieve&db=PubMed&list_uids=10542651&dopt=Abstract

- **Erectile dysfunction.**
  Author(s): Lewis JH, Rosen R, Goldstein I; Consensus Panel on Health Care Clinician Management of Erectile Dysfunction.
  Source: The American Journal of Nursing. 2003 October; 103(10): 48-57; Quiz 57-8. Review.
  http://www.ncbi.nlm.nih.gov:80/entrez/query.fcgi?cmd=Retrieve&db=PubMed&list_uids=14530708&dopt=Abstract

- **Erectile dysfunction. A guide to diagnosis and management.**
  Author(s): Arduca P.
  Source: Aust Fam Physician. 2003 June; 32(6): 414-20. Review.
  http://www.ncbi.nlm.nih.gov:80/entrez/query.fcgi?cmd=Retrieve&db=PubMed&list_uids=12833766&dopt=Abstract

- **Erectile dysfunction: getting to the root of the problem.**
  Author(s): Hurn W.
  Source: Community Nurse. 2000 April; 6(3): 11-4. No Abstract Available.
  http://www.ncbi.nlm.nih.gov:80/entrez/query.fcgi?cmd=Retrieve&db=PubMed&list_uids=12778500&dopt=Abstract

- **Erectile dysfunction: prevalence and relationship to depression, alcohol abuse and panic disorder.**
  Author(s): Okulate G, Olayinka O, Dogunro AS.
  Source: General Hospital Psychiatry. 2003 May-June; 25(3): 209-13.
  http://www.ncbi.nlm.nih.gov:80/entrez/query.fcgi?cmd=Retrieve&db=PubMed&list_uids=12748034&dopt=Abstract

- **Erectile dysfunction—diagnostic approach and treatment options.**
  Author(s): Hilz MJ.
  Source: Suppl Clin Neurophysiol. 2000; 53: 234-6. Review. No Abstract Available.
  http://www.ncbi.nlm.nih.gov:80/entrez/query.fcgi?cmd=Retrieve&db=PubMed&list_uids=12741004&dopt=Abstract

- **Erectile physiological and pathophysiological pathways involved in erectile dysfunction.**
  Author(s): Andersson KE.
  Source: The Journal of Urology. 2003 August; 170(2 Pt 2): S6-13; Discussion S13-4. Review.
  http://www.ncbi.nlm.nih.gov:80/entrez/query.fcgi?cmd=Retrieve&db=PubMed&list_uids=12853766&dopt=Abstract

- **Evaluation and therapeutic regulation of erectile dysfunction with visual stimulation test. An objective approach by using sildenafil citrate test.**
  Author(s): Erbagci A, Yagci F, Sarica K, Ozbek E, Topcu O.
  Source: Urologia Internationalis. 2002; 69(1): 21-6.
  http://www.ncbi.nlm.nih.gov:80/entrez/query.fcgi?cmd=Retrieve&db=PubMed&list_uids=12119434&dopt=Abstract

- **Factors predicting efficacy of phentolamine-papaverine intracorporeal injection for treatment of erectile dysfunction in diabetic male.**
  Author(s): Bell DS, Cutter GR, Hayne VB, Lloyd LK.
  Source: Urology. 1992 July; 40(1): 36-40.
  http://www.ncbi.nlm.nih.gov:80/entrez/query.fcgi?cmd=Retrieve&db=PubMed&list_uids=1621310&dopt=Abstract

- **Feasibility of multi-slice computed tomography in the diagnosis of arteriogenic erectile dysfunction.**
  Author(s): Kawanishi Y, Lee KS, Kimura K, Kojima K, Yamamoto A, Numata A.
  Source: Bju International. 2001 September; 88(4): 390-5.
  http://www.ncbi.nlm.nih.gov:80/entrez/query.fcgi?cmd=Retrieve&db=PubMed&list_uids=11564028&dopt=Abstract

- **Fibrinogen, lipoprotein (a) and lipids in patients with erectile dysfunction. A preliminary study.**
  Author(s): Sullivan ME, Miller MA, Bell CR, Jagroop IA, Thompson CS, Khan MA, Morgan RJ, Mikhailidis DP.
  Source: International Angiology : a Journal of the International Union of Angiology. 2001 September; 20(3): 195-9.
  http://www.ncbi.nlm.nih.gov:80/entrez/query.fcgi?cmd=Retrieve&db=PubMed&list_uids=11573052&dopt=Abstract

- **Financial implications of an erectile dysfunction clinic in a Trust hospital.**
  Author(s): Harris JR.
  Source: International Journal of Std & Aids. 1996; 7 Suppl 3: 22-3.
  http://www.ncbi.nlm.nih.gov:80/entrez/query.fcgi?cmd=Retrieve&db=PubMed&list_uids=8876377&dopt=Abstract

- **First international conference on the management of erectile dysfunction. Overview consensus statement.**
  Author(s): Eid JF, Nehra A, Andersson KE, Heaton J, Lewis RW, Morales A, Moreland RB, Mulcahy JJ, Porst H, Pryor JL, Sharlip ID, Wagner G, Wyllie M.
  Source: International Journal of Impotence Research : Official Journal of the International Society for Impotence Research. 2000 October; 12 Suppl 4: S2-5. Review.
  http://www.ncbi.nlm.nih.gov:80/entrez/query.fcgi?cmd=Retrieve&db=PubMed&list_uids=11035379&dopt=Abstract

- **First-line therapies for erectile dysfunction.**
  Author(s): Ensign C.
  Source: Jaapa. 2001 October; 14(10): 17-20. Review. No Abstract Available.
  http://www.ncbi.nlm.nih.gov:80/entrez/query.fcgi?cmd=Retrieve&db=PubMed&list_uids=11715672&dopt=Abstract

- **Fluvoxamine-induced erectile dysfunction responding to sildenafil.**
  Author(s): Balon R.
  Source: Journal of Sex & Marital Therapy. 1998 October-December; 24(4): 313-7.
  http://www.ncbi.nlm.nih.gov:80/entrez/query.fcgi?cmd=Retrieve&db=PubMed&list_uids=9805292&dopt=Abstract

- **Follow-up of vacuum and nonvacuum constriction devices as treatments for erectile dysfunction.**
  Author(s): Schuetz-Mueller D, Tiefer L, Melman A.
  Source: Journal of Sex & Marital Therapy. 1995 Winter; 21(4): 229-38.
  http://www.ncbi.nlm.nih.gov:80/entrez/query.fcgi?cmd=Retrieve&db=PubMed&list_uids=8789504&dopt=Abstract

- **Followup results of a combination of calcitonin gene-related peptide and prostaglandin E1 in the treatment of erectile dysfunction.**
  Author(s): Djamilian M, Stief CG, Kuczyk M, Jonas U.
  Source: The Journal of Urology. 1993 May; 149(5 Pt 2): 1296-8.
  http://www.ncbi.nlm.nih.gov:80/entrez/query.fcgi?cmd=Retrieve&db=PubMed&list_uids=8479019&dopt=Abstract

- **Four cases of erectile dysfunction in substance abusers treated with sildenafil.**
  Author(s): Telias ID, Kadmon-Telias A.
  Source: Addiction (Abingdon, England). 2002 November; 97(11): 1473-4.
  http://www.ncbi.nlm.nih.gov:80/entrez/query.fcgi?cmd=Retrieve&db=PubMed&list_uids=12410787&dopt=Abstract

- **Fournier's gangrene in a patient with erectile dysfunction following use of a mechanical erection aid device.**
  Author(s): Theiss M, Hofmockel G, Frohmuller HG.
  Source: The Journal of Urology. 1995 June; 153(6): 1921-2.
  http://www.ncbi.nlm.nih.gov:80/entrez/query.fcgi?cmd=Retrieve&db=PubMed&list_uids=7752355&dopt=Abstract

- **Frequency and determinants of erectile dysfunction in Italy.**
  Author(s): Parazzini F, Menchini Fabris F, Bortolotti A, Calabro A, Chatenoud L, Colli E, Landoni M, Lavezzari M, Turchi P, Sessa A, Mirone V.
  Source: European Urology. 2000 January; 37(1): 43-9.
  http://www.ncbi.nlm.nih.gov:80/entrez/query.fcgi?cmd=Retrieve&db=PubMed&list_uids=10671784&dopt=Abstract

- **Functional electromyostimulation of the corpus cavernosum penis—preliminary results of a novel therapeutic option for erectile dysfunction.**
  Author(s): Stief CG, Weller E, Noack T, Djamilian M, Meschi M, Truss M, Jonas U.
  Source: World Journal of Urology. 1995; 13(4): 243-7.
  http://www.ncbi.nlm.nih.gov:80/entrez/query.fcgi?cmd=Retrieve&db=PubMed&list_uids=8528300&dopt=Abstract

- **Future considerations: advances in the surgical management of erectile dysfunction.**
  Author(s): Montague DK, Angermeier KW.
  Source: International Journal of Impotence Research : Official Journal of the International Society for Impotence Research. 2000 October; 12 Suppl 4: S140-3. Review.
  http://www.ncbi.nlm.nih.gov:80/entrez/query.fcgi?cmd=Retrieve&db=PubMed&list_uids=11035402&dopt=Abstract

- **Gap junctions and ion channels: relevance to erectile dysfunction.**
  Author(s): Christ GJ.
  Source: International Journal of Impotence Research : Official Journal of the International Society for Impotence Research. 2000 October; 12 Suppl 4: S15-25. Review.
  http://www.ncbi.nlm.nih.gov:80/entrez/query.fcgi?cmd=Retrieve&db=PubMed&list_uids=11035382&dopt=Abstract

- **Gene therapy for erectile dysfunction: where is it going?**
  Author(s): Christ GJ.
  Source: Current Opinion in Urology. 2002 November; 12(6): 497-501. Review.
  http://www.ncbi.nlm.nih.gov:80/entrez/query.fcgi?cmd=Retrieve&db=PubMed&list_uids=12409880&dopt=Abstract

- **Gene therapy: future therapy for erectile dysfunction.**
  Author(s): Schenk G, Melman A, Christ G.
  Source: Curr Urol Rep. 2001 December; 2(6): 480-7. Review.
  http://www.ncbi.nlm.nih.gov:80/entrez/query.fcgi?cmd=Retrieve&db=PubMed&list_uids=12084235&dopt=Abstract

- **Gene-polymorphisms of angiotensin converting enzyme and endothelial nitric oxide synthase in patients with erectile dysfunction.**
  Author(s): Park JK, Kim W, Kim SW, Koh GY, Park SK.
  Source: International Journal of Impotence Research : Official Journal of the International Society for Impotence Research. 1999 October; 11(5): 273-6.
  http://www.ncbi.nlm.nih.gov:80/entrez/query.fcgi?cmd=Retrieve&db=PubMed&list_uids=10553806&dopt=Abstract

- **Genital plus audiovisual sexual stimulation following intracavernous vasoactive injection versus re-dosing for erectile dysfunction—results of a prospective study.**
  Author(s): Montorsi F, Guazzoni G, Barbieri L, Ferini-Strambi L, Iannaccone S, Calori G, Nava L, Rigatti P, Pizzini G, Miani A.
  Source: The Journal of Urology. 1998 January; 159(1): 113-5.
  http://www.ncbi.nlm.nih.gov:80/entrez/query.fcgi?cmd=Retrieve&db=PubMed&list_uids=9400449&dopt=Abstract

- **Global perspectives and controversies in the epidemiology of male erectile dysfunction.**
  Author(s): Nehra A, Kulaksizoglu H.
  Source: Current Opinion in Urology. 2002 November; 12(6): 493-6. Review.
  http://www.ncbi.nlm.nih.gov:80/entrez/query.fcgi?cmd=Retrieve&db=PubMed&list_uids=12409879&dopt=Abstract

- **Goal-directed therapy for erectile dysfunction.**
  Author(s): Kuritzky L.
  Source: American Family Physician. 1997 August; 56(2): 379.
  http://www.ncbi.nlm.nih.gov:80/entrez/query.fcgi?cmd=Retrieve&db=PubMed&list_uids=9262519&dopt=Abstract

- **Group treatment of secondary erectile dysfunction.**
  Author(s): Kilmann PR, Milan RJ Jr, Boland JP, Nankin HR, Davidson E, West MO, Sabalis RF, Caid C, Devine JM.
  Source: Journal of Sex & Marital Therapy. 1987 Fall; 13(3): 168-82.
  http://www.ncbi.nlm.nih.gov:80/entrez/query.fcgi?cmd=Retrieve&db=PubMed&list_uids=3669078&dopt=Abstract

- **Group treatment of single males with erectile dysfunction.**
  Author(s): Lobitz WC, Baker EL Jr.
  Source: Archives of Sexual Behavior. 1979 March; 8(2): 127-38.
  http://www.ncbi.nlm.nih.gov:80/entrez/query.fcgi?cmd=Retrieve&db=PubMed&list_uids=475575&dopt=Abstract

- **Guidelines for treating erectile dysfunction issued.**
  Author(s): Skolnick AA.
  Source: Jama : the Journal of the American Medical Association. 1997 January 1; 277(1): 7-8.
  http://www.ncbi.nlm.nih.gov:80/entrez/query.fcgi?cmd=Retrieve&db=PubMed&list_uids=8980192&dopt=Abstract

- **Guidelines on erectile dysfunction.**
  Author(s): Wespes E, Amar E, Hatzichristou D, Montorsi F, Pryor J, Vardi Y; European Association of Urology.
  Source: European Urology. 2002 January; 41(1): 1-5.
  http://www.ncbi.nlm.nih.gov:80/entrez/query.fcgi?cmd=Retrieve&db=PubMed&list_uids=11999460&dopt=Abstract

- **Has the efficacy of penile arterial by-pass surgery in the treatment of arteriogenic erectile dysfunction been determined?**
  Author(s): Vickers KE, Vickers MA.
  Source: International Journal of Impotence Research : Official Journal of the International Society for Impotence Research. 1996 December; 8(4): 247-51; Discussion 251-3. Review.
  http://www.ncbi.nlm.nih.gov:80/entrez/query.fcgi?cmd=Retrieve&db=PubMed&list_uids=8981176&dopt=Abstract

- **Health care clinicians in sexual health medicine: focus on erectile dysfunction.**
  Author(s): Albaugh J, Amargo I, Capelson R, Flaherty E, Forest C, Goldstein I, Jensen PK, Jones K, Kloner R, Lewis J, Mullin S, Payton T, Rines B, Rosen R, Sadovsky R, Snow K, Vetrosky D; University of Medicine and Dentistry of New Jersey.
  Source: Urologic Nursing : Official Journal of the American Urological Association Allied. 2002 August; 22(4): 217-31; Quiz 232. Review.
  http://www.ncbi.nlm.nih.gov:80/entrez/query.fcgi?cmd=Retrieve&db=PubMed&list_uids=12242893&dopt=Abstract

- **Health outcomes variables important to patients in the treatment of erectile dysfunction.**
  Author(s): Hanson-Divers C, Jackson SE, Lue TF, Crawford SY, Rosen RC.
  Source: The Journal of Urology. 1998 May; 159(5): 1541-7.
  http://www.ncbi.nlm.nih.gov:80/entrez/query.fcgi?cmd=Retrieve&db=PubMed&list_uids=9554350&dopt=Abstract

- **Health-related quality of life in a UK-based population of men with erectile dysfunction.**
  Author(s): Guest JF, Das Gupta R.
  Source: Pharmacoeconomics. 2002; 20(2): 109-17.
  http://www.ncbi.nlm.nih.gov:80/entrez/query.fcgi?cmd=Retrieve&db=PubMed&list_uids=11888363&dopt=Abstract

- **Health-related quality of life in men with erectile dysfunction.**
  Author(s): Litwin MS, Nied RJ, Dhanani N.
  Source: Journal of General Internal Medicine : Official Journal of the Society for Research and Education in Primary Care Internal Medicine. 1998 March; 13(3): 159-66.
  http://www.ncbi.nlm.nih.gov:80/entrez/query.fcgi?cmd=Retrieve&db=PubMed&list_uids=9541372&dopt=Abstract

- **Hemodynamic effects of transurethral alprostadil measured by color duplex ultrasonography in men with erectile dysfunction.**
  Author(s): Tam PY, Keller T, Poppiti R, Gesundheit N, Padma-Nathan H.
  Source: The Journal of Urology. 1998 October; 160(4): 1321-4.
  http://www.ncbi.nlm.nih.gov:80/entrez/query.fcgi?cmd=Retrieve&db=PubMed&list_uids=9751345&dopt=Abstract

- **Hemodynamic evaluation of the penile arterial system in patients with erectile dysfunction using power Doppler imaging.**
  Author(s): Sakamoto H, Shimada M, Yoshida H.
  Source: Urology. 2002 September; 60(3): 480-4.
  http://www.ncbi.nlm.nih.gov:80/entrez/query.fcgi?cmd=Retrieve&db=PubMed&list_uids=12350490&dopt=Abstract

- **Hemodynamic insult by vascular risk factors and pharmacologic erection in men with erectile dysfunction: Doppler sonography study.**
  Author(s): Chung WS, Shim BS, Park YY.
  Source: World Journal of Urology. 2000 December; 18(6): 427-30.
  http://www.ncbi.nlm.nih.gov:80/entrez/query.fcgi?cmd=Retrieve&db=PubMed&list_uids=11204263&dopt=Abstract

- **Herpes zoster producing temporary erectile dysfunction.**
  Author(s): Rix GH, Carroll DN, MacFarlane JR.
  Source: International Journal of Impotence Research : Official Journal of the International Society for Impotence Research. 2001 December; 13(6): 352-3.
  http://www.ncbi.nlm.nih.gov:80/entrez/query.fcgi?cmd=Retrieve&db=PubMed&list_uids=11918252&dopt=Abstract

- **High dose sildenafil citrate as a salvage therapy for severe erectile dysfunction.**
  Author(s): McMahon CG.
  Source: International Journal of Impotence Research : Official Journal of the International Society for Impotence Research. 2002 December; 14(6): 533-8.
  http://www.ncbi.nlm.nih.gov:80/entrez/query.fcgi?cmd=Retrieve&db=PubMed&list_uids=12494291&dopt=Abstract

- **High prevalence of erectile dysfunction after renal transplantation.**
  Author(s): Malavaud B, Rostaing L, Rischmann P, Sarramon JP, Durand D.
  Source: Transplantation. 2000 May 27; 69(10): 2121-4.
  http://www.ncbi.nlm.nih.gov:80/entrez/query.fcgi?cmd=Retrieve&db=PubMed&list_uids=10852609&dopt=Abstract

- **High resolution ultrasonography and pulsed wave Doppler for detection of corporovenous incompetence in erectile dysfunction.**
  Author(s): Vickers MA Jr, Benson CB, Richie JP.
  Source: The Journal of Urology. 1990 June; 143(6): 1125-7.
  http://www.ncbi.nlm.nih.gov:80/entrez/query.fcgi?cmd=Retrieve&db=PubMed&list_uids=2188015&dopt=Abstract

- **Hormonal erectile dysfunction. Evaluation and management.**
  Author(s): Morales A, Heaton JP.
  Source: The Urologic Clinics of North America. 2001 May; 28(2): 279-88.
  http://www.ncbi.nlm.nih.gov:80/entrez/query.fcgi?cmd=Retrieve&db=PubMed&list_uids=11402581&dopt=Abstract

- **Hormonal variations during sleep in men with erectile dysfunction and normal controls.**
  Author(s): Schiavi RC, Fisher C, White D, Beers P, Fogel M, Szechter R.
  Source: Archives of Sexual Behavior. 1982 June; 11(3): 189-200.
  http://www.ncbi.nlm.nih.gov:80/entrez/query.fcgi?cmd=Retrieve&db=PubMed&list_uids=6814402&dopt=Abstract

- **Hyperlipidemia and erectile dysfunction.**
  Author(s): Kim SC.
  Source: Asian Journal of Andrology. 2000 September; 2(3): 161-6. Review.
  http://www.ncbi.nlm.nih.gov:80/entrez/query.fcgi?cmd=Retrieve&db=PubMed&list_uids=11225973&dopt=Abstract

- **Hypertension is associated with severe erectile dysfunction.**
  Author(s): Burchardt M, Burchardt T, Baer L, Kiss AJ, Pawar RV, Shabsigh A, de la Taille A, Hayek OR, Shabsigh R.
  Source: The Journal of Urology. 2000 October; 164(4): 1188-91.
  http://www.ncbi.nlm.nih.gov:80/entrez/query.fcgi?cmd=Retrieve&db=PubMed&list_uids=10992363&dopt=Abstract

- **Hypertension, anti-hypertensive drug therapy and erectile dysfunction in diabetes.**
  Author(s): Moulik PK, Hardy KJ.
  Source: Diabetic Medicine : a Journal of the British Diabetic Association. 2003 April; 20(4): 290-3.
  http://www.ncbi.nlm.nih.gov:80/entrez/query.fcgi?cmd=Retrieve&db=PubMed&list_uids=12675642&dopt=Abstract

- **Hypertension, erectile dysfunction, and occult sleep apnea.**
  Author(s): Hirshkowitz M, Karacan I, Gurakar A, Williams RL.
  Source: Sleep. 1989 June; 12(3): 223-32.
  http://www.ncbi.nlm.nih.gov:80/entrez/query.fcgi?cmd=Retrieve&db=PubMed&list_uids=2740693&dopt=Abstract

- **Hypertension, stress and erectile dysfunction: potential insights from the analysis of heart rate variability.**
  Author(s): Pagani M.
  Source: Current Medical Research and Opinion. 2000; 16 Suppl 1: S3-8. Review.
  http://www.ncbi.nlm.nih.gov:80/entrez/query.fcgi?cmd=Retrieve&db=PubMed&list_uids=11329819&dopt=Abstract

- **Hypothalamic-hypophyseal-testicular abnormalities and erectile dysfunction.**
  Author(s): Shah RS, Pardanani DS, Parulkar BG, Purohit SP, Bandivdekar AH, Sheth AR.
  Source: Archives of Andrology. 1988; 20(2): 137-40.
  http://www.ncbi.nlm.nih.gov:80/entrez/query.fcgi?cmd=Retrieve&db=PubMed&list_
  uids=3134861&dopt=Abstract

- **I am a male in my late 50s. I have heart disease and erectile dysfunction. Are the two related?**
  Author(s): Francis GS.
  Source: Heart Advis. 2002 September; 5(9): 8. No Abstract Available.
  http://www.ncbi.nlm.nih.gov:80/entrez/query.fcgi?cmd=Retrieve&db=PubMed&list_
  uids=12243149&dopt=Abstract

- **Identifying patients with type 2 diabetes with a higher likelihood of erectile dysfunction: the role of the interaction between clinical and psychological factors.**
  Author(s): De Berardis G, Pellegrini F, Franciosi M, Belfiglio M, Di Nardo B, Greenfield S, Kaplan SH, Rossi MC, Sacco M, Tognoni G, Valentini M, Nicolucci A; Quality of Care and Outcomes in Type 2 Diabetes Study Group.
  Source: The Journal of Urology. 2003 April; 169(4): 1422-8.
  http://www.ncbi.nlm.nih.gov:80/entrez/query.fcgi?cmd=Retrieve&db=PubMed&list_
  uids=12629376&dopt=Abstract

- **Impulse magnetic-field therapy for erectile dysfunction: a double-blind, placebo-controlled study.**
  Author(s): Pelka RB, Jaenicke C, Gruenwald J.
  Source: Adv Ther. 2002 January-February; 19(1): 53-60.
  http://www.ncbi.nlm.nih.gov:80/entrez/query.fcgi?cmd=Retrieve&db=PubMed&list_
  uids=12008861&dopt=Abstract

- **Incidence of erectile dysfunction and characteristics of patients before and after the introduction of sildenafil in the United Kingdom: cross sectional study with comparison patients.**
  Author(s): Kaye JA, Jick H.
  Source: Bmj (Clinical Research Ed.). 2003 February 22; 326(7386): 424-5.
  http://www.ncbi.nlm.nih.gov:80/entrez/query.fcgi?cmd=Retrieve&db=PubMed&list_
  uids=12595382&dopt=Abstract

- **Incidence of erectile dysfunction in men 40 to 69 years old: results from a population-based cohort study in Brazil.**
  Author(s): Moreira ED Jr, Lbo CF, Diament A, Nicolosi A, Glasser DB.
  Source: Urology. 2003 February; 61(2): 431-6.
  http://www.ncbi.nlm.nih.gov:80/entrez/query.fcgi?cmd=Retrieve&db=PubMed&list_
  uids=12597962&dopt=Abstract

- **Incidence, etiology, and therapy for erectile dysfunction after external beam radiotherapy for prostate cancer.**
  Author(s): Incrocci L, Slob AK.
  Source: Urology. 2002 July; 60(1): 1-7. Review.
  http://www.ncbi.nlm.nih.gov:80/entrez/query.fcgi?cmd=Retrieve&db=PubMed&list_uids=12100912&dopt=Abstract

- **Inhibition of tonic contraction—a novel way to approach erectile dysfunction.**
  Author(s): Mills TM, Lewis RW, Wingard CJ, Chitaley K, Webb RC.
  Source: Journal of Andrology. 2002 September-October; 23(5): S5-9. Review.
  http://www.ncbi.nlm.nih.gov:80/entrez/query.fcgi?cmd=Retrieve&db=PubMed&list_uids=12236171&dopt=Abstract

- **Insights into the management of erectile dysfunction: Part II.**
  Author(s): Lewis JH, Albaugh J.
  Source: Urologic Nursing : Official Journal of the American Urological Association Allied. 2000 February; 20(1): 29-36, 53; Quiz 37, 40. Review.
  http://www.ncbi.nlm.nih.gov:80/entrez/query.fcgi?cmd=Retrieve&db=PubMed&list_uids=11998039&dopt=Abstract

- **Interactions between drugs for erectile dysfunction and drugs for cardiovascular disease.**
  Author(s): Simonsen U.
  Source: International Journal of Impotence Research : Official Journal of the International Society for Impotence Research. 2002 June; 14(3): 178-88. Review.
  http://www.ncbi.nlm.nih.gov:80/entrez/query.fcgi?cmd=Retrieve&db=PubMed&list_uids=12058245&dopt=Abstract

- **Intracavernosal alprostadil is effective for the treatment of erectile dysfunction in diabetic men.**
  Author(s): Heaton JP, Lording D, Liu SN, Litonjua AD, Guangwei L, Kim SC, Kim JJ, Zhi-Zhou S, Israr D, Niazi D, Rajatanavin R, Suyono S, Benard F, Casey R, Brock G, Belanger A.
  Source: International Journal of Impotence Research : Official Journal of the International Society for Impotence Research. 2001 December; 13(6): 317-21.
  http://www.ncbi.nlm.nih.gov:80/entrez/query.fcgi?cmd=Retrieve&db=PubMed&list_uids=11918246&dopt=Abstract

- **Intracavernosal injection therapy and surgical therapy in diabetic patients with erectile dysfunction.**
  Author(s): Savoca G, Silvestre G, Belgrano E.
  Source: Diabetes Nutr Metab. 2002 February; 15(1): 53-7. Review. No Abstract Available.
  http://www.ncbi.nlm.nih.gov:80/entrez/query.fcgi?cmd=Retrieve&db=PubMed&list_uids=11942740&dopt=Abstract

- **Intracavernosal injection therapy with and without sexological counselling in men with erectile dysfunction.**
  Author(s): van der Windt F, Dohle GR, van der Tak J, Slob AK.
  Source: Bju International. 2002 June; 89(9): 901-4.
  http://www.ncbi.nlm.nih.gov:80/entrez/query.fcgi?cmd=Retrieve&db=PubMed&list_uids=12010236&dopt=Abstract

- **Intracavernous injection as an option for aging men with erectile dysfunction.**
  Author(s): Wespes E.
  Source: The Aging Male : the Official Journal of the International Society for the Study of the Aging Male. 2002 September; 5(3): 177-80. Review.
  http://www.ncbi.nlm.nih.gov:80/entrez/query.fcgi?cmd=Retrieve&db=PubMed&list_uids=12471778&dopt=Abstract

- **Intracavernous injection during diagnostic screening for erectile dysfunction; five-year experience with over 600 patients.**
  Author(s): Slob AK, Verhulst AC, Gijs L, Maksimovic PA, van der Werff ten Bosch JJ.
  Source: Journal of Sex & Marital Therapy. 2002 January-February; 28(1): 61-70.
  http://www.ncbi.nlm.nih.gov:80/entrez/query.fcgi?cmd=Retrieve&db=PubMed&list_uids=11928180&dopt=Abstract

- **Intracavernous injections for erectile dysfunction in patients with cardiovascular diseases and failure or contraindications for sildenafil citrate.**
  Author(s): Israilov S, Niv E, Livne PM, Shmueli J, Engelstein D, Segenreich E, Baniel J.
  Source: International Journal of Impotence Research : Official Journal of the International Society for Impotence Research. 2002 February; 14(1): 38-43.
  http://www.ncbi.nlm.nih.gov:80/entrez/query.fcgi?cmd=Retrieve&db=PubMed&list_uids=11896476&dopt=Abstract

- **Introduction. The management of erectile dysfunction (ED).**
  Author(s): Padma-Nathan H.
  Source: Urology. 2002 September; 60(2 Suppl 2): 1-3.
  http://www.ncbi.nlm.nih.gov:80/entrez/query.fcgi?cmd=Retrieve&db=PubMed&list_uids=12414328&dopt=Abstract

- **Investigating the effect of erectile dysfunction on the lives of men: a qualitative research study.**
  Author(s): Pontin D, Porter T, McDonagh R.
  Source: Journal of Clinical Nursing. 2002 March; 11(2): 264-72.
  http://www.ncbi.nlm.nih.gov:80/entrez/query.fcgi?cmd=Retrieve&db=PubMed&list_uids=11903726&dopt=Abstract

- **Is quality of life different for men with erectile dysfunction and prostate cancer compared to men with erectile dysfunction due to other causes? Results from the ExCEED data base.**
  Author(s): Penson DF, Latini DM, Lubeck DP, Wallace K, Henning JM, Lue T.
  Source: The Journal of Urology. 2003 April; 169(4): 1458-61.
  http://www.ncbi.nlm.nih.gov:80/entrez/query.fcgi?cmd=Retrieve&db=PubMed&list_uids=12629383&dopt=Abstract

- **Is smoking a cause of erectile dysfunction? A literature review.**
  Author(s): Dorey G.
  Source: British Journal of Nursing (Mark Allen Publishing). 2001 April 12-25; 10(7): 455-65. Review.
  http://www.ncbi.nlm.nih.gov:80/entrez/query.fcgi?cmd=Retrieve&db=PubMed&list_uids=12070390&dopt=Abstract

- **Is there any relation between serum levels of total testosterone and the severity of erectile dysfunction?**
  Author(s): Rhoden EL, Teloken C, Mafessoni R, Souto CA.
  Source: International Journal of Impotence Research : Official Journal of the International Society for Impotence Research. 2002 June; 14(3): 167-71.
  http://www.ncbi.nlm.nih.gov:80/entrez/query.fcgi?cmd=Retrieve&db=PubMed&list_uids=12058243&dopt=Abstract

- **K channels as molecular targets for the treatment of erectile dysfunction.**
  Author(s): Christ GJ.
  Source: Journal of Andrology. 2002 September-October; 23(5): S10-9. Review.
  http://www.ncbi.nlm.nih.gov:80/entrez/query.fcgi?cmd=Retrieve&db=PubMed&list_uids=12236168&dopt=Abstract

- **Ketanserin plus prostaglandin E1 (PGE-1) as intracavernosal therapy for patients with erectile dysfunction unresponsive to PGE-1 alone.**
  Author(s): Mirone V, Imbimbo C, Fabrizio F, Longo N, Palmieri A.
  Source: British Journal of Urology. 1996 May; 77(5): 736-9.
  http://www.ncbi.nlm.nih.gov:80/entrez/query.fcgi?cmd=Retrieve&db=PubMed&list_uids=8689122&dopt=Abstract

- **Laboratory evaluations of erectile dysfunction: an evidence based approach.**
  Author(s): Bodie J, Lewis J, Schow D, Monga M.
  Source: The Journal of Urology. 2003 June; 169(6): 2262-4.
  http://www.ncbi.nlm.nih.gov:80/entrez/query.fcgi?cmd=Retrieve&db=PubMed&list_uids=12771765&dopt=Abstract

- **Lack of diagnostic tools to prove erectile dysfunction: consequences for reimbursement?**
  Author(s): Lehmann K, Eichlisberger R, Gasser TC.
  Source: The Journal of Urology. 2000 January; 163(1): 91-4.
  http://www.ncbi.nlm.nih.gov:80/entrez/query.fcgi?cmd=Retrieve&db=PubMed&list_uids=10604322&dopt=Abstract

- **Lack of sexual activity from erectile dysfunction is associated with a reversible reduction in serum testosterone.**
  Author(s): Jannini EA, Screponi E, Carosa E, Pepe M, Lo Giudice F, Trimarchi F, Benvenga S.
  Source: International Journal of Andrology. 1999 December; 22(6): 385-92.
  http://www.ncbi.nlm.nih.gov:80/entrez/query.fcgi?cmd=Retrieve&db=PubMed&list_uids=10624607&dopt=Abstract

- **Lecture 4: psychogenic erectile dysfunction-a theoretical approach.**
  Author(s): Bancroft J.
  Source: International Journal of Impotence Research : Official Journal of the International Society for Impotence Research. 2000 September; 12 Suppl 3: S46-8.
  http://www.ncbi.nlm.nih.gov:80/entrez/query.fcgi?cmd=Retrieve&db=PubMed&list_uids=11002401&dopt=Abstract

- **Lecture 5: erectile dysfunction in the HIV-positive male: a review of medical, legal and ethical considerations in the age of oral pharmacotherapy.**
  Author(s): Sadeghi-Nejad H, Watson R, Irwin R, Nokes K, Gern A, Price D.
  Source: International Journal of Impotence Research : Official Journal of the International Society for Impotence Research. 2000 September; 12 Suppl 3: S49-53.
  http://www.ncbi.nlm.nih.gov:80/entrez/query.fcgi?cmd=Retrieve&db=PubMed&list_uids=11002402&dopt=Abstract

- **Lipid-lowering drugs and erectile dysfunction.**
  Author(s): Blanker MH, Verhagen AP.
  Source: Family Practice. 2002 October; 19(5): 567.
  http://www.ncbi.nlm.nih.gov:80/entrez/query.fcgi?cmd=Retrieve&db=PubMed&list_uids=12356716&dopt=Abstract

- **Liposome encapsulated prostaglandin E1 in erectile dysfunction: correlation between in vitro delivery through foreskin and efficacy in patients.**
  Author(s): Foldvari M, Oguejiofor C, Afridi S, Kudel T, Wilson T.
  Source: Urology. 1998 November; 52(5): 838-43.
  http://www.ncbi.nlm.nih.gov:80/entrez/query.fcgi?cmd=Retrieve&db=PubMed&list_uids=9801110&dopt=Abstract

- **Longitudinal differences in disease specific quality of life in men with erectile dysfunction: results from the Exploratory Comprehensive Evaluation of Erectile Dysfunction study.**
  Author(s): Latini DM, Penson DF, Lubeck DP, Wallace KL, Henning JM, Lue TF.
  Source: The Journal of Urology. 2003 April; 169(4): 1437-42.
  http://www.ncbi.nlm.nih.gov:80/entrez/query.fcgi?cmd=Retrieve&db=PubMed&list_uids=12629379&dopt=Abstract

- **Long-term effect of sildenafil citrate on erectile dysfunction after radical prostatectomy: 3-year follow-up.**
  Author(s): Raina R, Lakin MM, Agarwal A, Sharma R, Goyal KK, Montague DK, Klein E, Zippe CD.
  Source: Urology. 2003 July; 62(1): 110-5. Review.
  http://www.ncbi.nlm.nih.gov:80/entrez/query.fcgi?cmd=Retrieve&db=PubMed&list_uids=12837433&dopt=Abstract

- **Long-term efficacy and safety of oral Viagra (sildenafil citrate) in men with erectile dysfunction and the effect of randomised treatment withdrawal.**
  Author(s): Christiansen E, Guirguis WR, Cox D, Osterloh IH; Sildenafil Multicentre Study Group.
  Source: International Journal of Impotence Research : Official Journal of the International Society for Impotence Research. 2000 June; 12(3): 177-82.
  http://www.ncbi.nlm.nih.gov:80/entrez/query.fcgi?cmd=Retrieve&db=PubMed&list_uids=11045912&dopt=Abstract

- **Long-term experience of self-injection therapy with prostaglandin E1 for erectile dysfunction.**
  Author(s): Lundberg L, Olsson JO, Kihl B.
  Source: Scandinavian Journal of Urology and Nephrology. 1996 October; 30(5): 395-7.
  http://www.ncbi.nlm.nih.gov:80/entrez/query.fcgi?cmd=Retrieve&db=PubMed&list_uids=8936629&dopt=Abstract

- **Long-term follow-up of patients receiving injection therapy for erectile dysfunction.**
  Author(s): Sundaram CP, Thomas W, Pryor LE, Sidi AA, Billups K, Pryor JL.
  Source: Urology. 1997 June; 49(6): 932-5.
  http://www.ncbi.nlm.nih.gov:80/entrez/query.fcgi?cmd=Retrieve&db=PubMed&list_uids=9187703&dopt=Abstract

- **Long-term follow-up of patients with erectile dysfunction commenced on self injection with intracavernosal papaverine with or without phentolamine.**
  Author(s): Flynn RJ, Williams G.
  Source: British Journal of Urology. 1996 October; 78(4): 628-31.
  http://www.ncbi.nlm.nih.gov:80/entrez/query.fcgi?cmd=Retrieve&db=PubMed&list_uids=8944522&dopt=Abstract

- **Long-term intracavernous self-injection with prostaglandin E1 for the treatment of erectile dysfunction.**
  Author(s): Canale D, Giorgi PM, Lencioni R, Morelli G, Gasperi M, Macchia E.
  Source: International Journal of Andrology. 1996 February; 19(1): 28-32.
  http://www.ncbi.nlm.nih.gov:80/entrez/query.fcgi?cmd=Retrieve&db=PubMed&list_uids=8698535&dopt=Abstract

- **Long-term results of dorsal penile vein ligation for symptomatic treatment of erectile dysfunction.**
  Author(s): Popken G, Katzenwadel A, Wetterauer U.
  Source: Andrologia. 1999; 31 Suppl 1: 77-82.
  http://www.ncbi.nlm.nih.gov:80/entrez/query.fcgi?cmd=Retrieve&db=PubMed&list_uids=10643523&dopt=Abstract

- **Long-term results of penile vein ligation for erectile dysfunction due to cavernovenous disease.**
  Author(s): Da Ros CT, Teloken C, Antonini CC, Sogari PR, Souto CA.
  Source: Tech Urol. 2000 September; 6(3): 172-4.
  http://www.ncbi.nlm.nih.gov:80/entrez/query.fcgi?cmd=Retrieve&db=PubMed&list_uids=10963480&dopt=Abstract

- **Long-term safety and efficacy of oral phentolamine mesylate (Vasomax) in men with mild to moderate erectile dysfunction.**
  Author(s): Padma-Nathan H, Goldstein I, Klimberg I, Coogan C, Auerbach S, Lammers P; Vasomax Study Group.
  Source: International Journal of Impotence Research : Official Journal of the International Society for Impotence Research. 2002 August; 14(4): 266-70.
  http://www.ncbi.nlm.nih.gov:80/entrez/query.fcgi?cmd=Retrieve&db=PubMed&list_uids=12152116&dopt=Abstract

- **Lower extremity above-knee prosthesis-associated erectile dysfunction.**
  Author(s): Munarriz R, Kulaksizoglu H, Hakim L, Gholami S, Nehra A, Goldstein I.
  Source: International Journal of Impotence Research : Official Journal of the International Society for Impotence Research. 2003 August; 15(4): 290-2.
  http://www.ncbi.nlm.nih.gov:80/entrez/query.fcgi?cmd=Retrieve&db=PubMed&list_uids=12934059&dopt=Abstract

- **Lower self-reported depression in patients with erectile dysfunction after treatment with sildenafil.**
  Author(s): Muller MJ, Benkert O.
  Source: Journal of Affective Disorders. 2001 October; 66(2-3): 255-61.
  http://www.ncbi.nlm.nih.gov:80/entrez/query.fcgi?cmd=Retrieve&db=PubMed&list_uids=11578679&dopt=Abstract

- **Low-flow priapism: risk factors for erectile dysfunction.**
  Author(s): El-Bahnasawy MS, Dawood A, Farouk A.
  Source: Bju International. 2002 February; 89(3): 285-90.
  http://www.ncbi.nlm.nih.gov:80/entrez/query.fcgi?cmd=Retrieve&db=PubMed&list_uids=11856112&dopt=Abstract

- **Malaysian cultural differences in knowledge, attitudes and practices related to erectile dysfunction: focus group discussions.**
  Author(s): Low WY, Wong YL, Zulkifli SN, Tan HM.
  Source: International Journal of Impotence Research : Official Journal of the International Society for Impotence Research. 2002 December; 14(6): 440-5.
  http://www.ncbi.nlm.nih.gov:80/entrez/query.fcgi?cmd=Retrieve&db=PubMed&list_uids=12494275&dopt=Abstract

- **Male infertility and erectile dysfunction in spinal cord injury: a review.**
  Author(s): Monga M, Bernie J, Rajasekaran M.
  Source: Archives of Physical Medicine and Rehabilitation. 1999 October; 80(10): 1331-9. Review.
  http://www.ncbi.nlm.nih.gov:80/entrez/query.fcgi?cmd=Retrieve&db=PubMed&list_uids=10527097&dopt=Abstract

- **Management of erectile dysfunction by combination therapy with testosterone and sildenafil in recipients of high-dose therapy for haematological malignancies.**
  Author(s): Chatterjee R, Kottaridis PD, McGarrigle HH, Linch DC.
  Source: Bone Marrow Transplantation. 2002 April; 29(7): 607-10.
  http://www.ncbi.nlm.nih.gov:80/entrez/query.fcgi?cmd=Retrieve&db=PubMed&list_uids=11979311&dopt=Abstract

- **Management of erectile dysfunction following radical prostatectomy.**
  Author(s): Zippe CD, Raina R, Thukral M, Lakin MM, Klein EA, Agarwal A.
  Source: Curr Urol Rep. 2001 December; 2(6): 495-503. Review.
  http://www.ncbi.nlm.nih.gov:80/entrez/query.fcgi?cmd=Retrieve&db=PubMed&list_
  uids=12084237&dopt=Abstract

- **Management of erectile dysfunction in diabetic patients.**
  Author(s): Ziegler D.
  Source: Diabetes Nutr Metab. 2002 February; 15(1): 58-65. Review. No Abstract
  Available.
  http://www.ncbi.nlm.nih.gov:80/entrez/query.fcgi?cmd=Retrieve&db=PubMed&list_
  uids=11942741&dopt=Abstract

- **Management of erectile dysfunction in diabetic subjects: results from a survey of 400
  diabetes centres in Italy.**
  Author(s): Fedele D, Coscelli C, Cucinotta D, Forti G, Santeusanio F, Fiori G, Velona T,
  Lavezzari M.
  Source: Diabetes Nutr Metab. 2001 October; 14(5): 277-82.
  http://www.ncbi.nlm.nih.gov:80/entrez/query.fcgi?cmd=Retrieve&db=PubMed&list_
  uids=11806468&dopt=Abstract

- **Management of erectile dysfunction in general practice.**
  Author(s): Sheehan E.
  Source: Ir Med J. 1999 August; 92(5): 356, 358. No Abstract Available.
  http://www.ncbi.nlm.nih.gov:80/entrez/query.fcgi?cmd=Retrieve&db=PubMed&list_
  uids=10522072&dopt=Abstract

- **Management of erectile dysfunction secondary to treatment for localized prostate
  cancer.**
  Author(s): Teloken C.
  Source: Cancer Control : Journal of the Moffitt Cancer Center. 2001 November-
  December; 8(6): 540-5. Review.
  http://www.ncbi.nlm.nih.gov:80/entrez/query.fcgi?cmd=Retrieve&db=PubMed&list_
  uids=11807424&dopt=Abstract

- **Management of erectile dysfunction.**
  Author(s): Ralph DJ.
  Source: International Journal of Std & Aids. 1999 March; 10(3): 209.
  http://www.ncbi.nlm.nih.gov:80/entrez/query.fcgi?cmd=Retrieve&db=PubMed&list_
  uids=10340205&dopt=Abstract

- **Management of premature ejaculation — a comparison of treatment outcome in
  patients with and without erectile dysfunction.**
  Author(s): Chia S.
  Source: International Journal of Andrology. 2002 October; 25(5): 301-5.
  http://www.ncbi.nlm.nih.gov:80/entrez/query.fcgi?cmd=Retrieve&db=PubMed&list_
  uids=12270028&dopt=Abstract

- **Managing erectile dysfunction.**
  Author(s): Hackett G.
  Source: The Practitioner. 1998 September; 242(1590): 632-6. Review.
  http://www.ncbi.nlm.nih.gov:80/entrez/query.fcgi?cmd=Retrieve&db=PubMed&list_
  uids=10534879&dopt=Abstract

- **Managing erectile dysfunction.**
  Author(s): Allen P.
  Source: Prof Nurse. 2003 January; 18(5): 253-4. No Abstract Available.
  http://www.ncbi.nlm.nih.gov:80/entrez/query.fcgi?cmd=Retrieve&db=PubMed&list_
  uids=12599953&dopt=Abstract

- **Managing erectile dysfunction.**
  Author(s): Hackett GI.
  Source: The Practitioner. 2001 October; 245(1627): 820, 823-4, 827-8. Review.
  http://www.ncbi.nlm.nih.gov:80/entrez/query.fcgi?cmd=Retrieve&db=PubMed&list_
  uids=11677897&dopt=Abstract

- **Masturbatory guilt leading to severe depression and erectile dysfunction.**
  Author(s): Chakrabarti N, Chopra VK, Sinha VK.
  Source: Journal of Sex & Marital Therapy. 2002 July-September; 28(4): 285-7.
  http://www.ncbi.nlm.nih.gov:80/entrez/query.fcgi?cmd=Retrieve&db=PubMed&list_
  uids=12082666&dopt=Abstract

- **Measurement of erectile dysfunction in population-based studies: the use of a single question self-assessment in the Massachusetts Male Aging Study.**
  Author(s): Derby CA, Araujo AB, Johannes CB, Feldman HA, McKinlay JB.
  Source: International Journal of Impotence Research : Official Journal of the International Society for Impotence Research. 2000 August; 12(4): 197-204.
  http://www.ncbi.nlm.nih.gov:80/entrez/query.fcgi?cmd=Retrieve&db=PubMed&list_
  uids=11079360&dopt=Abstract

- **Mechanical reliability of the AMS 700CXM inflatable penile prosthesis for the treatment of male erectile dysfunction.**
  Author(s): Deuk Choi Y, Jin Choi Y, Hwan Kim J, Ki Choi H.
  Source: The Journal of Urology. 2001 March; 165(3): 822-4.
  http://www.ncbi.nlm.nih.gov:80/entrez/query.fcgi?cmd=Retrieve&db=PubMed&list_
  uids=11176478&dopt=Abstract

- **Membrane bound guanylyl cyclase as a potential molecular target for the treatment of erectile dysfunction.**
  Author(s): Christ GJ.
  Source: The Journal of Urology. 2003 May; 169(5): 1923.
  http://www.ncbi.nlm.nih.gov:80/entrez/query.fcgi?cmd=Retrieve&db=PubMed&list_
  uids=12686874&dopt=Abstract

- **Mode of action of a new oral treatment for erectile dysfunction: apomorphine SL.**
  Author(s): Rampin O.
  Source: Bju International. 2001 October; 88 Suppl 3: 22-4. Review.
  http://www.ncbi.nlm.nih.gov:80/entrez/query.fcgi?cmd=Retrieve&db=PubMed&list_uids=11578275&dopt=Abstract

- **Modern pharmacotherapy for erectile dysfunction: evolving concepts with central and peripheral acting agents.**
  Author(s): Brock GB, Bochinski D.
  Source: Current Opinion in Urology. 2001 November; 11(6): 625-30. Review.
  http://www.ncbi.nlm.nih.gov:80/entrez/query.fcgi?cmd=Retrieve&db=PubMed&list_uids=11734700&dopt=Abstract

- **Multicentral clinical evaluation of the aetiology of erectile dysfunction: a survey report.**
  Author(s): Aydin S, Unal D, Erol H, Karaman I, Yilmaz Y, Sengul E, Bayrakli H.
  Source: International Urology and Nephrology. 2001; 32(4): 699-703.
  http://www.ncbi.nlm.nih.gov:80/entrez/query.fcgi?cmd=Retrieve&db=PubMed&list_uids=11989568&dopt=Abstract

- **Near infrared spectrophotometry for the diagnosis of vasculogenic erectile dysfunction.**
  Author(s): Burnett AL, Allen RP, Davis, Wright DC, Trueheart IN, Chance B.
  Source: International Journal of Impotence Research : Official Journal of the International Society for Impotence Research. 2000 October; 12(5): 247-54.
  http://www.ncbi.nlm.nih.gov:80/entrez/query.fcgi?cmd=Retrieve&db=PubMed&list_uids=11424961&dopt=Abstract

- **Neurogenic erectile dysfunction.**
  Author(s): Lue TF.
  Source: Clinical Autonomic Research : Official Journal of the Clinical Autonomic Research Society. 2001 October; 11(5): 285-94. Review.
  http://www.ncbi.nlm.nih.gov:80/entrez/query.fcgi?cmd=Retrieve&db=PubMed&list_uids=11758794&dopt=Abstract

- **Neurologic erectile dysfunction.**
  Author(s): Nehra A, Moreland RB.
  Source: The Urologic Clinics of North America. 2001 May; 28(2): 289-308. Review.
  http://www.ncbi.nlm.nih.gov:80/entrez/query.fcgi?cmd=Retrieve&db=PubMed&list_uids=11402582&dopt=Abstract

- **Neuropathy is a major contributing factor to diabetic erectile dysfunction.**
  Author(s): Hecht MJ, Neundorfer B, Kiesewetter F, Hilz MJ.
  Source: Neurological Research. 2001 September; 23(6): 651-4.
  http://www.ncbi.nlm.nih.gov:80/entrez/query.fcgi?cmd=Retrieve&db=PubMed&list_uids=11547937&dopt=Abstract

- **Neuroprotection and nerve grafts in the treatment of neurogenic erectile dysfunction.**
  Author(s): Burnett AL.
  Source: The Journal of Urology. 2003 August; 170(2 Pt 2): S31-4; Discussion S34. Review.
  http://www.ncbi.nlm.nih.gov:80/entrez/query.fcgi?cmd=Retrieve&db=PubMed&list_uids=12853770&dopt=Abstract

- **New concept parameters of RigiScan in differentiation of vascular erectile dysfunction: is it a useful test?**
  Author(s): Basar MM, Atan A, Tekdogan UY.
  Source: International Journal of Urology : Official Journal of the Japanese Urological Association. 2001 December; 8(12): 686-91.
  http://www.ncbi.nlm.nih.gov:80/entrez/query.fcgi?cmd=Retrieve&db=PubMed&list_uids=11851769&dopt=Abstract

- **New directions for erectile dysfunction therapies.**
  Author(s): Andersson KE, Hedlund P.
  Source: International Journal of Impotence Research : Official Journal of the International Society for Impotence Research. 2002 February; 14 Suppl 1: S82-92. Review.
  http://www.ncbi.nlm.nih.gov:80/entrez/query.fcgi?cmd=Retrieve&db=PubMed&list_uids=11850740&dopt=Abstract

- **New oral agents for erectile dysfunction: what is changing in our practice?**
  Author(s): Aversa A, Fabbri A.
  Source: Asian Journal of Andrology. 2001 September; 3(3): 175-9. Review.
  http://www.ncbi.nlm.nih.gov:80/entrez/query.fcgi?cmd=Retrieve&db=PubMed&list_uids=11561186&dopt=Abstract

- **New phosphodiesterase type 5 inhibitors in the management of erectile dysfunction.**
  Author(s): Mason RG.
  Source: J R Soc Health. 2003 June; 123(2): 79-80. No Abstract Available.
  http://www.ncbi.nlm.nih.gov:80/entrez/query.fcgi?cmd=Retrieve&db=PubMed&list_uids=12852189&dopt=Abstract

- **Nocturnal electrobioimpedance volumetric assessment of patients with erectile dysfunction.**
  Author(s): Knoll LD, Abrams JH.
  Source: Urology. 1999 June; 53(6): 1200-4.
  http://www.ncbi.nlm.nih.gov:80/entrez/query.fcgi?cmd=Retrieve&db=PubMed&list_uids=10367852&dopt=Abstract

- **Non-surgical treatment of erectile dysfunction.**
  Author(s): Papp G, Kopa Z.
  Source: Acta Chir Hung. 1998; 37(3-4): 183-93. Review.
  http://www.ncbi.nlm.nih.gov:80/entrez/query.fcgi?cmd=Retrieve&db=PubMed&list_uids=10379370&dopt=Abstract

- **Novel treatment options for overlapping yet distinct erectile dysfunction and andropause syndromes.**
  Author(s): Tan RS.
  Source: Curr Opin Investig Drugs. 2003 April; 4(4): 435-8. Review.
  http://www.ncbi.nlm.nih.gov:80/entrez/query.fcgi?cmd=Retrieve&db=PubMed&list_uids=12808883&dopt=Abstract

- **Onset and duration of action of sildenafil for the treatment of erectile dysfunction.**
  Author(s): Eardley I, Ellis P, Boolell M, Wulff M.
  Source: British Journal of Clinical Pharmacology. 2002; 53 Suppl 1: 61S-65S.
  http://www.ncbi.nlm.nih.gov:80/entrez/query.fcgi?cmd=Retrieve&db=PubMed&list_uids=11879261&dopt=Abstract

- **Optimizing treatment for diabetes mellitus induced erectile dysfunction.**
  Author(s): Costabile RA.
  Source: The Journal of Urology. 2003 August; 170(2 Pt 2): S35-8; Discussion S39. Review.
  http://www.ncbi.nlm.nih.gov:80/entrez/query.fcgi?cmd=Retrieve&db=PubMed&list_uids=12853771&dopt=Abstract

- **Oral agents for erectile dysfunction.**
  Author(s): Kalsi JS, Minhas S, Kell PD, Ralph DJ.
  Source: Hosp Med. 2003 May; 64(5): 292-5. Review.
  http://www.ncbi.nlm.nih.gov:80/entrez/query.fcgi?cmd=Retrieve&db=PubMed&list_uids=12789739&dopt=Abstract

- **Oral and injectable medications for the treatment of erectile dysfunction.**
  Author(s): Carson CC.
  Source: Curr Urol Rep. 2000 December; 1(4): 307-12. Review.
  http://www.ncbi.nlm.nih.gov:80/entrez/query.fcgi?cmd=Retrieve&db=PubMed&list_uids=12084309&dopt=Abstract

- **Oral and topical treatment of erectile dysfunction. Present and future.**
  Author(s): Morales A, Heaton JP, Johnston B, Adams M.
  Source: The Urologic Clinics of North America. 1995 November; 22(4): 879-86. Review.
  http://www.ncbi.nlm.nih.gov:80/entrez/query.fcgi?cmd=Retrieve&db=PubMed&list_uids=7483136&dopt=Abstract

- **Oral sildenafil in the treatment of erectile dysfunction. 1998.**
  Author(s): Goldstein I, Lue TF, Padma-Nathan H, Rosen RC, Steers WD, Wicker PA; Sildenafil Study Group.
  Source: The Journal of Urology. 2002 February; 167(2 Pt 2): 1197-203; Discussion 1204.
  http://www.ncbi.nlm.nih.gov:80/entrez/query.fcgi?cmd=Retrieve&db=PubMed&list_uids=11905901&dopt=Abstract

- **Oral testosterone undecanoate reverses erectile dysfunction associated with diabetes mellitus in patients failing on sildenafil citrate therapy alone.**
  Author(s): Kalinchenko SY, Kozlov GI, Gontcharov NP, Katsiya GV.
  Source: The Aging Male : the Official Journal of the International Society for the Study of the Aging Male. 2003 June; 6(2): 94-9.
  http://www.ncbi.nlm.nih.gov:80/entrez/query.fcgi?cmd=Retrieve&db=PubMed&list_uids=12898793&dopt=Abstract

- **Oral treatment of erectile dysfunction with apomorphine SL.**
  Author(s): Altwein JE, Keuler FU.
  Source: Urologia Internationalis. 2001; 67(4): 257-63. Review.
  http://www.ncbi.nlm.nih.gov:80/entrez/query.fcgi?cmd=Retrieve&db=PubMed&list_uids=11741126&dopt=Abstract

- **Outcome measures for erectile dysfunction 2: evaluation.**
  Author(s): Dorey G.
  Source: British Journal of Nursing (Mark Allen Publishing). 2002 January 24-February 13; 11(2): 120-5.
  http://www.ncbi.nlm.nih.gov:80/entrez/query.fcgi?cmd=Retrieve&db=PubMed&list_uids=11823739&dopt=Abstract

- **Outcome measures for erectile dysfunction. 1: Literature review.**
  Author(s): Dorey G.
  Source: British Journal of Nursing (Mark Allen Publishing). 2002 January 10-23; 11(1): 54-64. Review.
  http://www.ncbi.nlm.nih.gov:80/entrez/query.fcgi?cmd=Retrieve&db=PubMed&list_uids=11826321&dopt=Abstract

- **Penile axial rigidity and Doppler ultrasonography parameters in patients with erectile dysfunction: association with type 2 diabetes.**
  Author(s): El-Sakka AI.
  Source: Urology. 2003 September; 62(3): 525-31.
  http://www.ncbi.nlm.nih.gov:80/entrez/query.fcgi?cmd=Retrieve&db=PubMed&list_uids=12946761&dopt=Abstract

- **Pharmacological aspects of erectile dysfunction.**
  Author(s): Thomas JA.
  Source: Japanese Journal of Pharmacology. 2002 June; 89(2): 101-12. Review.
  http://www.ncbi.nlm.nih.gov:80/entrez/query.fcgi?cmd=Retrieve&db=PubMed&list_uids=12120751&dopt=Abstract

- **Pharmacological management of erectile dysfunction.**
  Author(s): Montorsi F, Salonia A, Deho' F, Cestari A, Guazzoni G, Rigatti P, Stief C.
  Source: Bju International. 2003 March; 91(5): 446-54. Review.
  http://www.ncbi.nlm.nih.gov:80/entrez/query.fcgi?cmd=Retrieve&db=PubMed&list_uids=12603396&dopt=Abstract

- **Preference for oral sildenafil or intracavernosal injection in patients with erectile dysfunction already using intracavernosal injection for > 1 year.**
  Author(s): Kim SC, Chang IH, Jeon HJ.
  Source: Bju International. 2003 August; 92(3): 277-80.
  http://www.ncbi.nlm.nih.gov:80/entrez/query.fcgi?cmd=Retrieve&db=PubMed&list_uids=12887483&dopt=Abstract

- **Preliminary report of association of chronic diseases and erectile dysfunction in middle-aged men in Japan.**
  Author(s): Naya Y, Mizutani Y, Ochiai A, Soh J, Kawauchi A, Fujito A, Nakamura N, Ono T, Iwamoto N, Aoki T, Marumo K, Murai M, Miki T.
  Source: Urology. 2003 September; 62(3): 532-6.
  http://www.ncbi.nlm.nih.gov:80/entrez/query.fcgi?cmd=Retrieve&db=PubMed&list_uids=12946762&dopt=Abstract

- **Prevalence and risk factors for erectile dysfunction in a population-based study in Iran.**
  Author(s): Safarinejad MR.
  Source: International Journal of Impotence Research : Official Journal of the International Society for Impotence Research. 2003 August; 15(4): 246-52.
  http://www.ncbi.nlm.nih.gov:80/entrez/query.fcgi?cmd=Retrieve&db=PubMed&list_uids=12934051&dopt=Abstract

- **Prevalence of erectile dysfunction and associated factors among men without concomitant diseases: a population study.**
  Author(s): Nicolosi A, Glasser DB, Moreira ED, Villa M; Erectile Dysfunction Epidemiology Cross National Study Group.
  Source: International Journal of Impotence Research : Official Journal of the International Society for Impotence Research. 2003 August; 15(4): 253-7.
  http://www.ncbi.nlm.nih.gov:80/entrez/query.fcgi?cmd=Retrieve&db=PubMed&list_uids=12934052&dopt=Abstract

- **Prevalence of erectile dysfunction and its correlates in Egypt: a community-based study.**
  Author(s): Seyam RM, Albakry A, Ghobish A, Arif H, Dandash K, Rashwan H.
  Source: International Journal of Impotence Research : Official Journal of the International Society for Impotence Research. 2003 August; 15(4): 237-45.
  http://www.ncbi.nlm.nih.gov:80/entrez/query.fcgi?cmd=Retrieve&db=PubMed&list_uids=12934050&dopt=Abstract

- **Prognostic factors for the vascular components of erectile dysfunction in patients on renal replacement therapy.**
  Author(s): Diemont WL, Hendriks JC, Lemmens WA, Langen H, Berden JH, Meuleman EJ.
  Source: International Journal of Impotence Research : Official Journal of the International Society for Impotence Research. 2003 February; 15(1): 44-52.
  http://www.ncbi.nlm.nih.gov:80/entrez/query.fcgi?cmd=Retrieve&db=PubMed&list_uids=12605240&dopt=Abstract

- **Prospective pilot study of sildenafil for treatment of postradiotherapy erectile dysfunction in patients with prostate cancer.**
  Author(s): Weber DC, Bieri S, Kurtz JM, Miralbell R.
  Source: Journal of Clinical Oncology : Official Journal of the American Society of Clinical Oncology. 1999 November; 17(11): 3444-9.
  http://www.ncbi.nlm.nih.gov:80/entrez/query.fcgi?cmd=Retrieve&db=PubMed&list_uids=10550140&dopt=Abstract

- **Quality control in the screening of erectile dysfunction--results of a survey.**
  Author(s): Hakim J, Subit M, Kandzari S, Zaslau S.
  Source: Urology. 2002 July; 60(1): 125-9.
  http://www.ncbi.nlm.nih.gov:80/entrez/query.fcgi?cmd=Retrieve&db=PubMed&list_uids=12100937&dopt=Abstract

- **Quality of life and erectile dysfunction.**
  Author(s): Althof SE.
  Source: Urology. 2002 June; 59(6): 803-10. Review.
  http://www.ncbi.nlm.nih.gov:80/entrez/query.fcgi?cmd=Retrieve&db=PubMed&list_uids=12031357&dopt=Abstract

- **Quality of life effects of alprostadil therapy for erectile dysfunction.**
  Author(s): Willke RJ, Glick HA, McCarron TJ, Erder MH, Althof SE, Linet OI.
  Source: The Journal of Urology. 1997 June; 157(6): 2124-8.
  http://www.ncbi.nlm.nih.gov:80/entrez/query.fcgi?cmd=Retrieve&db=PubMed&list_uids=9146597&dopt=Abstract

- **Quality of life effects of alprostadil therapy for erectile dysfunction: results of a trial in Europe and South Africa.**
  Author(s): Willke RJ, Yen W, Parkerson GR Jr, Linet OI, Erder MH, Glick HA.
  Source: International Journal of Impotence Research : Official Journal of the International Society for Impotence Research. 1998 December; 10(4): 239-46.
  http://www.ncbi.nlm.nih.gov:80/entrez/query.fcgi?cmd=Retrieve&db=PubMed&list_uids=9884920&dopt=Abstract

- **Quality of life in patients using self-administered intracavernous injections of prostaglandin E1 for erectile dysfunction.**
  Author(s): Gheorghiu S, Godschalk M, Gentili A, Mulligan T.
  Source: The Journal of Urology. 1996 July; 156(1): 80-1.
  http://www.ncbi.nlm.nih.gov:80/entrez/query.fcgi?cmd=Retrieve&db=PubMed&list_uids=8648844&dopt=Abstract

- **Quality of life in patients with spinal cord injury receiving Viagra (sildenafil citrate) for the treatment of erectile dysfunction.**
  Author(s): Hultling C, Giuliano F, Quirk F, Pena B, Mishra A, Smith MD.
  Source: Spinal Cord : the Official Journal of the International Medical Society of Paraplegia. 2000 June; 38(6): 363-70.
  http://www.ncbi.nlm.nih.gov:80/entrez/query.fcgi?cmd=Retrieve&db=PubMed&list_uids=10889565&dopt=Abstract

- **Quality of partnership in patients with erectile dysfunction after sildenafil treatment.**
  Author(s): Muller MJ, Ruof J, Graf-Morgenstern M, Porst H, Benkert O.
  Source: Pharmacopsychiatry. 2001 May; 34(3): 91-5.
  http://www.ncbi.nlm.nih.gov:80/entrez/query.fcgi?cmd=Retrieve&db=PubMed&list_uids=11434405&dopt=Abstract

- **Quality of Sexual Life Questionnaire (QVS): a reliable, sensitive and reproducible instrument to assess quality of life in subjects with erectile dysfunction.**
  Author(s): Costa P, Arnould B, Cour F, Boyer P, Marrel A, Jaudinot EO, Solesse de Gendre A.
  Source: International Journal of Impotence Research : Official Journal of the International Society for Impotence Research. 2003 June; 15(3): 173-84.
  http://www.ncbi.nlm.nih.gov:80/entrez/query.fcgi?cmd=Retrieve&db=PubMed&list_uids=12904803&dopt=Abstract

- **Quantitative analysis of penile ultrasonographic shape during the erectile cycle: a new diagnostic tool for erectile dysfunction? Repeatability of the method and preliminary results.**
  Author(s): Sforza C, Montorsi F, Bianchi A, Ferrario VF.
  Source: International Journal of Impotence Research : Official Journal of the International Society for Impotence Research. 1998 December; 10(4): 203-9.
  http://www.ncbi.nlm.nih.gov:80/entrez/query.fcgi?cmd=Retrieve&db=PubMed&list_uids=9884915&dopt=Abstract

- **Quantitative sensory and autonomic testing in male diabetic patients with erectile dysfunction.**
  Author(s): Wellmer A, Sharief MK, Knowles CH, Misra VP, Kopelman P, Ralph D, Anand P.
  Source: Bju International. 1999 January; 83(1): 66-70.
  http://www.ncbi.nlm.nih.gov:80/entrez/query.fcgi?cmd=Retrieve&db=PubMed&list_uids=10233454&dopt=Abstract

- **Randomized, double-blind, placebo-controlled trial of sildenafil (Viagra) for erectile dysfunction after rectal excision for cancer and inflammatory bowel disease.**
  Author(s): Lindsey I, George B, Kettlewell M, Mortensen N.
  Source: Diseases of the Colon and Rectum. 2002 June; 45(6): 727-32.
  http://www.ncbi.nlm.nih.gov:80/entrez/query.fcgi?cmd=Retrieve&db=PubMed&list_uids=12072621&dopt=Abstract

- **Rationale for combination therapy of intraurethral prostaglandin E(1) and sildenafil in the salvage of erectile dysfunction patients desiring noninvasive therapy.**
  Author(s): Nehra A, Blute ML, Barrett DM, Moreland RB.
  Source: International Journal of Impotence Research : Official Journal of the International Society for Impotence Research. 2002 February; 14 Suppl 1: S38-42.
  http://www.ncbi.nlm.nih.gov:80/entrez/query.fcgi?cmd=Retrieve&db=PubMed&list_uids=11850734&dopt=Abstract

- **Recent advances in the treatment of erectile dysfunction in patients with diabetes mellitus.**
  Author(s): Koppiker N, Boolell M, Price D.
  Source: Endocrine Practice : Official Journal of the American College of Endocrinology and the American Association of Clinical Endocrinologists. 2003 January-February; 9(1): 52-63. Review.
  http://www.ncbi.nlm.nih.gov:80/entrez/query.fcgi?cmd=Retrieve&db=PubMed&list_uids=12917094&dopt=Abstract

- **Relation of C-reactive protein and other cardiovascular risk factors to penile vascular disease in men with erectile dysfunction.**
  Author(s): Bank AJ, Billups KL, Kaiser DR, Kelly AS, Wetterling RA, Tsai MY, Hanson N.
  Source: International Journal of Impotence Research : Official Journal of the International Society for Impotence Research. 2003 August; 15(4): 231-6.
  http://www.ncbi.nlm.nih.gov:80/entrez/query.fcgi?cmd=Retrieve&db=PubMed&list_uids=12934049&dopt=Abstract

- **Relation of erectile dysfunction to angiographic coronary artery disease.**
  Author(s): Solomon H, Man JW, Wierzbicki AS, Jackson G.
  Source: The American Journal of Cardiology. 2003 January 15; 91(2): 230-1.
  http://www.ncbi.nlm.nih.gov:80/entrez/query.fcgi?cmd=Retrieve&db=PubMed&list_uids=12521639&dopt=Abstract

- **Relationship between patient self-assessment of erectile dysfunction and the sexual health inventory for men.**
  Author(s): Cappelleri JC, Siegel RL, Glasser DB, Osterloh IH, Rosen RC.
  Source: Clinical Therapeutics. 2001 October; 23(10): 1707-19.
  http://www.ncbi.nlm.nih.gov:80/entrez/query.fcgi?cmd=Retrieve&db=PubMed&list_uids=11726005&dopt=Abstract

- **Relaxation degree: a new concept in erectile dysfunction.**
  Author(s): Kayigil O, Metin A.
  Source: International Urology and Nephrology. 2001; 33(2): 391-4.
  http://www.ncbi.nlm.nih.gov:80/entrez/query.fcgi?cmd=Retrieve&db=PubMed&list_uids=12092664&dopt=Abstract

- **Reply to: Is there a role of radial rigidity in the evaluation of erectile dysfunction? By Ku JH, Song YS, Kim ME, Lee NK and Park YH.**
  Author(s): Udelson D, Goldstein I.
  Source: International Journal of Impotence Research : Official Journal of the International Society for Impotence Research. 2001 December; 13(6): 363-4.
  http://www.ncbi.nlm.nih.gov:80/entrez/query.fcgi?cmd=Retrieve&db=PubMed&list_uids=11918256&dopt=Abstract

- **Role of exercise treadmill testing in the management of erectile dysfunction: a joint cardiovascular/erectile dysfunction clinic.**
  Author(s): Solomon H, Man J, Martin E, Jackson G.
  Source: Heart (British Cardiac Society). 2003 June; 89(6): 671-2.
  http://www.ncbi.nlm.nih.gov:80/entrez/query.fcgi?cmd=Retrieve&db=PubMed&list_uids=12748235&dopt=Abstract

- **Role of penile vascular insufficiency in erectile dysfunction in renal transplant recipients.**
  Author(s): Abdel-Hamid IA, Eraky I, Fouda MA, Mansour OE.
  Source: International Journal of Impotence Research : Official Journal of the International Society for Impotence Research. 2002 February; 14(1): 32-7.
  http://www.ncbi.nlm.nih.gov:80/entrez/query.fcgi?cmd=Retrieve&db=PubMed&list_uids=11896475&dopt=Abstract

- **Safety and efficacy of vardenafil for the treatment of men with erectile dysfunction after radical retropubic prostatectomy.**
  Author(s): Brock G, Nehra A, Lipshultz LI, Karlin GS, Gleave M, Seger M, Padma-Nathan H.
  Source: The Journal of Urology. 2003 October; 170(4 Pt 1): 1278-83.
  http://www.ncbi.nlm.nih.gov:80/entrez/query.fcgi?cmd=Retrieve&db=PubMed&list_uids=14501741&dopt=Abstract

- **Selective phosphodiesterase type 5 inhibition using tadalafil for the treatment of erectile dysfunction.**
  Author(s): Kuan J, Brock G.
  Source: Expert Opinion on Investigational Drugs. 2002 November; 11(11): 1605-13. Review.
  http://www.ncbi.nlm.nih.gov:80/entrez/query.fcgi?cmd=Retrieve&db=PubMed&list_uids=12437506&dopt=Abstract

- **Sildenafil citrate for treatment of erectile dysfunction in men with type 1 diabetes: results of a randomized controlled trial.**
  Author(s): Stuckey BG, Jadzinsky MN, Murphy LJ, Montorsi F, Kadioglu A, Fraige F, Manzano P, Deerochanawong C.
  Source: Diabetes Care. 2003 February; 26(2): 279-84.
  http://www.ncbi.nlm.nih.gov:80/entrez/query.fcgi?cmd=Retrieve&db=PubMed&list_uids=12547849&dopt=Abstract

- **Sildenafil does not improve sexual function in men without erectile dysfunction but does reduce the postorgasmic refractory time.**
  Author(s): Mondaini N, Ponchietti R, Muir GH, Montorsi F, Di Loro F, Lombardi G, Rizzo M.
  Source: International Journal of Impotence Research : Official Journal of the International Society for Impotence Research. 2003 June; 15(3): 225-8.
  http://www.ncbi.nlm.nih.gov:80/entrez/query.fcgi?cmd=Retrieve&db=PubMed&list_uids=12904810&dopt=Abstract

- **Sildenafil effects on exercise, neurohormonal activation, and erectile dysfunction in congestive heart failure: a double-blind, placebo-controlled, randomized study followed by a prospective treatment for erectile dysfunction.**
  Author(s): Bocchi EA, Guimaraes G, Mocelin A, Bacal F, Bellotti G, Ramires JF.
  Source: Circulation. 2002 August 27; 106(9): 1097-103.
  http://www.ncbi.nlm.nih.gov:80/entrez/query.fcgi?cmd=Retrieve&db=PubMed&list_uids=12196335&dopt=Abstract

- **Sildenafil test: changes in the diagnostic and therapeutic management of erectile dysfunction.**
  Author(s): Perimenis P, Athanasopoulos A, Gyftopoulos K, Barbalias G.
  Source: International Urology and Nephrology. 2001; 33(2): 387-9.
  http://www.ncbi.nlm.nih.gov:80/entrez/query.fcgi?cmd=Retrieve&db=PubMed&list_uids=12092663&dopt=Abstract

- **Sildenafil use in patients with olanzapine-induced erectile dysfunction.**
  Author(s): Atmaca M, Kuloglu M, Tezcan E.
  Source: International Journal of Impotence Research : Official Journal of the International Society for Impotence Research. 2002 December; 14(6): 547-9.
  http://www.ncbi.nlm.nih.gov:80/entrez/query.fcgi?cmd=Retrieve&db=PubMed&list_uids=12494295&dopt=Abstract

- **Spinal schwannoma as a cause of erectile dysfunction with urinary incontinence and groin and testicular pain.**
  Author(s): Kawsar M, Goh BT.
  Source: International Journal of Std & Aids. 2002 August; 13(8): 584-5.
  http://www.ncbi.nlm.nih.gov:80/entrez/query.fcgi?cmd=Retrieve&db=PubMed&list_uids=12194747&dopt=Abstract

- **Structured interview on erectile dysfunction (SIEDY): a new, multidimensional instrument for quantification of pathogenetic issues on erectile dysfunction.**
  Author(s): Petrone L, Mannucci E, Corona G, Bartolini M, Forti G, Giommi R, Maggi M.
  Source: International Journal of Impotence Research : Official Journal of the International Society for Impotence Research. 2003 June; 15(3): 210-20.
  http://www.ncbi.nlm.nih.gov:80/entrez/query.fcgi?cmd=Retrieve&db=PubMed&list_uids=12904808&dopt=Abstract

- **Sustained efficacy and tolerability of vardenafil, a highly potent selective phosphodiesterase type 5 inhibitor, in men with erectile dysfunction: results of a randomized, double-blind, 26-week placebo-controlled pivotal trial.**
  Author(s): Hellstrom WJ, Gittelman M, Karlin G, Segerson T, Thibonnier M, Taylor T, Padma-Nathan H; Vardenafil Study Group.
  Source: Urology. 2003 April; 61(4 Suppl 1): 8-14.
  http://www.ncbi.nlm.nih.gov:80/entrez/query.fcgi?cmd=Retrieve&db=PubMed&list_uids=12657355&dopt=Abstract

- **Test retest reliability of anal pressure measurements in men with erectile dysfunction.**
  Author(s): Dorey G, Swinkels A.
  Source: Urologic Nursing : Official Journal of the American Urological Association Allied. 2003 June; 23(3): 204-12.
  http://www.ncbi.nlm.nih.gov:80/entrez/query.fcgi?cmd=Retrieve&db=PubMed&list_uids=12861738&dopt=Abstract

- **The ageing male and erectile dysfunction.**
  Author(s): Montorsi F, Salonia A, Deho F, Briganti A, Rigatti P.
  Source: World Journal of Urology. 2002 May; 20(1): 28-35. Review.
  http://www.ncbi.nlm.nih.gov:80/entrez/query.fcgi?cmd=Retrieve&db=PubMed&list_uids=12088186&dopt=Abstract

- **The ageing male and erectile dysfunction.**
  Author(s): Montorsi F, Briganti A, Salonia A, Deho' F, Zanni G, Cestari A, Guazzoni G, Rigatti P, Stief C.
  Source: Bju International. 2003 September; 92(5): 516-20. Review.
  http://www.ncbi.nlm.nih.gov:80/entrez/query.fcgi?cmd=Retrieve&db=PubMed&list_uids=12930410&dopt=Abstract

- **The association of ED (erectile dysfunction) with ED (endothelial dysfunction) in the International Journal of Impotence Research: The Journal of Sexual Medicine.**
  Author(s): Goldstein I.
  Source: International Journal of Impotence Research : Official Journal of the International Society for Impotence Research. 2003 August; 15(4): 229-30.
  http://www.ncbi.nlm.nih.gov:80/entrez/query.fcgi?cmd=Retrieve&db=PubMed&list_uids=12934048&dopt=Abstract

- **The epidemiology of erectile dysfunction: results from the National Health and Social Life Survey.**
  Author(s): Laumann EO, Paik A, Rosen RC.
  Source: International Journal of Impotence Research : Official Journal of the International Society for Impotence Research. 1999 September; 11 Suppl 1: S60-4. Review.
  http://www.ncbi.nlm.nih.gov:80/entrez/query.fcgi?cmd=Retrieve&db=PubMed&list_uids=10554933&dopt=Abstract

- **The epidemiology, anatomy, physiology, and treatment of erectile dysfunction in chronic renal failure patients.**
  Author(s): Carson CC, Patel MP.
  Source: Adv Ren Replace Ther. 1999 October; 6(4): 296-309. Review.
  http://www.ncbi.nlm.nih.gov:80/entrez/query.fcgi?cmd=Retrieve&db=PubMed&list_uids=10543709&dopt=Abstract

- **The Second International Consultation on Erectile Dysfunction: highlights from the pharmaceutical industry.**
  Author(s): Wyllie MG.
  Source: Bju International. 2003 October; 92(6): 645-6.
  http://www.ncbi.nlm.nih.gov:80/entrez/query.fcgi?cmd=Retrieve&db=PubMed&list_
  uids=14511053&dopt=Abstract

- **The treatment of erectile dysfunction in the elderly.**
  Author(s): Gholami SS, Graziottin TM, Lue TF.
  Source: Curr Urol Rep. 2001 February; 2(1): 1-2. No Abstract Available.
  http://www.ncbi.nlm.nih.gov:80/entrez/query.fcgi?cmd=Retrieve&db=PubMed&list_
  uids=12084288&dopt=Abstract

- **Time dependent patient satisfaction with sildenafil for erectile dysfunction (ED) after nerve-sparing radical retropubic prostatectomy (RRP).**
  Author(s): Hong EK, Lepor H, McCullough AR.
  Source: International Journal of Impotence Research : Official Journal of the International Society for Impotence Research. 1999 September; 11 Suppl 1: S15-22.
  http://www.ncbi.nlm.nih.gov:80/entrez/query.fcgi?cmd=Retrieve&db=PubMed&list_
  uids=10554925&dopt=Abstract

- **Tissue engineering applications for erectile dysfunction.**
  Author(s): Atala A.
  Source: International Journal of Impotence Research : Official Journal of the International Society for Impotence Research. 1999 September; 11 Suppl 1: S41-7. Review.
  http://www.ncbi.nlm.nih.gov:80/entrez/query.fcgi?cmd=Retrieve&db=PubMed&list_
  uids=10554929&dopt=Abstract

- **UK management guidelines for erectile dysfunction.**
  Author(s): Ralph D, McNicholas T.
  Source: Bmj (Clinical Research Ed.). 2000 August 19-26; 321(7259): 499-503. Review.
  http://www.ncbi.nlm.nih.gov:80/entrez/query.fcgi?cmd=Retrieve&db=PubMed&list_
  uids=10948037&dopt=Abstract

- **Ultrastructual changes of corpora cavernosa in vascular erectile dysfunction.**
  Author(s): Aydos K, Baltaci S, Saglam M, Tanyolac A, Anafarta K, Beduk Y, Gogus O.
  Source: International Urology and Nephrology. 1996; 28(3): 375-85.
  http://www.ncbi.nlm.nih.gov:80/entrez/query.fcgi?cmd=Retrieve&db=PubMed&list_
  uids=8899479&dopt=Abstract

- **Unilateral adrenal tumor, erectile dysfunction and infertility in a patient with 21-hydroxylase deficiency: effects of glucocorticoid treatment and surgery.**
  Author(s): Scaroni C, Favia G, Lumachi F, Opocher G, Bonanni G, Mantero F, Armanini D.
  Source: Experimental and Clinical Endocrinology & Diabetes : Official Journal, German Society of Endocrinology [and] German Diabetes Association. 2003 February; 111(1): 41-3.
  http://www.ncbi.nlm.nih.gov:80/entrez/query.fcgi?cmd=Retrieve&db=PubMed&list_
  uids=12605349&dopt=Abstract

- **Update on male erectile dysfunction.**
  Author(s): Wagner G, Saenz de Tejada I.
  Source: Bmj (Clinical Research Ed.). 1998 February 28; 316(7132): 678-82. Review.
  http://www.ncbi.nlm.nih.gov:80/entrez/query.fcgi?cmd=Retrieve&db=PubMed&list_
  uids=9522795&dopt=Abstract

- **Use of intracavernosal alprostadil in erectile dysfunction.**
  Author(s): Gingell C.
  Source: Hosp Med. 1998 October; 59(10): 777.
  http://www.ncbi.nlm.nih.gov:80/entrez/query.fcgi?cmd=Retrieve&db=PubMed&list_
  uids=9850293&dopt=Abstract

- **Use of medications for erectile dysfunction in the United States, 1996 through 2001.**
  Author(s): Wysowski DK, Swann J.
  Source: The Journal of Urology. 2003 March; 169(3): 1040-2.
  http://www.ncbi.nlm.nih.gov:80/entrez/query.fcgi?cmd=Retrieve&db=PubMed&list_
  uids=12576841&dopt=Abstract

- **Use of nocturnal penile tumescence and rigidity in the evaluation of male erectile dysfunction.**
  Author(s): Levine LA, Lenting EL.
  Source: The Urologic Clinics of North America. 1995 November; 22(4): 775-88. Review.
  http://www.ncbi.nlm.nih.gov:80/entrez/query.fcgi?cmd=Retrieve&db=PubMed&list_
  uids=7483128&dopt=Abstract

- **Use of oral sildenafil (Viagra) in the treatment of erectile dysfunction.**
  Author(s): Licht MR.
  Source: Compr Ther. 1999 February; 25(2): 90-4. Review.
  http://www.ncbi.nlm.nih.gov:80/entrez/query.fcgi?cmd=Retrieve&db=PubMed&list_
  uids=10091013&dopt=Abstract

- **Use of sildenafil citrate in treatment of Taiwanese men with erectile dysfunction: a single center experience.**
  Author(s): Huang ST.
  Source: Chang Gung Med J. 2001 February; 24(2): 91-6.
  http://www.ncbi.nlm.nih.gov:80/entrez/query.fcgi?cmd=Retrieve&db=PubMed&list_
  uids=11360407&dopt=Abstract

- **Usefulness of power Doppler ultrasonography in evaluating erectile dysfunction.**
  Author(s): Golubinski AJ, Sikorski A.
  Source: Bju International. 2002 May; 89(7): 779-82.
  http://www.ncbi.nlm.nih.gov:80/entrez/query.fcgi?cmd=Retrieve&db=PubMed&list_
  uids=11966647&dopt=Abstract

- **Vacuum constriction and external erection devices in erectile dysfunction.**
  Author(s): Levine LA, Dimitriou RJ.
  Source: The Urologic Clinics of North America. 2001 May; 28(2): 335-41, Ix-X. Review.
  http://www.ncbi.nlm.nih.gov:80/entrez/query.fcgi?cmd=Retrieve&db=PubMed&list_
  uids=11402585&dopt=Abstract

- **Vacuum constriction devices for erectile dysfunction: a long-term, prospective study of patients with mild, moderate, and severe dysfunction.**
  Author(s): Dutta TC, Eid JF.
  Source: Urology. 1999 November; 54(5): 891-3.
  http://www.ncbi.nlm.nih.gov:80/entrez/query.fcgi?cmd=Retrieve&db=PubMed&list_
  uids=10565753&dopt=Abstract

- **Validation of the German version of the International Index of Erectile Function (IIEF) in patients with erectile dysfunction, Peyronie's disease and controls.**
  Author(s): Wiltink J, Hauck EW, Phadayanon M, Weidner W, Beutel ME.
  Source: International Journal of Impotence Research : Official Journal of the International Society for Impotence Research. 2003 June; 15(3): 192-7.
  http://www.ncbi.nlm.nih.gov:80/entrez/query.fcgi?cmd=Retrieve&db=PubMed&list_
  uids=12904805&dopt=Abstract

- **Vardenafil for treatment of men with erectile dysfunction: efficacy and safety in a randomized, double-blind, placebo-controlled trial.**
  Author(s): Hellstrom WJ, Gittelman M, Karlin G, Segerson T, Thibonnier M, Taylor T, Padma-Nathan H.
  Source: Journal of Andrology. 2002 November-December; 23(6): 763-71.
  http://www.ncbi.nlm.nih.gov:80/entrez/query.fcgi?cmd=Retrieve&db=PubMed&list_
  uids=12399521&dopt=Abstract

- **Vardenafil increases penile rigidity and tumescence in men with erectile dysfunction after a single oral dose.**
  Author(s): Stark S, Sachse R, Liedl T, Hensen J, Rohde G, Wensing G, Horstmann R, Schrott KM.
  Source: European Urology. 2001 August; 40(2): 181-8; Discussion 189-90.
  http://www.ncbi.nlm.nih.gov:80/entrez/query.fcgi?cmd=Retrieve&db=PubMed&list_
  uids=11528196&dopt=Abstract

- **Vardenafil, a new phosphodiesterase type 5 inhibitor, in the treatment of erectile dysfunction in men with diabetes: a multicenter double-blind placebo-controlled fixed-dose study.**
  Author(s): Goldstein I, Young JM, Fischer J, Bangerter K, Segerson T, Taylor T; Vardenafil Diabetes Study Group.
  Source: Diabetes Care. 2003 March; 26(3): 777-83.
  http://www.ncbi.nlm.nih.gov:80/entrez/query.fcgi?cmd=Retrieve&db=PubMed&list_
  uids=12610037&dopt=Abstract

- **Vascular risk factors and erectile dysfunction.**
  Author(s): Sullivan ME, Keoghane SR, Miller MA.
  Source: Bju International. 2001 June; 87(9): 838-45. Review.
  http://www.ncbi.nlm.nih.gov:80/entrez/query.fcgi?cmd=Retrieve&db=PubMed&list_
  uids=11412223&dopt=Abstract

- **Vasculogenic erectile dysfunction: newer therapeutic strategies.**
  Author(s): Siroky MB, Azadzoi KM.
  Source: The Journal of Urology. 2003 August; 170(2 Pt 2): S24-9; Discussion S29-30. Review.
  http://www.ncbi.nlm.nih.gov:80/entrez/query.fcgi?cmd=Retrieve&db=PubMed&list_uids=12853769&dopt=Abstract

- **Vasomax for the treatment of male erectile dysfunction.**
  Author(s): Goldstein I, Carson C, Rosen R, Islam A.
  Source: World Journal of Urology. 2001 February; 19(1): 51-6.
  http://www.ncbi.nlm.nih.gov:80/entrez/query.fcgi?cmd=Retrieve&db=PubMed&list_uids=11289571&dopt=Abstract

- **Viability and safety of combination drug therapies for erectile dysfunction.**
  Author(s): Steers WD.
  Source: The Journal of Urology. 2003 August; 170(2 Pt 2): S20-3; Discussion S23. Review.
  http://www.ncbi.nlm.nih.gov:80/entrez/query.fcgi?cmd=Retrieve&db=PubMed&list_uids=12853768&dopt=Abstract

- **What does duplex ultrasound add to sexual history, nocturnal penile tumescence and intracavernosal injection of smooth muscle relaxant, in the diagnosis of erectile dysfunction?**
  Author(s): Gutierrez P, Pye S, Bancroft J.
  Source: International Journal of Impotence Research : Official Journal of the International Society for Impotence Research. 1993 September; 5(3): 123-31; Discussion 132.
  http://www.ncbi.nlm.nih.gov:80/entrez/query.fcgi?cmd=Retrieve&db=PubMed&list_uids=8124430&dopt=Abstract

- **Withered Yang: a review of traditional Chinese medical treatment of male infertility and erectile dysfunction.**
  Author(s): Crimmel AS, Conner CS, Monga M.
  Source: Journal of Andrology. 2001 March-April; 22(2): 173-82. Review.
  http://www.ncbi.nlm.nih.gov:80/entrez/query.fcgi?cmd=Retrieve&db=PubMed&list_uids=11229790&dopt=Abstract

- **Yohimbine and pentoxifylline in the treatment of erectile dysfunction.**
  Author(s): Nessel MA.
  Source: The American Journal of Psychiatry. 1994 March; 151(3): 453.
  http://www.ncbi.nlm.nih.gov:80/entrez/query.fcgi?cmd=Retrieve&db=PubMed&list_uids=8109665&dopt=Abstract

- **Yohimbine for erectile dysfunction.**
  Author(s): Witt DK.
  Source: The Journal of Family Practice. 1998 April; 46(4): 282-3.
  http://www.ncbi.nlm.nih.gov:80/entrez/query.fcgi?cmd=Retrieve&db=PubMed&list_uids=9564368&dopt=Abstract

- **Yohimbine for erectile dysfunction: a systematic review and meta-analysis of randomized clinical trials.**
  Author(s): Ernst E, Pittler MH.
  Source: The Journal of Urology. 1998 February; 159(2): 433-6.
  http://www.ncbi.nlm.nih.gov:80/entrez/query.fcgi?cmd=Retrieve&db=PubMed&list_uids=9649257&dopt=Abstract

- **Yohimbine in erectile dysfunction: the facts.**
  Author(s): Morales A.
  Source: International Journal of Impotence Research : Official Journal of the International Society for Impotence Research. 2000 March; 12 Suppl 1: S70-74. Review.
  http://www.ncbi.nlm.nih.gov:80/entrez/query.fcgi?cmd=Retrieve&db=PubMed&list_uids=10845767&dopt=Abstract

- **Yohimbine in erectile dysfunction: would an orphan drug ever be properly assessed?**
  Author(s): Morales A.
  Source: World Journal of Urology. 2001 August; 19(4): 251-5. Review.
  http://www.ncbi.nlm.nih.gov:80/entrez/query.fcgi?cmd=Retrieve&db=PubMed&list_uids=11550783&dopt=Abstract

- **Yohimbine in the treatment of male erectile dysfunction.**
  Author(s): Ashton AK.
  Source: The American Journal of Psychiatry. 1994 September; 151(9): 1397.
  http://www.ncbi.nlm.nih.gov:80/entrez/query.fcgi?cmd=Retrieve&db=PubMed&list_uids=8067505&dopt=Abstract

CHAPTER 2. NUTRITION AND ERECTILE DYSFUNCTION

Overview

In this chapter, we will show you how to find studies dedicated specifically to nutrition and erectile dysfunction.

Finding Nutrition Studies on Erectile Dysfunction

The National Institutes of Health's Office of Dietary Supplements (ODS) offers a searchable bibliographic database called the IBIDS (International Bibliographic Information on Dietary Supplements; National Institutes of Health, Building 31, Room 1B29, 31 Center Drive, MSC 2086, Bethesda, Maryland 20892-2086, Tel: 301-435-2920, Fax: 301-480-1845, E-mail: ods@nih.gov). The IBIDS contains over 460,000 scientific citations and summaries about dietary supplements and nutrition as well as references to published international, scientific literature on dietary supplements such as vitamins, minerals, and botanicals.[7] The IBIDS includes references and citations to both human and animal research studies.

As a service of the ODS, access to the IBIDS database is available free of charge at the following Web address: **http://ods.od.nih.gov/databases/ibids.html** After entering the search area, you have three choices: (1) IBIDS Consumer Database, (2) Full IBIDS Database, or (3) Peer Reviewed Citations Only.

Now that you have selected a database, click on the "Advanced" tab. An advanced search allows you to retrieve up to 100 fully explained references in a comprehensive format. Type "erectile dysfunction" (or synonyms) into the search box, and click "Go." To narrow the search, you can also select the "Title" field.

---

[7] Adapted from **http://ods.od.nih.gov**. IBIDS is produced by the Office of Dietary Supplements (ODS) at the National Institutes of Health to assist the public, healthcare providers, educators, and researchers in locating credible, scientific information on dietary supplements. IBIDS was developed and will be maintained through an interagency partnership with the Food and Nutrition Information Center of the National Agricultural Library, U.S. Department of Agriculture.

The following information is typical of that found when using the "Full IBIDS Database" to search for "erectile dysfunction" (or a synonym):

- **A clinical comparative study on effects of intracavernous injection of sodium nitroprusside and papaverine/phentolamine in erectile dysfunction patients.**
  Author(s): Department of Urology, the Ninth People's Hospital, Shanghai Second Medical University, Shanghai 200011, China. james-fu@citiz.net
  Source: Fu, Q Yao, D H Jiang, Y Q Asian-J-Androl. 2000 December; 2(4): 301-3

- **A double-blind, placebo-controlled, efficacy and safety study of topical gel formulation of 1% alprostadil (Topiglan) for the in-office treatment of erectile dysfunction.**
  Author(s): Department of Urology, Boston University School of Medicine, Boston, Massachusetts, USA.
  Source: Goldstein, I Payton, T R Schechter, P J Urology. 2001 February; 57(2): 301-5 1527-9995

- **A European multicentre study to evaluate the tolerability of apomorphine sublingual administered in a forced dose-escalation regimen in patients with erectile dysfunction.**
  Author(s): Urology Practice, Krummbogen, Marburg, Germany.
  Source: Von Keitz, A T Stroberg, P Bukofzer, S Mallard, N Hibberd, M BJU-Int. 2002 March; 89(4): 409-15 1464-4096

- **A goal-oriented, cost-effective approach to the diagnosis and treatment of 24 male erectile dysfunction.**
  Author(s): Department of Surgery, University of Louisville School of Medicine, KY 40292, USA.
  Source: Long, R L Sherman, L S Lombardi, T J J-Ky-Med-Assoc. 1995 November; 93(11): 500-8 0023-0294

- **An international comparison of the reliability and responsiveness of the Duke Health Profile for measuring health-related quality of life of patients treated with alprostadil for erectile dysfunction.**
  Author(s): Department of Community and Family Medicine, Duke University Medical Center, Durham, NC 27710, USA. parke001@mc.duke.edu
  Source: Parkerson, G R Willke, R J Hays, R D Med-Care. 1999 January; 37(1): 56-67 0025-7079

- **Coincidence of induratio penis plastica and erectile dysfunction.**
  Author(s): Department of Urology, University of Jena, Germany.
  Source: Wunderlich, H Werner, W Schubert, J Urol-Int. 1998; 60(2): 97-100 0042-1138

- **Combination therapy using oral alpha-blockers and intracavernosal injection in men with erectile dysfunction.**
  Author(s): Department of Urology, College of Physicians and Surgeons, Columbia University, New York, New York 10032, USA.
  Source: Kaplan, S A Reis, R B Kohn, I J Shabsigh, R Te, A E Urology. 1998 November; 52(5): 739-43 0090-4295

- **Comparative evaluation of treatments for erectile dysfunction in patients with prostate cancer after radical retropubic prostatectomy.**
  Author(s): Institute of Urology, Rabin Medical Center, Beilinson Campus, Petah Tiqva, Israel.
  Source: Baniel, J Israilov, S Segenreich, E Livne, P M BJU-Int. 2001 July; 88(1): 58-62 1464-4096

- **Current concepts in erectile dysfunction.**
  Source: Mulhall, J P Am-J-Manag-Care. 2000 August; 6(12 Suppl): S625-31 1096-1860

- **Dehydroepiandrosterone in the treatment of erectile dysfunction: a prospective, double-blind, randomized, placebo-controlled study.**
  Author(s): Department of Urology, University of Vienna, Austria.
  Source: Reiter, W J Pycha, A Schatzl, G Pokorny, A Gruber, D M Huber, J C Marberger, M Urology. 1999 Mar; 53(3): 590-4; discussion 594-5 0090-4295

- **Diagnosis and therapy of erectile dysfunction using papaverine and phentolamine.**
  Author(s): Byk Gulden Lomberg, Department of Clinical Development, Konstanz, FRG.
  Source: Zentgraf, M Baccouche, M Junemann, K P Urol-Int. 1988; 43(2): 65-75 0042-1138

- **Dietary supplements and other alternative medicines for erectile dysfunction. What do I tell my patients?**
  Author(s): Department of Urology, University of Michigan Medical Center, 1500 East Medical Center Drive, Ann Arbor, MI 48109-0330, USA. moyad@umich.edu
  Source: Moyad, Mark A Urol-Clin-North-Am. 2002 February; 29(1): 11-22, vii 0094-0143

- **Economic aspects of medical erectile dysfunction therapies.**
  Author(s): Department of Urology, College of Physicians and Surgeons of Columbia University, 161 Fort Washington Avenue, Dana Atchley Pavilion, 11th Floor, New York, NY 10032, USA.
  Source: Anastasiadis, A G Ghafar, M A Burchardt, M Shabsigh, R Expert-Opin-Pharmacother. 2002 March; 3(3): 257-63 1465-6566

- **Effect of nitric oxide-donor, linsidomine chlorhydrate, in treatment of human erectile dysfunction caused by venous leakage.**
  Author(s): Department of Urology, Universitatsklinikum Steglitz, Freie Universitat Berlin, Germany.
  Source: Wegner, H E Knispel, H H Urology. 1993 October; 42(4): 409-11 0090-4295

- **Effect of oral administration of high-dose nitric oxide donor L-arginine in men with organic erectile dysfunction: results of a double-blind, randomized, placebo-controlled study.**
  Author(s): Department of Urology, Tel Aviv Sourasky Medical Center, Sackler Faculty of Medicine, Tel Aviv University, Tel Aviv, Israel.
  Source: Chen, J Wollman, Y Chernichovsky, T Iaina, A Sofer, M Matzkin, H BJU-Int. 1999 February; 83(3): 269-73 1464-4096

- **Effect of testosterone administration on sexual behavior and mood in men with erectile dysfunction.**
  Author(s): Department of Psychiatry, Mount Sinai School of Medicine, New York, New York 10029, USA.
  Source: Schiavi, R C White, D Mandeli, J Levine, A C Arch-Sex-Behavolume 1997 June; 26(3): 231-41 0004-0002

- **Effectiveness of oral L-arginine in first-line treatment of erectile dysfunction in a controlled crossover study.**
  Author(s): Department of Urology, University of Cologne, Germany. tklotz@t-online.de
  Source: Klotz, T Mathers, M J Braun, M Bloch, W Engelmann, U Urol-Int. 1999; 63(4): 220-3 0042-1138

- **Efficacy and safety of fixed-dose and dose-optimization regimens of sublingual apomorphine versus placebo in men with erectile dysfunction. The Apomorphine Study Group.**
  Author(s): West Coast Clinical Research, Van Nuys, California, USA.

Source: Dula, E Keating, W Siami, P F Edmonds, A O'neil, J Buttler, S Urology. 2000 July; 56(1): 130-5 0090-4295

- **Erectile dysfunction in diabetes.**
  Author(s): Center for the Study of Male Sexual Dysfunction, Hospital of the University of Pennsylvania.
  Source: Broderick, G A Schwartz, S Hosp-Pract-(Off-Ed). 1991 August 15; 26(8): 139-42, 147-55 8750-2836

- **Evaluation and treatment of erectile dysfunction following spinal cord injury: a review.**
  Author(s): University of Medicine and Dentistry of New Jersey.
  Source: Linsenmeyer, T A J-Am-Paraplegia-Soc. 1991 April; 14(2): 43-51 0195-2307

- **Evaluation of transurethal alprostadil for safety and efficacy in men with erectile dysfunction.**
  Author(s): Department of Urology, Faculty of Medicine, Chulalongkorn, University, Bangkok, Thailand.
  Source: Kongkanand, Apichat Ratana Olarn, Krisda Wuddhikarn, Supoj Luengwattanakit, Sombun Tantiwong, Anupun Ruengdilokrat, Satit Opanuraks, Julin Sripalakit, Supon J-Med-Assoc-Thai. 2002 February; 85(2): 223-8 0125-2208

- **Evaluation, treatment, and management of erectile dysfunction: an overview.**
  Author(s): Virginia Mason Medical Center, Department of Urology, Seattle, WA, USA.
  Source: Colpo, L M Urol-Nurs. 1998 June; 18(2): 100-6 1053-816X

- **Factors predicting efficacy of phentolamine-papaverine intracorporeal injection for treatment of erectile dysfunction in diabetic male.**
  Author(s): Division of Endocrinology and Metabolism, University of Alabama, Birmingham School of Medicine.
  Source: Bell, D S Cutter, G R Hayne, V B Lloyd, L K Urology. 1992 July; 40(1): 36-40 0090-4295

- **First-line therapies for erectile dysfunction.**
  Author(s): Urology Clinic of Utah Valley, Provo, Utah, USA.
  Source: Ensign, C JAAPA. 2001 October; 14(10): 17-20

- **Hemodynamic evaluation of the penile arterial system in patients with erectile dysfunction using power Doppler imaging.**
  Author(s): Department of Urology, Showa University School of Medicine, Tokyo, Japan.
  Source: Sakamoto, H Shimada, M Yoshida, H Urology. 2002 September; 60(3): 480-4 1527-9995

- **Hormonal erectile dysfunction. Evaluation and management.**
  Author(s): Department of Urology, Queen's University, Kingston, Ontario, Canada.
  Source: Morales, A Heaton, J P Urol-Clin-North-Am. 2001 May; 28(2): 279-88 0094-0143

- **Intracavernosal injection and intraurethral therapy for erectile dysfunction.**
  Author(s): Department of Urology, Tulane University Health Sciences Center, New Orleans, Louisiana, USA.
  Source: Leungwattanakij, S Flynn, V Jr Hellstrom, W J Urol-Clin-North-Am. 2001 May; 28(2): 343-54 0094-0143

- **Intracavernous alprostadil alfadex (EDEX/VIRIDAL) is effective and safe in patients with erectile dysfunction after failing sildenafil (Viagra).**
  Author(s): Columbia-Presbyterian Medical Center, New York, New York, USA.
  Source: Shabsigh, R Padma Nathan, H Gittleman, M McMurray, J Kaufman, J Goldstein, I Urology. 2000 April; 55(4): 477-80 0090-4295

- **Intracavernous injection as an option for aging men with erectile dysfunction.**
  Author(s): Department of Urology, CHU de Charleroi, Boulevard Zoe Drion Drion, 1 6000 Charleroi, Belgium.
  Source: Wespes, E Aging-Male. 2002 September; 5(3): 177-80 1368-5538

- **Intracavernous pharmacotherapy for management of erectile dysfunction in spinal cord injury.**
  Author(s): Urological Rehabilitation and Research Center, Spain Rehabilitation Center, University of Alabama, Birmingham 35294.
  Source: Lloyd, L K Richards, J S Paraplegia. 1989 December; 27(6): 457-64 0031-1758

- **Intracavernous prostaglandin E1 in erectile dysfunction.**
  Author(s): Upjohn Company, Kalamazoo.
  Source: Linet, O I Neff, L L Clin-Investig. 1994 January; 72(2): 139-49 0941-0198

- **Intracavernous self-injection of prostaglandin E1 in the therapy of erectile dysfunction.**
  Source: Porst, H van Ahlen, H Block, T Halbig, W Hautmann, R Lochner Ernst, D Rudnick, J Staehler, G Weber, H M Weidner, W et al. Vasa-Suppl. 1989; 2850-6 0251-1029

- **Intraurethral alprostadil for treatment of erectile dysfunction in patients with spinal cord injury.**
  Author(s): Cleveland Veterans Affairs Medical Center, Case Western Reserve University, Ohio 44106-5046, USA.
  Source: Bodner, D R Haas, C A Krueger, B Seftel, A D Urology. 1999 January; 53(1): 199-202 0090-4295

- **Intraurethral prostaglandin E-2 cream: a possible alternative treatment for erectile dysfunction.**
  Author(s): Department of Surgery, Harbor-UCLA Medical Center, UCLA School of Medicine, Torrance.
  Source: Wolfson, B Pickett, S Scott, N E DeKernion, J B Rajfer, J Urology. 1993 July; 42(1): 73-5 0090-4295

- **Liposome encapsulated prostaglandin E1 in erectile dysfunction: correlation between in vitro delivery through foreskin and efficacy in patients.**
  Author(s): College of Pharmacy and Nutrition, Department of Surgery, College of Medicine, University of Saskatchewan, Saskatoon, Canada.
  Source: Foldvari, M Oguejiofor, C Afridi, S Kudel, T Wilson, T Urology. 1998 November; 52(5): 838-43 0090-4295

- **Long-term experience of self-injection therapy with prostaglandin E1 for erectile dysfunction.**
  Author(s): Section of Urology, Department of Surgery, Central Hospital, Karlstad, Sweden.
  Source: Lundberg, L Olsson, J O Kihl, B Scand-J-Urol-Nephrol. 1996 October; 30(5): 395-7 0036-5599

- **Long-term results of corpus cavernosum autoinjection therapy for chronic erectile dysfunction.**
  Author(s): Abteilung Dermatologie, Bundeswehrkrankenhaus, Ulm, Germany.
  Source: Gall, H Sparwasser, C Bahren, W Scherb, W Irion, R Andrologia. 1992 Sep-October; 24(5): 285-92 0303-4569

- **Management of erectile dysfunction by combination therapy with testosterone and sildenafil in recipients of high-dose therapy for haematological malignancies.**
  Author(s): Department of Obstetrics and Gynaecology, University College London Hospital, London, UK.
  Source: Chatterjee, R Kottaridis, P D McGarrigle, H H Linch, D C Bone-Marrow-Transplant. 2002 April; 29(7): 607-10 0268-3369

- **Mid-term results of autoinjection therapy for erectile dysfunction.**
  Author(s): Department of Urology, Academic Hospital, University of Ulm, West Germany.
  Source: Stief, C G Gall, H Scherb, W Bahren, W Urology. 1988 June; 31(6): 483-5 0090-4295

- **New oral agents for erectile dysfunction: what is changing in our practice?**
  Author(s): AFaR-CRCCS, Fatebenefratelli-Isola Tiberina Hospital, University of Rome Tor Vergata, Italy. amfaversa@yahoo.com
  Source: Aversa, A Fabbri, A Asian-J-Androl. 2001 September; 3(3): 175-9

- **New treatment for erectile dysfunction.**
  Author(s): Department of Psychiatry, MetroHealth Medical Center, 2500 MetroHealth Drive, Cleveland, OH 44109, USA. rsegraves@metrohealth.org
  Source: Segraves, R T Curr-Psychiatry-Repage 2000 June; 2(3): 206-10 1523-3812

- **New treatment options for erectile dysfunction.**
  Author(s): Australian Centre for Sexual Health, St Luke's Hospital, Sydney, NSW.
  Source: McMahon, C G Aust-Fam-Physician. 1999 August; 28(8): 783-7, 789-90 0300-8495

- **Non-prosthetic surgery in the treatment of erectile dysfunction. A retrospective study of 45 impotent patients in the University of Oulu.**
  Author(s): Division of Urology, Oulu University Central Hospital, Finland.
  Source: Lukkarinen, O Tonttila, P Hellstrom, P Leinonen, S Scand-J-Urol-Nephrol. 1998 February; 32(1): 42-6 0036-5599

- **Non-surgical treatment of erectile dysfunction.**
  Author(s): Clinic of Urology Center of Andrology, Semmelweis Medical School, Budapest, Hungary.
  Source: Papp, G Kopa, Z Acta-Chir-Hung. 1998; 37(3-4): 183-93 0231-4614

- **Oral treatment of erectile dysfunction with apomorphine SL.**
  Author(s): Department of Urology, Krankenhaus der Barmherzigen Bruder, Munich, Germany. dr.bartha@t-online.de
  Source: Altwein, J E Keuler, F U Urol-Int. 2001; 67(4): 257-63 0042-1138

- **Oral treatments for erectile dysfunction.**
  Author(s): Human Sexuality Unit, St George's Hospital Medical School, London, UK.
  Source: Riley, A Int-J-STD-AIDS. 1996; 7 Suppl 316-8 0956-4624

- **Pharmacologic erection programs: a treatment option for erectile dysfunction.**
  Source: Williams, L Rehabil-Nurs. 1989 Sep-October; 14(5): 264-8 0278-4807

- **Pharmacological treatment of erectile dysfunction.**
  Author(s): Unidada de Urologicay Andrologia, Hospital Ruber Internacional, Madrid, Spain.
  Source: Moncada Iribarren, I Saenz de Tejada, I Curr-Opin-Urol. 1999 November; 9(6): 547-51 0963-0643

- **Pilot study of the transdermal application of testosterone gel to the penile skin for the treatment of hypogonadotropic men with erectile dysfunction.**
  Author(s): Department of Urology, Medizinische Hochschule Hannover, Germany. schlutheiss.dirk@mh-hannover.de
  Source: Schultheiss, D Hiltl, D M Meschi, M R Machtens, S A Truss, M C Stief, C G Jonas, U World-J-Urol. 2000 December; 18(6): 431-5 0724-4983

- **Prostaglandin E(1)-based vasoactive cocktails in erectile dysfunction: how environmental conditions affect PGE(1) efficacy.**
  Author(s): Department of Urology, University of Bologna, Italy. bertacc@tin.it
  Source: Bertaccini, A Gotti, R Soli, M Carparelli, F Ceccarelli, R Cavrini, V Martorana, G Urol-Int. 2002; 68(4): 251-4 0042-1138

- **Prostaglandin E1 in the medical management of erectile dysfunction in a genito-urinary medicine clinic.**
  Author(s): Genito-Urinary Medicine Clinic, Royal Victoria Hospital, Belfast.
  Source: Armstrong, D K Convery, A Dinsmore, W W Ulster-Med-J. 1994 April; 63(1): 18-22 0041-6193

- **Prostaglandin E1 long-term self-injection programme for treatment of erectile dysfunction—a follow-up of at least 5 years.**
  Author(s): Department of Urology, Justus Liebig University, Giessen, Germany.
  Source: Hauck, E W Altinkilic, B M Schroeder Printzen, I Rudnick, J Weidner, W Andrologia. 1999; 31 Suppl 199-103 0303-4569

- **Prostaglandin E1 versus linsidomine chlorhydrate in erectile dysfunction.**
  Author(s): Department of Urology, Universitatsklinikum Steglitz, Freie Universitat Berlin, Germany.
  Source: Wegner, H E Knispel, H H Klan, R Meier, T Miller, K Urol-Int. 1994; 53(4): 214-6 0042-1138

- **Role of radionuclide phallogram in therapeutic decision-making for erectile dysfunction.**
  Author(s): Department of Radiology, Eastern Virginia Medical School, Norfolk, USA.
  Source: Smith, E M Netto, I C Gladden, K H Chaudhuri, T K Fink, S Kolm, P Urology. 1998 May; 51(5A Suppl): 175-8 0090-4295

- **Severe penile erosion after use of a vacuum suction device for management of erectile dysfunction in a spinal cord injured patient. Case report.**
  Author(s): Department of Urologic Surgery, University of Minnesota Hospital and Clinic, Minneapolis 55455.
  Source: LeRoy, S C Pryor, J L Paraplegia. 1994 February; 32(2): 120-3 0031-1758

- **Spontaneous erections in a patient with erectile dysfunction after palliative chemotherapy for non-small cell lung cancer.**
  Author(s): Department of Internal Medicine I, Division of Oncology, University Hospital, Vienna, Austria. michael.hejna@akh-wien.ac.at
  Source: Hejna, M Fiebiger, W C Reiter, W J Raderer, M Urol-Int. 2001; 67(2): 163-4 0042-1138

- **The clinical effectiveness of self-injection and external vacuum devices in the treatment of erectile dysfunction: a six-month comparison.**
  Author(s): Department of Psychiatry, Case Western Reserve University School of Medicine, Cleveland, Ohio.
  Source: Turner, L A Althof, S E Psychiatr-Med. 1992; 10(2): 283-93 0732-0868

- **The incidence of pharmacologically induced priapism in the diagnostic and therapeutic management of 685 men with erectile dysfunction.**
  Author(s): Department of Urology, Medical School, University of Patras, Greece.
  Source: Perimenis, P Athanasopoulos, A Geramoutsos, I Barbalias, G Urol-Int. 2001; 66(1): 27-9 0042-1138

- **The interaction of homocysteine and copper markedly inhibits the relaxation of rabbit corpus cavernosum: new risk factors for angiopathic erectile dysfunction?**
  Author(s): Department of Urology, Royal Free and University College Medical School (University College London), Royal Free Campus & The Royal Free Hampstead NHS Trust, London, UK.
  Source: Khan, M A Thompson, C S Emsley, A M Mumtaz, F H Mikhailidis, D P Angelini, G D Morgan, R J Jeremy, J Y BJU-Int. 1999 October; 84(6): 720-4 1464-4096

- **The management of erectile dysfunction following spinal cord injury.**
  Author(s): University of Southern California School of Medicine, Los Angeles.
  Source: Padma Nathan, H Kanellos, A Semin-Urol. 1992 May; 10(2): 133-7 0730-9147

- **Three-year outcome of a progressive treatment program for erectile dysfunction with intracavernous injections of vasoactive drugs.**
  Author(s): Institute of Urology, Rabin Medical Center, Beilinson Campus, Petah Tiqva and Sackler Faculty of Medicine, Tel Aviv University, Tel Aviv, Israel.
  Source: Baniel, J Israilov, S Engelstein, D Shmueli, J Segenreich, E Livne, P M Urology. 2000 October 1; 56(4): 647-52 1527-9995

- **Topical alprostadil cream for the treatment of erectile dysfunction: a combined analysis of the phase II program.**
  Author(s): Northeast Indiana Research, Fort Wayne, Indiana, USA.
  Source: Steidle, C Padma Nathan, H Salem, S Tayse, N Thwing, D Fendl, J Yeager, J Harning, R Urology. 2002 December; 60(6): 1077-82 1527-9995

- **Transcutaneous nitroglycerin in the treatment of erectile dysfunction in spinal cord injured.**
  Author(s): Department of Urology, Rigshospitalet, University of Copenhagen, Denmark.
  Source: Sonksen, J Biering Sorensen, F Paraplegia. 1992 August; 30(8): 554-7 0031-1758

- **Treating men with predominantly nonpsychogenic erectile dysfunction with intracavernosal vasoactive intestinal polypeptide and phentolamine mesylate in a novel auto-injector system: a multicentre double-blind placebo-controlled study.**
  Author(s): Department of Genito-Urinary Medicine, Royal Victoria Hospital, Belfast, Northern Ireland.
  Source: Dinsmore, W W Gingell, C Hackett, G Kell, P Savage, D Oakes, R Frentz, G D BJU-Int. 1999 February; 83(3): 274-9 1464-4096

- **Twelve-month comparison of two treatments for erectile dysfunction: self-injection versus external vacuum devices.**
  Author(s): Department of Psychiatry, Case Western Reserve University School of Medicine, University Hospitals of Cleveland, Ohio.
  Source: Turner, L A Althof, S E Levine, S B Bodner, D R Kursh, E D Resnick, M I Urology. 1992 February; 39(2): 139-44 0090-4295

- **Use of intracavernosal alprostadil in erectile dysfunction.**
  Author(s): Bristol Urological Institute, Southmead Hospital.
  Source: Gingell, C Hosp-Med. 1998 October; 59(10): 777 1462-3935

- **Use of intracavernous injection of prostaglandin E1 for neuropathic erectile dysfunction.**
  Author(s): Department of Urology, Jefferson Medical College, Philadelphia, PA 19107.
  Source: Hirsch, I H Smith, R L Chancellor, M B Bagley, D H Carsello, J Staas, W E Paraplegia. 1994 October; 32(10): 661-4 0031-1758

- **Usefulness of power Doppler ultrasonography in evaluating erectile dysfunction.**
  Author(s): Department of Urology, Pomeranian Academy of Medicine, ul. Powstancow Wlkp. 72, 70-111 Szczecin, Poland. golubinski@interia.com.pl
  Source: Golubinski, A J Sikorski, A BJU-Int. 2002 May; 89(7): 779-82 1464-4096

- **Variable response to intracavernous prostaglandin E1 testing for erectile dysfunction.**
  Author(s): Urologic Clinic, University of Basel, Kantonsspital, Switzerland.
  Source: Lehmann, K John, H Kacl, G Hauri, D Gasser, T C Urology. 1999 September; 54(3): 539-43 0090-4295

Federal Resources on Nutrition

In addition to the IBIDS, the United States Department of Health and Human Services (HHS) and the United States Department of Agriculture (USDA) provide many sources of information on general nutrition and health. Recommended resources include:

- healthfinder®, HHS's gateway to health information, including diet and nutrition: **http://www.healthfinder.gov/scripts/SearchContext.asp?topic=238&page=0**

- The United States Department of Agriculture's Web site dedicated to nutrition information: **www.nutrition.gov**

- The Food and Drug Administration's Web site for federal food safety information: **www.foodsafety.gov**

- The National Action Plan on Overweight and Obesity sponsored by the United States Surgeon General: **http://www.surgeongeneral.gov/topics/obesity/**

- The Center for Food Safety and Applied Nutrition has an Internet site sponsored by the Food and Drug Administration and the Department of Health and Human Services: **http://vm.cfsan.fda.gov/**

- Center for Nutrition Policy and Promotion sponsored by the United States Department of Agriculture: **http://www.usda.gov/cnpp/**

- Food and Nutrition Information Center, National Agricultural Library sponsored by the United States Department of Agriculture: **http://www.nal.usda.gov/fnic/**

- Food and Nutrition Service sponsored by the United States Department of Agriculture: **http://www.fns.usda.gov/fns/**

Additional Web Resources

A number of additional Web sites offer encyclopedic information covering food and nutrition. The following is a representative sample:

- AOL: **http://search.aol.com/cat.adp?id=174&layer=&from=subcats**

- Family Village: **http://www.familyvillage.wisc.edu/med_nutrition.html**

- Google: **http://directory.google.com/Top/Health/Nutrition/**

- Healthnotes: **http://www.healthnotes.com/**

- Open Directory Project: **http://dmoz.org/Health/Nutrition/**

- Yahoo.com: **http://dir.yahoo.com/Health/Nutrition/**

- WebMD®Health: **http://my.webmd.com/nutrition**

- WholeHealthMD.com: **http://www.wholehealthmd.com/reflib/0,1529,00.html**

The following is a specific Web list relating to erectile dysfunction; please note that any particular subject below may indicate either a therapeutic use, or a contraindication (potential danger), and does not reflect an official recommendation:

- **Minerals**

    Paroxetine
    Source: Healthnotes, Inc.; www.healthnotes.com

CHAPTER 3. ALTERNATIVE MEDICINE AND ERECTILE DYSFUNCTION

Overview

In this chapter, we will begin by introducing you to official information sources on complementary and alternative medicine (CAM) relating to erectile dysfunction. At the conclusion of this chapter, we will provide additional sources.

The Combined Health Information Database

The Combined Health Information Database (CHID) is a bibliographic database produced by health-related agencies of the U.S. federal government (mostly from the National Institutes of Health) that can offer concise information for a targeted search. The CHID database is updated four times a year at the end of January, April, July, and October. Check the titles, summaries, and availability of CAM-related information by using the "Simple Search" option at the following Web site: **http://chid.nih.gov/simple/simple.html**. In the drop box at the top, select "Complementary and Alternative Medicine." Then type "erectile dysfunction" (or synonyms) in the second search box. We recommend that you select 100 "documents per page" and to check the "whole records" options. The following was extracted using this technique:

- **Saw Palmetto Extracts for Treatment of Benign Prostatic Hyperplasia: A Systematic Review**

  Source: JAMA. Journal of the American Medical Association. 280(18): 1604-1609. November 11, 1998.

  Summary: This journal article reviews the research on the efficacy and safety of saw palmetto extract (Serenoa repens) in men with symptomatic benign prostatic hyperplasia (BPH). A comprehensive search of the literature identified 18 randomized controlled trials involving 2,393 men who met inclusion criteria. Studies were included if the participants had symptomatic BPH, the intervention was a preparation of Serenoa repens alone or in combination with other phytotherapeutic agents, a control group received a placebo or other pharmacological therapies for BPH, and the treatment duration was at least 30 days. Results from doctor and participant assessments showed that Serenoa repens was superior to a placebo and comparable with finasteride in improving urinary tract symptom scores, nocturia, peak and mean urine flow rates, and residual urine volume. Adverse effects due to Serenoa repens generally were mild and comparable with a placebo. **Erectile dysfunction** was more common with finasteride (4.9 percent) than with S repens (1.1 percent). The withdrawal rates in men receiving Serenoa repens, a placebo, and finasteride were 9.1 percent, 7 percent, and 11.2 percent, respectively. The authors conclude that Serenoa repens appears to improve urologic symptoms and flow measures in men with BPH; its efficacy is similar to that of finasteride but with fewer adverse effects. The article has 4 figures and 51 references.

National Center for Complementary and Alternative Medicine

The National Center for Complementary and Alternative Medicine (NCCAM) of the National Institutes of Health (**http://nccam.nih.gov/**) has created a link to the National Library of Medicine's databases to facilitate research for articles that specifically relate to erectile dysfunction and complementary medicine. To search the database, go to the following Web site: **http://www.nlm.nih.gov/nccam/camonpubmed.html**. Select "CAM on PubMed." Enter "erectile dysfunction" (or synonyms) into the search box. Click "Go." The following references provide information on particular aspects of complementary and alternative medicine that are related to erectile dysfunction:

- **A double-blind crossover study evaluating the efficacy of korean red ginseng in patients with erectile dysfunction: a preliminary report.**
  Author(s): Hong B, Ji YH, Hong JH, Nam KY, Ahn TY.
  Source: The Journal of Urology. 2002 November; 168(5): 2070-3.
  http://www.ncbi.nlm.nih.gov:80/entrez/query.fcgi?cmd=Retrieve&db=PubMed&list_uids=12394711&dopt=Abstract

- **A shared care approach to the management of erectile dysfunction in the community.**
  Author(s): Wagner G, Claes H, Costa P, Cricelli C, De Boer J, Debruyne FM, Dean J, Dinsmore WW, Fitzpatrick JM, Ralph DJ, Hackett GI, Heaton JP, Hatzichristou DG, Mendive J, Meuleman EJ, Mirone V, Montorsi F, Raineri F, Schulman CC, Stief CG, Von Keitz AT, Wright PJ; Lygon Arms Group.
  Source: International Journal of Impotence Research : Official Journal of the International Society for Impotence Research. 2002 June; 14(3): 189-94. Review.
  http://www.ncbi.nlm.nih.gov:80/entrez/query.fcgi?cmd=Retrieve&db=PubMed&list_uids=12058246&dopt=Abstract

- **Acupuncture in the treatment of psychogenic erectile dysfunction: first results of a prospective randomized placebo-controlled study.**
  Author(s): Engelhardt PF, Daha LK, Zils T, Simak R, Konig K, Pfluger H.
  Source: International Journal of Impotence Research : Official Journal of the International Society for Impotence Research. 2003 October; 15(5): 343-6.
  http://www.ncbi.nlm.nih.gov:80/entrez/query.fcgi?cmd=Retrieve&db=PubMed&list_uids=14562135&dopt=Abstract

- **Assessment and management of erectile dysfunction in men with diabetes.**
  Author(s): Spollett GR.

Source: Diabetes Educ. 1999 January-February; 25(1): 65-73; Quiz 75. Review.
http://www.ncbi.nlm.nih.gov:80/entrez/query.fcgi?cmd=Retrieve&db=PubMed&list_uids=10232182&dopt=Abstract

- **Biofeedback and facilitation of erection in men with erectile dysfunction.**
  Author(s): Reynolds BS.
  Source: Archives of Sexual Behavior. 1980 April; 9(2): 101-13.
  http://www.ncbi.nlm.nih.gov:80/entrez/query.fcgi?cmd=Retrieve&db=PubMed&list_uids=6156665&dopt=Abstract

- **Clinical efficacy of Korean red ginseng for erectile dysfunction.**
  Author(s): Choi HK, Seong DH, Rha KH.
  Source: International Journal of Impotence Research : Official Journal of the International Society for Impotence Research. 1995 September; 7(3): 181-6.
  http://www.ncbi.nlm.nih.gov:80/entrez/query.fcgi?cmd=Retrieve&db=PubMed&list_uids=8750052&dopt=Abstract

- **Clinical trial of Butea superba, an alternative herbal treatment for erectile dysfunction.**
  Author(s): Cherdshewasart W, Nimsakul N.
  Source: Asian Journal of Andrology. 2003 September; 5(3): 243-6.
  http://www.ncbi.nlm.nih.gov:80/entrez/query.fcgi?cmd=Retrieve&db=PubMed&list_uids=12937809&dopt=Abstract

- **Conservative treatment of erectile dysfunction. 2: Clinical trials.**
  Author(s): Dorey G.
  Source: British Journal of Nursing (Mark Allen Publishing). 2000 June 22-July 12; 9(12): 755-62. Review.
  http://www.ncbi.nlm.nih.gov:80/entrez/query.fcgi?cmd=Retrieve&db=PubMed&list_uids=11235296&dopt=Abstract

- **Conservative treatment of erectile dysfunction. 3: Literature review.**
  Author(s): Dorey G.
  Source: British Journal of Nursing (Mark Allen Publishing). 2000 July 13-26; 9(13): 859-63. Review.
  http://www.ncbi.nlm.nih.gov:80/entrez/query.fcgi?cmd=Retrieve&db=PubMed&list_uids=11261059&dopt=Abstract

- **Dietary supplements and other alternative medicines for erectile dysfunction. What do I tell my patients?**
  Author(s): Moyad MA.
  Source: The Urologic Clinics of North America. 2002 February; 29(1): 11-22, Vii.
  http://www.ncbi.nlm.nih.gov:80/entrez/query.fcgi?cmd=Retrieve&db=PubMed&list_uids=12109338&dopt=Abstract

- **Effect of a Chinese herbal medicine mixture on a rat model of hypercholesterolemic erectile dysfunction.**
  Author(s): Bakircioglu ME, Hsu K, El-Sakka A, Sievert KD, Lin CS, Lue TF.

Source: The Journal of Urology. 2000 November; 164(5): 1798-801.
http://www.ncbi.nlm.nih.gov:80/entrez/query.fcgi?cmd=Retrieve&db=PubMed&list_
uids=11025772&dopt=Abstract

- **Effect of oral administration of prostaglandin E1 on erectile dysfunction.**
  Author(s): Sato Y, Horita H, Adachi H, Suzuki N, Tanda H, Kumamoto Y, Tsukamoto T.
  Source: British Journal of Urology. 1997 November; 80(5): 772-5.
  http://www.ncbi.nlm.nih.gov:80/entrez/query.fcgi?cmd=Retrieve&db=PubMed&list_
  uids=9393301&dopt=Abstract

- **Effects of visual sexual stimuli and apomorphine SL on cerebral activity in men with erectile dysfunction.**
  Author(s): Hagemann JH, Berding G, Bergh S, Sleep DJ, Knapp WH, Jonas U, Stief CG.
  Source: European Urology. 2003 April; 43(4): 412-20.
  http://www.ncbi.nlm.nih.gov:80/entrez/query.fcgi?cmd=Retrieve&db=PubMed&list_
  uids=12667723&dopt=Abstract

- **Erectile dysfunction with chemotherapy.**
  Author(s): van Basten JP, van Driel MF, Hoekstra HJ, Sleijfer DT.
  Source: Lancet. 2000 July 8; 356(9224): 169.
  http://www.ncbi.nlm.nih.gov:80/entrez/query.fcgi?cmd=Retrieve&db=PubMed&list_
  uids=10963279&dopt=Abstract

- **Erectile dysfunctions: assessment and care.**
  Author(s): Mason DR.
  Source: The Nurse Practitioner. 1989 December; 14(12): 23, 27-30, 32-34.
  http://www.ncbi.nlm.nih.gov:80/entrez/query.fcgi?cmd=Retrieve&db=PubMed&list_
  uids=2601903&dopt=Abstract

- **Evidence based assessment of erectile dysfunction.**
  Author(s): Broderick GA.
  Source: International Journal of Impotence Research : Official Journal of the International Society for Impotence Research. 1998 May; 10 Suppl 2: S64-73; Discussion S77-9. Review.
  http://www.ncbi.nlm.nih.gov:80/entrez/query.fcgi?cmd=Retrieve&db=PubMed&list_
  uids=9647964&dopt=Abstract

- **Global perspectives and controversies in the epidemiology of male erectile dysfunction.**
  Author(s): Nehra A, Kulaksizoglu H.
  Source: Current Opinion in Urology. 2002 November; 12(6): 493-6. Review.
  http://www.ncbi.nlm.nih.gov:80/entrez/query.fcgi?cmd=Retrieve&db=PubMed&list_
  uids=12409879&dopt=Abstract

- **Injured external anal sphincter in erectile dysfunction.**
  Author(s): Shafik A.
  Source: Andrologia. 2001 January; 33(1): 35-41.
  http://www.ncbi.nlm.nih.gov:80/entrez/query.fcgi?cmd=Retrieve&db=PubMed&list_
  uids=11167517&dopt=Abstract

- **Korean red ginseng effective for treatment of erectile dysfunction.**
  Author(s): Price A, Gazewood J.
  Source: The Journal of Family Practice. 2003 January; 52(1): 20-1.
  http://www.ncbi.nlm.nih.gov:80/entrez/query.fcgi?cmd=Retrieve&db=PubMed&list_
  uids=12540305&dopt=Abstract

- **Magnetic stimulation of the cavernous nerve for the treatment of erectile dysfunction in humans.**
  Author(s): Shafik A, el-Sibai O, Shafik AA.
  Source: International Journal of Impotence Research : Official Journal of the International Society for Impotence Research. 2000 June; 12(3): 137-41; Discussion 141-2.
  http://www.ncbi.nlm.nih.gov:80/entrez/query.fcgi?cmd=Retrieve&db=PubMed&list_
  uids=11045905&dopt=Abstract

- **Malaysian cultural differences in knowledge, attitudes and practices related to erectile dysfunction: focus group discussions.**
  Author(s): Low WY, Wong YL, Zulkifli SN, Tan HM.
  Source: International Journal of Impotence Research : Official Journal of the International Society for Impotence Research. 2002 December; 14(6): 440-5.
  http://www.ncbi.nlm.nih.gov:80/entrez/query.fcgi?cmd=Retrieve&db=PubMed&list_
  uids=12494275&dopt=Abstract

- **Manually assisted ejaculation in a stallion with erectile dysfunction subsequent to paraphimosis.**
  Author(s): Love CC, McDonnell SM, Kenney RM.
  Source: J Am Vet Med Assoc. 1992 May 1; 200(9): 1357-9.
  http://www.ncbi.nlm.nih.gov:80/entrez/query.fcgi?cmd=Retrieve&db=PubMed&list_
  uids=1601723&dopt=Abstract

- **Oral treatment of erectile dysfunction: from herbal remedies to designer drugs.**
  Author(s): Guirguis WR.
  Source: Journal of Sex & Marital Therapy. 1998 April-June; 24(2): 69-73. Review.
  http://www.ncbi.nlm.nih.gov:80/entrez/query.fcgi?cmd=Retrieve&db=PubMed&list_
  uids=9611686&dopt=Abstract

- **Pelvic floor muscle exercises and manometric biofeedback for erectile dysfunction and postmicturition dribble: three case studies.**
  Author(s): Dorey G, Feneley RC, Speakman MJ, Robinson JP, Paterson J.
  Source: Journal of Wound, Ostomy, and Continence Nursing : Official Publication of the Wound, Ostomy and Continence Nurses Society / Wocn. 2003 January; 30(1): 44-51; Discussion 51-2.
  http://www.ncbi.nlm.nih.gov:80/entrez/query.fcgi?cmd=Retrieve&db=PubMed&list_
  uids=12529593&dopt=Abstract

- **Running an erectile dysfunction clinic.**
  Author(s): Duckworth K.
  Source: Prof Nurse. 1997 August; 12(11): 775-8.
  http://www.ncbi.nlm.nih.gov:80/entrez/query.fcgi?cmd=Retrieve&db=PubMed&list_
  uids=9287859&dopt=Abstract

- **Spontaneous erections in a patient with erectile dysfunction after palliative chemotherapy for non-small cell lung cancer.**
  Author(s): Hejna M, Fiebiger WC, Reiter WJ, Raderer M.
  Source: Urologia Internationalis. 2001; 67(2): 163-4.
  http://www.ncbi.nlm.nih.gov:80/entrez/query.fcgi?cmd=Retrieve&db=PubMed&list_uids=11490213&dopt=Abstract

- **Systematic review of randomised controlled trials of sildenafil (Viagra) in the treatment of male erectile dysfunction.**
  Author(s): Burls A, Gold L, Clark W.
  Source: The British Journal of General Practice : the Journal of the Royal College of General Practitioners. 2001 December; 51(473): 1004-12. Review.
  http://www.ncbi.nlm.nih.gov:80/entrez/query.fcgi?cmd=Retrieve&db=PubMed&list_uids=11766850&dopt=Abstract

- **The effect of vascular endothelial growth factor on a rat model of traumatic arteriogenic erectile dysfunction.**
  Author(s): Lee MC, El-Sakka AI, Graziottin TM, Ho HC, Lin CS, Lue TF.
  Source: The Journal of Urology. 2002 February; 167(2 Pt 1): 761-7.
  http://www.ncbi.nlm.nih.gov:80/entrez/query.fcgi?cmd=Retrieve&db=PubMed&list_uids=11792968&dopt=Abstract

- **The false organic-psychogenic distinction and related problems in the classification of erectile dysfunction.**
  Author(s): Sachs BD.
  Source: International Journal of Impotence Research : Official Journal of the International Society for Impotence Research. 2003 February; 15(1): 72-8. Review.
  http://www.ncbi.nlm.nih.gov:80/entrez/query.fcgi?cmd=Retrieve&db=PubMed&list_uids=12605243&dopt=Abstract

- **The limited practical value of color Doppler sonography in the differential diagnosis of men with erectile dysfunction.**
  Author(s): Slob AK, Cornelissen S, Dohle GR, Gijs L, van der Werff ten Bosch JJ.
  Source: International Journal of Impotence Research : Official Journal of the International Society for Impotence Research. 2002 June; 14(3): 201-3.
  http://www.ncbi.nlm.nih.gov:80/entrez/query.fcgi?cmd=Retrieve&db=PubMed&list_uids=12058250&dopt=Abstract

- **The use of acupuncture in the treatment of erectile dysfunction.**
  Author(s): Kho HG, Sweep CG, Chen X, Rabsztyn PR, Meuleman EJ.
  Source: International Journal of Impotence Research : Official Journal of the International Society for Impotence Research. 1999 February; 11(1): 41-6.
  http://www.ncbi.nlm.nih.gov:80/entrez/query.fcgi?cmd=Retrieve&db=PubMed&list_uids=10098953&dopt=Abstract

- **Traumatic arteriogenic erectile dysfunction: a rat model.**
  Author(s): El-Sakka A, Yen TS, Lin CS, Lue TF.

Source: International Journal of Impotence Research : Official Journal of the International Society for Impotence Research. 2001 June; 13(3): 162-71.
http://www.ncbi.nlm.nih.gov:80/entrez/query.fcgi?cmd=Retrieve&db=PubMed&list_uids=11525315&dopt=Abstract

- **Treatment of erectile dysfunction by an external ischiocavernous muscle stimulator.**
  Author(s): Derouet H, Nolden W, Jost WH, Osterhage J, Eckert RE, Ziegler M.
  Source: European Urology. 1998 October; 34(4): 355-9.
  http://www.ncbi.nlm.nih.gov:80/entrez/query.fcgi?cmd=Retrieve&db=PubMed&list_uids=9748685&dopt=Abstract

- **Treatment of erectile dysfunction by perineal exercise, electromyographic biofeedback, and electrical stimulation.**
  Author(s): Van Kampen M, De Weerdt W, Claes H, Feys H, De Maeyer M, Van Poppel H.
  Source: Physical Therapy. 2003 June; 83(6): 536-43.
  http://www.ncbi.nlm.nih.gov:80/entrez/query.fcgi?cmd=Retrieve&db=PubMed&list_uids=12775199&dopt=Abstract

- **Validation of a psychophysiological waking erectile assessment (WEA) for the diagnosis of male erectile disorder.**
  Author(s): Janssen E, Everaerd W, Van Lunsen RH, Oerlemans S.
  Source: Urology. 1994 May; 43(5): 686-95; Discussion 695-6.
  http://www.ncbi.nlm.nih.gov:80/entrez/query.fcgi?cmd=Retrieve&db=PubMed&list_uids=8165769&dopt=Abstract

- **Withered Yang: a review of traditional Chinese medical treatment of male infertility and erectile dysfunction.**
  Author(s): Crimmel AS, Conner CS, Monga M.
  Source: Journal of Andrology. 2001 March-April; 22(2): 173-82. Review.
  http://www.ncbi.nlm.nih.gov:80/entrez/query.fcgi?cmd=Retrieve&db=PubMed&list_uids=11229790&dopt=Abstract

Additional Web Resources

A number of additional Web sites offer encyclopedic information covering CAM and related topics. The following is a representative sample:

- Alternative Medicine Foundation, Inc.: **http://www.herbmed.org/**

- AOL: **http://search.aol.com/cat.adp?id=169&layer=&from=subcats**

- Chinese Medicine: **http://www.newcenturynutrition.com/**

- drkoop.com®: **http://www.drkoop.com/InteractiveMedicine/IndexC.html**

- Family Village: **http://www.familyvillage.wisc.edu/med_altn.htm**

- Google: **http://directory.google.com/Top/Health/Alternative/**

- Healthnotes: **http://www.healthnotes.com/**

- MedWebPlus:
  http://medwebplus.com/subject/Alternative_and_Complementary_Medicine

- Open Directory Project: **http://dmoz.org/Health/Alternative/**

- HealthGate: **http://www.tnp.com/**

- WebMD®Health: **http://my.webmd.com/drugs_and_herbs**

- WholeHealthMD.com: **http://www.wholehealthmd.com/reflib/0,1529,00.html**

- Yahoo.com: **http://dir.yahoo.com/Health/Alternative_Medicine/**

The following is a specific Web list relating to erectile dysfunction; please note that any particular subject below may indicate either a therapeutic use, or a contraindication (potential danger), and does not reflect an official recommendation:

- **General Overview**

    Benign Prostatic Hyperplasia
    Source: Healthnotes, Inc.; www.healthnotes.com

    Erectile Dysfunction
    Source: Healthnotes, Inc.; www.healthnotes.com

    Impotence
    Source: Prima Communications, Inc.www.personalhealthzone.com

    Peripheral Vascular Disease
    Source: Healthnotes, Inc.; www.healthnotes.com

- **Alternative Therapy**

    Acupuncture
    Source: Healthnotes, Inc.; www.healthnotes.com

- **Homeopathy**

    Agnus Castus
    Source: Healthnotes, Inc.; www.healthnotes.com

    Argentum Nitricum
    Source: Healthnotes, Inc.; www.healthnotes.com

    Caladium
    Source: Healthnotes, Inc.; www.healthnotes.com

    Causticum
    Source: Healthnotes, Inc.; www.healthnotes.com

    Lycopodium
    Source: Healthnotes, Inc.; www.healthnotes.com

Selenium Metallicum
Source: Healthnotes, Inc.; www.healthnotes.com

Staphysagria
Source: Healthnotes, Inc.; www.healthnotes.com

- **Herbs and Supplements**

  Androstenedione
  Source: Healthnotes, Inc.; www.healthnotes.com

  Arginine
  Source: Healthnotes, Inc.; www.healthnotes.com

  Asian Ginseng
  Alternative names: Panax ginseng
  Source: Healthnotes, Inc.; www.healthnotes.com

  Asian Ginseng
  Alternative names: Panax ginseng
  Source: Integrative Medicine Communications; www.drkoop.com

  Damiana
  Alternative names: Turnera diffusa
  Source: Healthnotes, Inc.; www.healthnotes.com

  Dehydroepiandrosterone (DHEA)
  Source: Healthnotes, Inc.; www.healthnotes.com

  DHEA (dehydroepiandrosterone)
  Source: Prima Communications, Inc.www.personalhealthzone.com

  Fo-ti
  Alternative names: Polygonum multiflorum
  Source: Healthnotes, Inc.; www.healthnotes.com

  Ginkgo Biloba
  Source: Healthnotes, Inc.; www.healthnotes.com

  Ginkgo Biloba
  Alternative names: Maidenhair Tree
  Source: Integrative Medicine Communications; www.drkoop.com

  Ginkgo Biloba
  Source: WholeHealthMD.com, LLC.; www.wholehealthmd.com
  Hyperlink:
  http://www.wholehealthmd.com/refshelf/substances_view/0,1525,788,00.html

  Maidenhair Tree
  Alternative names: Ginkgo Biloba
  Source: Integrative Medicine Communications; www.drkoop.com

Panax
Alternative names: Ginseng; Panax ginseng
Source: Alternative Medicine Foundation, Inc.; www.amfoundation.org

Panax Ginseng
Source: Integrative Medicine Communications; www.drkoop.com

Sertraline
Source: Healthnotes, Inc.; www.healthnotes.com

Sildenafil
Source: Healthnotes, Inc.; www.healthnotes.com

Yohimbe
Alternative names: Pausinystalia yohimbe
Source: Healthnotes, Inc.; www.healthnotes.com

Yohimbe
Source: WholeHealthMD.com, LLC.; www.wholehealthmd.com
Hyperlink:
http://www.wholehealthmd.com/refshelf/substances_view/0,1525,830,00.html

General References

A good place to find general background information on CAM is the National Library of Medicine. It has prepared within the MEDLINEplus system an information topic page dedicated to complementary and alternative medicine. To access this page, go to the MEDLINEplus site at **http://www.nlm.nih.gov/medlineplus/alternativemedicine.html** This Web site provides a general overview of various topics and can lead to a number of general sources.

CHAPTER 4. DISSERTATIONS ON ERECTILE DYSFUNCTION

Overview

In this chapter, we will give you a bibliography on recent dissertations relating to erectile dysfunction. We will also provide you with information on how to use the Internet to stay current on dissertations. **IMPORTANT NOTE:** When following the search strategy described below, you may discover <u>non-medical dissertations</u> that use the generic term "erectile dysfunction" (or a synonym) in their titles. To accurately reflect the results that you might find while conducting research on erectile dysfunction, <u>we have not necessarily excluded non-medical dissertations</u> in this bibliography.

Dissertations on Erectile Dysfunction

ProQuest Digital Dissertations, the largest archive of academic dissertations available, is located at the following Web address: **http://wwwlib.umi.com/dissertations**. From this archive, we have compiled the following list covering dissertations devoted to erectile dysfunction. You will see that the information provided includes the dissertation's title, its author, and the institution with which the author is associated. The following covers recent dissertations found when using this search procedure:

- **A Clinical Trial of Two Treatment Interventions with Nonpartnered Men Experiencing Erectile Dysfunction** by Altman, Ian; PhD from The University of Manitoba (Canada), 1986
  http://wwwlib.umi.com/dissertations/fullcit/NL33543

- **A Twin Study of Erectile Dysfunction in the Vietnam Era Twin (VET) Registry** by Fischer, Mary Ellen; PhD from University of Illinois at Chicago, Health Sciences Center, 2002, 75 pages
  http://wwwlib.umi.com/dissertations/fullcit/3058233

- **Erectile Dysfunction Following a Long-Distance Cycling Event: Is There an Increased Risk and What Bicycle Characteristics Might Contribute?** by Dettori, Joseph Raymond; PhD from University of Washington, 2002, 39 pages
  http://wwwlib.umi.com/dissertations/fullcit/3053492

- **The Effects of a Sex and Aging Workshop Highlighting Permission and Limited Information on the Sexual Knowledge, Attitudes, Behaviors and Satisfaction of a**

Group of Older Heterosexual Couples Experiencing Erectile Dysfunction: a Quasi-experimental and Qua by Goldman, Arlene, PhD from University of Pennsylvania, 1989, 278 pages
http://wwwlib.umi.com/dissertations/fullcit/9004786

- **The Enhancing Effects of Manualized Treatment for Erectile Dysfunction among Men Using Sildenafil: a Preliminary Investigation** by Bach Dilello, Amy K.; PhD from Boston University, 2002, 221 pages
http://wwwlib.umi.com/dissertations/fullcit/3090397

Keeping Current

Ask the medical librarian at your library if it has full and unlimited access to the *ProQuest Digital Dissertations* database. From the library, you should be able to do more complete searches via **http://wwwlib.umi.com/dissertations**.

CHAPTER 5. CLINICAL TRIALS AND ERECTILE DYSFUNCTION

Overview

In this chapter, we will show you how to keep informed of the latest clinical trials concerning erectile dysfunction.

Recent Trials on Erectile Dysfunction

The following is a list of recent trials dedicated to erectile dysfunction.[8] Further information on a trial is available at the Web site indicated.

- **Effects of Yohimbine and Naltrexone on Sexual Function**

  Condition(s): Erectile Dysfunction

  Study Status: This study is currently recruiting patients.

  Sponsor(s): National Institute of Mental Health (NIMH)

  Purpose - Excerpt: The purpose of this study is to evaluate the safety and effectiveness of the drugs yohimbine and naltrexone in treating men with **erectile dysfunction** (ED) (the inability to achieve or maintain penile erection for satisfactory sexual performance).

  Study Type: Observational

  Contact(s): see Web site below

  Web Site: http://clinicaltrials.gov/ct/show/NCT00042536

- **Sildenafil in Treating Erectile Dysfunction in Patients With Prostate Cancer**

  Condition(s): sexual dysfunction and infertility; sexuality and reproductive issues; radiation toxicity; stage II prostate cancer; stage III prostate cancer; psychosocial effects/treatment

  Study Status: This study is currently recruiting patients.

  Sponsor(s): Radiation Therapy Oncology Group; National Cancer Institute (NCI)

---

[8] These are listed at **www.ClinicalTrials.gov**.

Purpose - Excerpt: RATIONALE: Sildenafil may be effective in helping patients who have undergone treatment for prostate cancer to have an erection for sexual activity and may improve sexual satisfaction and quality of life. PURPOSE: Randomized clinical trial to study the effectiveness of sildenafil in treating erectile dysfunction in patients who have undergone radiation therapy and hormone therapy for prostate cancer in clinical trial RTOG-9910.

Study Type: Interventional

Contact(s): see Web site below

Web Site: http://clinicaltrials.gov/ct/show/NCT00057759

Keeping Current on Clinical Trials

The U.S. National Institutes of Health, through the National Library of Medicine, has developed ClinicalTrials.gov to provide current information about clinical research across the broadest number of diseases and conditions.

The site was launched in February 2000 and currently contains approximately 5,700 clinical studies in over 59,000 locations worldwide, with most studies being conducted in the United States. ClinicalTrials.gov receives about 2 million hits per month and hosts approximately 5,400 visitors daily. To access this database, simply go to the Web site at **http://www.clinicaltrials.gov/** and search by "erectile dysfunction" (or synonyms).

While ClinicalTrials.gov is the most comprehensive listing of NIH-supported clinical trials available, not all trials are in the database. The database is updated regularly, so clinical trials are continually being added. The following is a list of specialty databases affiliated with the National Institutes of Health that offer additional information on trials:

- For clinical studies at the Warren Grant Magnuson Clinical Center located in Bethesda, Maryland, visit their Web site: **http://clinicalstudies.info.nih.gov/**

- For clinical studies conducted at the Bayview Campus in Baltimore, Maryland, visit their Web site: **http://www.jhbmc.jhu.edu/studies/index.html**

- For cancer trials, visit the National Cancer Institute: **http://cancertrials.nci.nih.gov/**

- For eye-related trials, visit and search the Web page of the National Eye Institute: **http://www.nei.nih.gov/neitrials/index.htm**

- For heart, lung and blood trials, visit the Web page of the National Heart, Lung and Blood Institute: **http://www.nhlbi.nih.gov/studies/index.htm**

- For trials on aging, visit and search the Web site of the National Institute on Aging: **http://www.grc.nia.nih.gov/studies/index.htm**

- For rare diseases, visit and search the Web site sponsored by the Office of Rare Diseases: **http://ord.aspensys.com/asp/resources/rsch_trials.asp**

- For alcoholism, visit the National Institute on Alcohol Abuse and Alcoholism: **http://www.niaaa.nih.gov/intramural/Web_dicbr_hp/particip.htm**

- For trials on infectious, immune, and allergic diseases, visit the site of the National Institute of Allergy and Infectious Diseases: **http://www.niaid.nih.gov/clintrials/**

- For trials on arthritis, musculoskeletal and skin diseases, visit newly revised site of the National Institute of Arthritis and Musculoskeletal and Skin Diseases of the National Institutes of Health: **http://www.niams.nih.gov/hi/studies/index.htm**

- For hearing-related trials, visit the National Institute on Deafness and Other Communication Disorders: **http://www.nidcd.nih.gov/health/clinical/index.htm**

- For trials on diseases of the digestive system and kidneys, and diabetes, visit the National Institute of Diabetes and Digestive and Kidney Diseases: **http://www.niddk.nih.gov/patient/patient.htm**

- For drug abuse trials, visit and search the Web site sponsored by the National Institute on Drug Abuse: **http://www.nida.nih.gov/CTN/Index.htm**

- For trials on mental disorders, visit and search the Web site of the National Institute of Mental Health: **http://www.nimh.nih.gov/studies/index.cfm**

- For trials on neurological disorders and stroke, visit and search the Web site sponsored by the National Institute of Neurological Disorders and Stroke of the NIH: **http://www.ninds.nih.gov/funding/funding_opportunities.htm#Clinical_Trials**

CHAPTER 6. PATENTS ON ERECTILE DYSFUNCTION

Overview

Patents can be physical innovations (e.g. chemicals, pharmaceuticals, medical equipment) or processes (e.g. treatments or diagnostic procedures). The United States Patent and Trademark Office defines a patent as a grant of a property right to the inventor, issued by the Patent and Trademark Office.[9] Patents, therefore, are intellectual property. For the United States, the term of a new patent is 20 years from the date when the patent application was filed. If the inventor wishes to receive economic benefits, it is likely that the invention will become commercially available within 20 years of the initial filing. It is important to understand, therefore, that an inventor's patent does not indicate that a product or service is or will be commercially available. The patent implies only that the inventor has "the right to exclude others from making, using, offering for sale, or selling" the invention in the United States. While this relates to U.S. patents, similar rules govern foreign patents.

In this chapter, we show you how to locate information on patents and their inventors. If you find a patent that is particularly interesting to you, contact the inventor or the assignee for further information. **IMPORTANT NOTE:** When following the search strategy described below, you may discover non-medical patents that use the generic term "erectile dysfunction" (or a synonym) in their titles. To accurately reflect the results that you might find while conducting research on erectile dysfunction, we have not necessarily excluded non-medical patents in this bibliography.

Patents on Erectile Dysfunction

By performing a patent search focusing on erectile dysfunction, you can obtain information such as the title of the invention, the names of the inventor(s), the assignee(s) or the company that owns or controls the patent, a short abstract that summarizes the patent, and a few excerpts from the description of the patent. The abstract of a patent tends to be more technical in nature, while the description is often written for the public. Full patent descriptions contain much more information than is presented here (e.g. claims, references, figures, diagrams, etc.). We will tell you how to obtain this information later in the chapter.

---

[9] Adapted from the United States Patent and Trademark Office: http://www.uspto.gov/web/offices/pac/doc/general/whatis.htm.

The following is an example of the type of information that you can expect to obtain from a patent search on erectile dysfunction:

- **2-phenyl substituted imidazotriazinones as phosphodiesterase inhibitors**

  Inventor(s): Bischoff; Erwin (Wuppertal, DE), Dembowsky; Klaus (Boston, MA), Es-Sayed; Mazen (Langenfeld, DE), Haning; Helmut (Wuppertal, DE), Keldenich; Jorg (Wuppertal, DE), Niewohner; Ulrich (Wermelskirchen, DE), Nowakowski; Marc (Wuppertal, DE), Perzborn; Elisabeth (Wuppertal, DE), Schenke; Thomas (Gladbach, DE), Schlemmer; Karl-Heinz (Wuppertal, DE), Serno; Peter (Gladbach, DE)

  Assignee(s): Bayer Aktiengesellschaft (Leverkusen, DE)

  Patent Number: 6,362,178

  Date filed: July 21, 2000

  Abstract: The 2-phenyl-substituted imidazotriazinones having short, unbranched alkyl radicals in the 9-position are prepared from the corresponding 2-phenyl-imidazotriazinones by chlorosulphonation and subsequent reaction with the amines. The compounds inhibit cGMP-metabolizing phosphodiesterases and are suitable for use as active compounds in pharmaceuticals, for the treatment of cardiovascular and cerebrovascular disorders and/or disorders of the urogenital system, in particular for the treatment of **erectile dysfunction.**

  Excerpt(s): The present invention relates to 2-phenyl-substituted imidazotriazinones, to processes for their preparation and to their use as pharmaceuticals, in particular as inhibitors of cGMP-metabolizing phosphodiesterases. The published specification DE 28 11 780 describes imidazotriazines as bronchodilators having spasmolytic activity and inhibitory activity against phosphodiesterases which metabolize cyclic adenosin monophosphate (cAMP-PDEs, nomenclature according to Beavo: PDE-III and PDE-IV). An inhibitory action against phosphodiesterases which metabolize cyclic guanosin monophosphate (cGMP-PDEs, nomenclature according to Beavo and Reifsnyder (Trends in Pharmacol. Sci. 11, 150-155, 1990) PDE-I, PDE-II and PDE-V) has not been described. Compounds having a sulphonamide group in the aryl radical in the 2-position are not claimed. Furthermore, FR 22 13 058, CH 59 46 71, DE 22 55 172, DE 23 64 076 and EP 000 9384 describe imidazotriazinones which do not have a substituted aryl radical in the 2-position and are likewise said to be bronchodilators having cAMP-PDE inhibitory action. The compounds according to the invention are potent inhibitors either of one or of more of the phosphodiesterases which metabolize cyclic guanosin 3',5'-monophosphate (cGMP-PDEs). According to the nomenclature of Beavo and Reifsnyder (Trends in Pharmacol. Sci. 11, 150-155, 1990) these are the phosphodiesterase isoenzymes PDE-I, PDE-II and PDE-V.

  Web site: http://www.delphion.com/details?pn=US06362178__

- **Bicyclic heterocyclic compounds for the treatment of impotence**

  Inventor(s): Campbell; Simon Fraser (Sandwich, GB)

  Assignee(s): Pfizer Inc. (New York, NY)

  Patent Number: 6,534,511

  Date filed: April 3, 2000

Abstract: The use of certain 6-arylpyrazolo[3,4-d]pyrimidin-4-ones, 2 arylquinazolin-4-ones, 2-arylpurin-6-ones and 2-arylpyrido[3,2-d]pyrimidin-4-ones, or a pharmaceutically acceptable salt thereof, or a pharmaceutical composition containing either entity, for the manufacture of a medicament for the curative or prophylactic treatment of **erectile dysfunction** in a male animal, including man; a pharmaceutical composition for said treatment; and a method of said treatment of said animal with said pharmaceutical composition or with said either entity.

Excerpt(s): This invention relates to the use of certain pyrazolo[4,3-d]pyrimidin-7-ones, pyrazolo[3,4-d]pyrimidin-4-ones, quinazolin-4-ones, purin-6-ones and pyrido[3,2-d]pyrimidin-4-ones for the treatment of impotence. Impotence can be defined literally as a lack of power, in the male, to copulate and may involve an inability to achieve penile erection or ejaculation, or both. More specifically, erectile impotence or dysfunction may be defined as an inability to obtain or sustain an erection adequate for intercourse. Its prevalence is claimed to be between 2 and 7% of the human male population, increasing with age, up to 50 years, and between 18 and 75% between 55 and 80 years of age. In the USA alone, for example, it has been estimated that there are up to 10 million impotent males, with the majority suffering from problems of organic rather than of psychogenic origin. Reports of well-controlled clinical trials in man are few and the efficacy of orally administered drugs is low. Although many different drugs have been shown to induce penile erection, they are only effective after direct injection into the penis, e.g. intraurethrally or intracavernosally (i.c.), and are not approved for **erectile dysfunction.** Current medical treatment is based on the i.c injection of vasoactive substances and good results have been claimed with phenoxybenzamine, phentolamine, papaverine and prostaglandin E.sub.1, either alone or in combination; however, pain, priapism and fibrosis of the penis are associated with the i.c. administration of some of these agents. Potassium channel openers (KCO) and vasoactive intestinal polypeptide (VIP) have also been shown to be active i.c., but cost and stability issues could limit development of the latter. An alternative to the i.c. route is the use of glyceryl trinitrate (GTN) patches applied to the penis, which has been shown to be effective but produces side-effects in both patient and partner.

Web site: http://www.delphion.com/details?pn=US06534511___

- **Composition and method for topically treating Peyronie's Disease, Dupuytren's hand contracture, Ledderhose Fibrosis, erectile dysfunction arising from plaque accumulations, and scarring**

Inventor(s): Easterling; W. Jerry (c/o Prescription Dispensing Laboratories, Inc., 8400 Blanco Rd., San Antonio, TX 78216)

Assignee(s): none reported

Patent Number: 6,353,028

Date filed: October 1, 1999

Abstract: The invention is of a topical medicament and associated methodology for use thereof, through the use of which fibrotic or connective tissue disorders involving scarring, sub-dermal plaque accumulations or fibrosis of muscle tissue may be effectively, cost effectively, and painlessly treated. One or more calcium channel blocker agents serve as the primary active ingredient of the present compositions, with carrier agents facilitating non-invasive transdermal delivery of the calcium channel blocker(s) to subdermal disease sites.

Excerpt(s): Applicant's invention relates to medicaments and treatment procedures relating to connective tissue disorders manifested by sub-dermal plaque accumulations as well as to fibrosis of muscle tissues, some example of which result in total or partial **erectile dysfunction.** Representative examples of such sub-dermal plaque accumulation disorders include Peyronie's Disease, Ledderhose Fibrosis, Dupuytren's contracture of the hand and certain forms of **erectile dysfunction.** An initial focus of the present invention--Peyronie's disease--has likely plagued men for time immemorial, but has been recognized as a distinct malady for no less than 400 years. Peyronie's disease was first described in 1743 by a French surgeon, Francois de la Peyronie. The disease was written about as early as 1687 and was oftentimes associated with impotence. Peyronie's disease often occurs in a mild form and heals spontaneously in 6 to 15 months. However, in severe cases, the hardened plaque substantially reduces penile flexibility and causes excruciating pain as the penis is forced into a highly arcuate or even serpentine configuration. A plaque on the top of the shaft (most common) causes the penis to bed upward; a plaque on the underside causes it to bend downward. In some cases, the plague develops on both top and bottom, leading to indentation and shortening of the penis.

Web site: http://www.delphion.com/details?pn=US06353028__

- **Compositions for nasal administration**

Inventor(s): Illum; Lisbeth (Nottingham, GB), Watts; Peter James (Nottingham, GB)

Assignee(s): West Pharmaceutical Services Drug Delivery & Clinical Research Centre (Nottingham, GB)

Patent Number: 6,342,251

Date filed: June 2, 2000

Abstract: There is provided a composition for the nasal delivery of a drug suitable for the treatment of **erectile dysfunction** to a mammal wherein the composition is adapted to provide an initial rise in plasma level followed by a sustained plasma level of the drug.

Excerpt(s): This invention relates to compositions for nasal administration of drugs and particularly to compositions for nasal administration of drugs for treating **erectile dysfunction,** such as apomorphine. The invention also relates to the nasal administration of drugs for treating **erectile dysfunction.** Erectile dysfunction is a major medical problem in middle-aged males. A variety of medical treatments has been proposed including local injections as well as hormone therapy. The prostaglandins have been especially useful in this regard. Other drugs suitable for the treatment of dysfunction include alpha-adrenoreceptor antagonists, e.g. phentolamine, phenoxybenzamine, yohimbine, moxislyte delaquamine; compounds with central D_2-receptor antagonist activity, e.g. apomorphine; compounds that act primarily by blocking the re-uptake of serotonin into nerve terminals, e.g. tadone and chlorophenylpiperazine; competitive and selective inhibitors of c-GMP type V phosphodiesterases, e.g. sildenafil; L-arginine; and papaverine.

Web site: http://www.delphion.com/details?pn=US06342251__

- **Compositions for the treatment of male erectile dysfunction**

Inventor(s): Podolski; Joseph S. (The Woodlands, TX)

Assignee(s): Zonagen, Inc. (The Woodlands, TX)

Patent Number: 6,482,426

Date filed: September 17, 1998

Abstract: Improved drug compositions and methods useful in the treatment of male **erectile dysfunction.** An optimized mixture of the drugs phentolamine mesylate, papaverine hydrochloride, and alprostadil in a buffer containing L-arginine and glycine is to be injected into the penile tissue to produce an erection in otherwise impotent men.

Excerpt(s): This invention relates to improved drug compositions useful in the treatment of male **erectile dysfunction** and also to methods of treatment. More particularly, this invention discloses specific formulations containing the pharmacological agents phentolamine mesylate, papaverine hydrochloride, and alprostadil (prostaglandin E1) in a novel buffer and the administration of such formulations to mammals (including humans) to treat male impotence. Impotence is a common medical disorder affecting about 20 million men in the U.S. alone. Male **erectile dysfunction** has been defined as the inability to achieve or maintain an erection sufficient for intercourse (Impotence, National Institutes of Health Consensus Development Panel on Impotence Conference, JAMA 1993, 270 83-90). The dominant etiology for this condition is arterial insufficiency associated with cardiovascular disease. Male **erectile dysfunction** adversely impacts the quality of life, being frequently associated with depression, anxiety, and low self-esteem. Although male **erectile dysfunction** represents a major clinical problem, treatment for this condition remains problematic and unsatisfactory. One of the least invasive therapies available entails the use of a vacuum constriction device on the penis to produce an erection. The physiology of the penis is such that blood flows in through arteries deep within the tissue while blood flows out through veins near the skin surface. By placing a plastic cylinder over the shaft of the penis and employing a vacuum pump to restrict venous blood flow from the penis, the corpus cavernosum penile tissue becomes engorged with trapped blood and an erection is produced. Common patient complaints are that this device is interruptive to the sex act, has a short duration of effectiveness, and can cause tissue damage to the penis, such as necrosis, with extended use.

Web site: http://www.delphion.com/details?pn=US06482426__

- **Compounds, compositions and methods for treating erectile dysfunction**

Inventor(s): Shoemaker; James D. (Clayton, MO)

Assignee(s): Saint Louis University (St. Louis, MO)

Patent Number: 6,365,590

Date filed: August 18, 2000

Abstract: Vasoactive compounds are described for the treatment of **erectile dysfunction** and impotence. The compounds are reaction products of an anionic or negatively charged vasoactive or erection-inducing component (such as alprostadil) and a cationic or positively charged vasoactive or erection-inducing component (such as prazosin) or a local anesthetic (such as lidocaine). These components are combined as acids and bases to form an organic salt or ionically bonded compound. The compounds have advantageous solubility characteristics and efficacy. A compound of the invention is combined with a pharmaceutical vehicle to form a composition which preferably includes an emulsifier. A local anesthetic and/or androgenic steroids may also be included. Compositions of the invention may also include more than one vasoactive organic salt compound. The composition can be advantageously formulated and administered to allow self-adjusted dosing, while minimizing or preventing overdosing.

Excerpt(s): This invention relates to compounds for the treatment of **erectile dysfunction,** including impotence. In particular, the invention relates to vasoactive compounds and their production, and treatments for impotence and the enhancement of sexual performance in men. The invention also includes a vehicle, delivery system and emulsifier for treating impotence. Erectile dysfunction or impotence is characterized by the inability to achieve or maintain erection or tumescence of the penis. Impotence can be secondary to a wide variety of causes and may be physiological or psychological in origin. This condition is estimated to affect approximately 10-20 million American men chronically, but affects all men occasionally. For example, erection of the penis is inhibited in normal men due to anxiety, exertion or sexual disinterest. Sexual activity includes physical exertion and as men age, the inhibitory effects of exertion may overcome normal arousal mechanisms. The etiology of chronic impotence may be psychogenic (32%), mixed psychogenic and organic (14%), organic (41%) or anatomical (13%). Organic causes include arterial insufficiency (27%), cavernous leakage (28%), neurological damage (13%), endocrinological defects (2.3%) and Peyronie's disease (13.1%). Govier, F. E. Timing of Penile Color Flow Duplex Ultrasonography Using a Triple Drug Mixture. J. Urol, Vol. 153(5) (May 1995), pp.1472-1475. Thus, about 30% of all cases of impotence are primarily vascular in origin.

Web site: http://www.delphion.com/details?pn=US06365590__

- **Device for treatment of erectile dysfunction**

  Inventor(s): Bonthuys; Barend Willem (P.O. Box 39385, Moreletapark, 0044, ZA)

  Assignee(s): none reported

  Patent Number: 6,458,073

  Date filed: August 30, 2000

  Abstract: A device for the treatment of **erectile dysfunction** or for penile exercise includes a vessel defining an elongated vacuum chamber and a mouth opening leading into the vacuum chamber. An annular pumping sleeve is mounted on, and slidingly displaceable relative to the vessel. The device includes valving arranged such that reciprocation of the sleeve relative to the vessel serves to pump air out of the vacuum chamber. The device further includes a constriction ring which is sealingly and dismountably mountable on the vessel, and which is configured sealingly to engage with an outer surface of a human penis inserted into the vacuum chamber.

  Excerpt(s): A problem that occasionally occurs in human male s is the inability to attain an erection of the penis. One manner which has been used to alleviate this problem is by subjecting the penis to a negative pressure thereby inducing blood to flow into the erectile tissue of the penis and cause an erection. In order to retain the blood in the erected penis, a constriction ring is used to inhibit the flow of blood from the erect penis and thereby retain the erection of the penis. Various vacuum devices have been proposed which operate in this fashion, Inter alia, U.S. Pat. Nos. 5,213,563, 6,095,895, 5,421,808, 4,602,625 and CH 3473007. It will be appreciated; that a device in accordance with the invention is normally used in an intimate situation. A major disadvantage with the prior art devices is that they are cumbersome and fairly time consuming to use which is not ideal in an intimate situation.

Web site: http://www.delphion.com/details?pn=US06458073__

- **Fully implantable neurostimulator for cavernous nerve stimulation as a therapy for erectile dysfunction and other sexual dysfunction**

Inventor(s): McGivern; James P. (Stevenson Ranch, CA), Whitehurst; Todd K. (Sherman Oaks, CA)

Assignee(s): Advanced Bionics Corporation (Sylmar, CA)

Patent Number: 6,650,943

Date filed: March 6, 2001

Abstract: An implantable stimulator(s) with at least two electrodes, which is small enough to have the electrodes located adjacent to a cavernous nerve(s) or other nerve(s) innervating the reproductive organs, uses a power source/storage device, such as a rechargeable battery. Periodic recharging of such a battery is accomplished, for example, by inductive coupling with an external appliance. The small stimulator provides means of stimulating a nerve(s) when desired, without the need for external appliances during the stimulation session. When necessary, external appliances are used for the transmission of data to and/or from the stimulator(s) and for the transmission of power. In a preferred embodiment, the system is capable of open-and closed-loop operation. In closed-loop operation, at least one implant includes a sensor, and the sensed condition is used to adjust stimulation parameters.

Excerpt(s): The present invention generally relates to implantable stimulator systems, and more particularly relates to an implantable stimulator system utilizing one or more implantable microstimulators as a therapy for **erectile dysfunction.** Recent estimates suggest that the number of U.S. men with **erectile dysfunction** may be near 10 to 20 million, and inclusion of individuals with partial **erectile dysfunction** increases the estimate to about 30 million. The male erectile response is initiated by the action of neurons, or nerve cells (i.e., neuronal action), and maintained by a complex interplay between events involving blood vessels (i.e., vascular events) and events involving the nervous system (i.e., neurological events). The part of the nervous system that regulates involuntary action (e.g., the intestines, heart, glands) is called the autonomic nervous system. The autonomic nervous system is divided into two mutually antagonistic, physiologically and anatomically distinct systems: the sympathetic nervous system and the parasympathetic nervous system. The sympathetic nervous system originates in the thoracic and lumbar regions of the spinal cord, and in general, opposes the physiological affects of the parasympathetic nervous system. For instance, the sympathetic nervous system will tend to reduce digestive secretions or speed up the heart, usually when an individual is in an active state. The parasympathetic nervous system originates in the brain stem and the lower part of the spinal cord, and, in general, opposes the physiological effects of the sympathetic nervous system. Thus, the parasympathetic nervous system will tend to stimulate digestive secretions or slow the heart usually when an individual is in a relaxed state.

Web site: http://www.delphion.com/details?pn=US06650943__

- **Image forms and method for ameliorating male erectile dysfunction**

    Inventor(s): Clarke; Anthony (Henley-on-Thames, GB), Green; Richard David (Marlborough, GB), Johnson; Edward Stewart (Ruscombe, GB)

    Assignee(s): R.P. Scherer Limited (GB)

    Patent Number: 6,342,246

    Date filed: July 12, 1999

    Abstract: The use of a pharmaceutical composition for oral administration comprising a carrier and active ingredient selected from a dopamine agonist, testosterone and mixtures thereof, the composition being in the form of a fast-dispersing dosage form designed to release the active ingredient rapidly in the oral cavity for the manufacture of a medicament for treatment of male **erectile dysfunction.**

    Excerpt(s): This invention relates to dosage forms and methods for ameliorating **erectile dysfunction** in male patients. More particularly, this invention relates to the use of fast-dispersing dosage forms of drugs for amelioration of **erectile dysfunction** in male patients. A normal erection occurs as a result of a coordinated vascular event in the penis. This is usually triggered neurally and consists of vasodilatation and smooth muscle relaxation in the penis and its supplying arterial vessels. Arterial inflow causes enlargement of the substance of the corpora cavernosa. Venous outflow is trapped by this enlargement, permitting sustained high blood pressures in the penis sufficient to cause rigidity. Muscles in the perineum also assist in creating and maintaining penile rigidity. Erection may be induced centrally in the nervous system by sexual thoughts or fantasy, and is usually reinforced locally by reflex mechanisms. Male **erectile dysfunction** (MED) is defined as the inability to achieve and sustain an erection sufficient for intercourse. In any given case this can result from psychological disturbances (psychogenic), from physiological abnormalities in general (organic), from neurological disturbances (neurogenic), hormonal deficiencies (endocrine) or from a combination of the foregoing.

    Web site: http://www.delphion.com/details?pn=US06342246__

- **Magnetic therapy devices and methods**

    Inventor(s): Paturu; Sumathi (307 Brooke-Lyn Ter., Pleasant Grove, AL 35127)

    Assignee(s): none reported

    Patent Number: 6,589,159

    Date filed: April 12, 2001

    Abstract: Static and electromagnetic therapeutic devices are disclosed for increasing the blood circulation to areas of the body subject to magnetic field induction. The therapeutic devices are useful in the treatment of various diseases and aliments of the human body, such as **erectile dysfunction,** peripheral vascular disease, cerebral insufficiency and certain vascular pathologies. The disclosure contemplates that the beneficial effects of the induced magnetic fields are the result of the interaction of certain constituents of the blood with the magnetic fields.

    Excerpt(s): This invention relates generally to the use of magnets in the treatment of human diseases and ailments and devices for carrying out this treatment. The study of magnetic therapy to treat human disease can be traced back as far as the early 16th century. Over the years, magnetic therapy has been alleged as a cure for diverse diseases and ailments ranging from cancer to chronic pain. The popularity of magnetic therapy continues today. However, despite the prevalence and popularity of magnetic therapy treatments, the physiological effects of magnetic therapy is still unsettled. Magnetic fields have been historically described in relation to electric current. This relationship to electric current forms the basis of understanding the properties of magnets. All atoms are composed of protons and neutrons, which reside in the nucleus of the atom, and electrons which move rapidly about the nucleus of the atom. As the electrons are negatively charged, each electron generates its own magnetic moment, or magnetic dipole. These magnetic dipoles can be oriented in either of two opposing directions. However, not all atoms demonstrate magnetic properties. This is because many atoms have electrons that are paired with electrons of opposite magnetic dipoles, the net effect being the cancellation of the magnetic dipoles. These atoms are referred to as diamagnetic. Other atoms have unpaired electrons and possess a net magnetic dipole. These atoms do exhibit magnetic properties and are referred to as paramagnetic. Iron is an example of a paramagnetic atom. However, in some cases, the individual magnetic dipoles behave cooperatively and align themselves in the same direction to form magnetic domains. The compounds composed of these atoms demonstrate strong magnetic properties and are referred to as ferromagnetic. Ferromagnetic compounds include iron, cobalt, nickel, samarium, dysprosium and gadolinium.

Web site: http://www.delphion.com/details?pn=US06589159__

- **Melanocortin receptor-3 ligands to treat sexual dysfunction**

  Inventor(s): Dines; Kevin C. (Poway, CA), Gahman; Timothy C. (Encinitas, CA), Girten; Beverly E. (Sunnyvale, CA), Hitchin; Douglas L. (San Diego, CA), Holme; Kevin R. (San Diego, CA), Lang; Hengyuan (San Diego, CA), Pei; Yazhong (San Diego, CA), Slivka; Sandra R. (San Diego, CA), Tuttle; Ronald R. (Escondido, CA), Watson-Straughan; Karen J. (Encinitas, CA)

  Assignee(s): Lion Bioscience AG (Heidelberg, DE)

  Patent Number: 6,534,503

  Date filed: July 13, 2000

  Abstract: Methods for treating sexual dysfunction, such as **erectile dysfunction** or sexual arousal disorder, with a compound having the generic formula X.sub.1 --X.sub.2 - (D)Phe-Arg-(D)Trp-X.sub.3. A particularly useful compound is HP-228, which has the formula Ac-Nle-Gln-His-(D)Phe-Arg-(D)Trp-Gly-NH.sub.2. The invention also provides methods for selecting melanocortin receptor-3 ligands by determining whether a compound modulates the activity of MC-3 as an agonist or antagonist. These methods can be used to screen compound libraries for ligands to treat MC-3-associated conditions. Such conditions include sexual dysfunction, including **erectile dysfunction** and sexual arousal disorder.

  Excerpt(s): The present invention relates to melanocortin receptors and more specifically to the treatment of sexual dysfunction using melanocortin receptor 3 ligands. Sexual dysfunction can be due to several physiological, as well as psychological, factors. In males, **erectile dysfunction** can be associated with diseases such as diabetes mellitus, syphilis, alcoholism, drug dependency, hypopituitarism and hypothyroidism. **Erectile dysfunction** can also be caused by vascular and neurogenic disorders, or be a side effect of drugs such as hypertensives, sedatives, tranquilizers and amphetamines. In all, **erectile dysfunction** is estimated to affect up to 10 million men in the United States, with its incidence increasing with age up to 25% of men at age 65. While various pharmaceutical treatments are commercially available or being developed, the underlying physiological bases for sexual dysfunction are not well understood. Attention has recently been drawn to melanocortin (MC) receptors, which are a group of cell surface proteins that mediate a variety of physiological effects. The MC receptors have been implicated in the regulation of adrenal gland function such as production of the glucocorticoid cortisol and aldosterone, control of melanocyte growth and pigment production, control of feeding, thermoregulation, immunomodulation, inflammation and analgesia. Five distinct MC receptors have been cloned, although the specific role of each MC receptor is still unclear.

Web site: http://www.delphion.com/details?pn=US06534503__

- **Method and composition for treatment of erectile dysfunction**

  Inventor(s): Resul; Bahram (Uppsala, SE), Stjernschantz; Johan (Uppsala, SE)

  Assignee(s): Synphora AB (Uppsala, SE)

  Patent Number: 6,476,074

  Date filed: April 10, 2000

  Abstract: Compositions and methods for treatment of impotence or **erectile dysfunction** employ prostaglandins that are selective EP.sub.2 or EP.sub.4 prostanoid receptor agonists. The compositions can be formulated for intracavernous injection, or for transurethral or transdermal application.

  Excerpt(s): The present invention relates to the treatment of impotence or **erectile dysfunction,** and more particularly to a novel prostaglandin based composition therefore and the use thereof for treating impotence or **erectile dysfunction.** Erectile dysfunction is a disorder characterized by the inability of the male to develop and maintain erection for satisfactory sexual intercourse. **Erectile dysfunction** is a frequent disorder particularly amongst elderly men which may lead to reduced quality of life and psychological problems. It is estimated that there may be as many as 10-20 million people in the United States suffering from **erectile dysfunction,** and an estimated 30 million males with at least partial **erectile dysfunction** (NIH Consensus Conference 1993). The prevalence of **erectile dysfunction** has been reported to be about 5% at age 40, and up to 25% at age 65 or older. Thus **erectile dysfunction** is a major clinical challenge of increasing importance with the increased standard of living and demand of a better quality of life. The ethiology of **erectile dysfunction** may be psychogenic or organic. The latter seems to account for the majority of cases. Such organic causes include vascular, endocrinological, and neurological diseases as well as trauma. Patients suffering from diabetes are typically at risk. While in many cases **erectile dysfunction** caused by, psychogenic factors may be reversible, impotence caused by organic factors needs adequate therapy. Such therapy comprises surgical intervention, devices and medical treatment. With more effective and better tolerated drugs there is a clear tendency towards medical therapy in the treatment of **erectile dysfunction.** The main modalities of medical therapy consist of systemic medication, usually peroral, and local medication in the genitourinary tract. Typical drugs given orally include e.g. yohimbine, an alpha-2 adrenergic antagonist, and testosterone, the male sex hormone. Furthermore bromocriptine has also been used, as well as antiserdtoninergic agents such as trazodone, ketanserin and mianserin. Recently, a selective type 5-phosphodiesterase inhibitor sildenafil (Viagra.TM.) has been approved for clinical use. In addition there are many other drugs that have been tested and used for the treatment of **erectile dysfunction.** Drugs given locally include e.g. papaverine, a smooth muscle relaxing agent, and phentol amine, an alpha-adrenergic antagonist as well as prostaglandins, particularly prostaglandin E.sub.1 (PGE.sub.1; alprostadil).These drugs relax smooth muscle, thus promoting the development of erection, and are given by local injection into the cavernous tissue of the penis. Formulations for intraurethral (transurethral) administration of prostaglandins have also been developed (Wolfson et al., 1993; Bradley et al., 1996) and are described in several patents and patent applications, for instance in WO 93/00894, WO 91/16021 and EP-A-357581.

Web site: http://www.delphion.com/details?pn=US06476074__

- **Method for the synthesis of compounds of formula I and their uses thereof**

Inventor(s): Avor; Kwasi S. (High Point, NC), Gopalaswamy; Ramesh (Greensboro, NC), Mjalli; Adnan M. M. (Jamestown, NC), Patron; Andrew (San Diego, CA), Wysong; Christopher L. (Winston-Salem, NC)

Assignee(s): TransTech Pharma, Inc. (High Point, NC)

Patent Number: 6,613,801

Date filed: March 5, 2001

Abstract: This invention provides certain compounds, methods of their preparation, pharmaceutical compositions comprising the compounds, their use in treating human or animal disorders. The compounds of the invention are useful as modulators of the interaction between the receptor for advanced glycated end products (RAGE) and its ligands, such as advanced glycated end products (AGEs), S100/calgranulin/EN-RAGE,.beta.-amyloid and amphoterin, and for the management, treatment, control, or as an adjunct treatment for diseases in humans caused by RAGE. Such diseases or disease states include acute and chronic inflammation, the development of diabetic late complications such as increased vascular permeability, nephropathy, atherosclerosis, and retinopathy, the development of Alzheimer's disease, **erectile dysfunction,** and tumor invasion and metastasis.

Excerpt(s): This invention relates to compounds which are modulators of the receptor for advanced glycated end products (RAGE) and interaction with its ligands such as advanced glycated end products (AGEs), S100/calgranulin/EN-RAGE,.beta.-amyloid and amphoterin, for the management, treatment, control, or as an adjunct treatment of diseases caused by RAGE. Incubation of proteins or lipids with aldose sugars results in nonenzymatic glycation and oxidation of amino groups on proteins to form Amadori adducts. Over time, the adducts undergo additional rearrangements, dehydrations, and cross-linking with other proteins to form complexes known as Advanced Glycosylation End Products (AGEs). Factors which promote formation of AGEs included delayed protein turnover (e.g. as in amyloidoses), accumulation of macromolecules having high lysine content, and high blood glucose levels (e.g. as in diabetes) (Hori et al., J. Biol. Chem. 270: 25752-761, (1995)). AGEs have implicated in a variety of disorders including complications associated with diabetes and normal aging. In addition to AGEs, other compounds can bind to, and modulate RAGE. In normal development, RAGE interacts with amphoterin, a polypeptide which mediates neurite outgrowth in cultured embryonic neurons (Hori et al., 1995). RAGE has also been shown to interact with EN-RAGE, a protein having substantial similarity to calgranulin (Hofmann et al., Cell 97:889-901 (1999)). RAGE has also been shown to interact with.beta.-amyloid (Yan et al., Nature 389:589-595, (1997); Yan et al., Nature 382:685-691 (1996); Yan et al., Proc. Natl.Acad. Sci., 94:5296-5301 (1997)).

Web site: http://www.delphion.com/details?pn=US06613801__

- **Method of ameliorating erectile dysfunction**

Inventor(s): Adams; Michael A. (Kingston, CA), Banting; James D. (Kingston, CA), Heaton; Jeremy P. W. (Gananoque, CA)

Assignee(s): Queen's University at Kingston (Kingston, CA)

Patent Number: 6,586,391

Date filed: July 18, 2000

Abstract: The mechanism of hypertension following acute NO synthase blockage is via endothelin-mediated vasoconstriction. Thus, NO appears to inhibit endothelin activity by blocking its expression and not as a chronic direct acting vasodilator. Administration of an endothelin antagonist to a patient in a `normal` physiological state may result in specific regional vasodilation. This treatment finds utility in the treatment of **erectile dysfunction.**

Excerpt(s): This invention relates to methods for down-regulating local endothelin-mediated vasoconstrictor and/or vascular growth activity in "apparently" normal physiological conditions in order to re-establish normal control in specific regions of the circulation which demonstrate pathophysiology. More particularly this invention relates to the administration of agents which antagonize the expression or activity of endothelin for the treatment of abnormalities of specific regions of the vasculature such as in **erectile dysfunction** in male patients. Endothelins were first described in 1988 and have been shown to be powerful vasoconstrictors, predominantly found in the vascular endothelium and, since that time, numerous endothelin antagonists and pharmaceutically acceptable salts thereof have been identified and can be obtained commercially (e.g., Sigma, American Peptides). Attention is also directed to U.S. Pat. No. 5,284,828 issued Feb. 8, 1994 to Hemmi et al., U.S. Pat. No. 5,378,715 issued Jan. 3, 1995 to Stein et al. and U.S. Pat. No. 5,382,569 issued Jan. 17, 1995 to Cody et al., which describe in detail the chemical structures of various endothelin antagonists, and to U.S. Pat. No. 5,338,726 issued Aug. 16, 1994 to Shinosaki et al., which describes the chemical structure of endothelin converting enzyme inhibitors, the disclosures of which are incorporated herein by reference. To date, however, antagonists of endothelin have not been approved for therapeutic use, although a number of investigators have postulated that endothelin antagonists could be used for conditions ranging from renal failure, endotoxic shock, asthma, angina, or diabetes to pulmonary hypertension and possibly other indications. Under normal physiological conditions, endothelin can be found in almost all parts of the circulation at very low levels. In general, in the normal rodent circulation endothelin (ET) is not found in elevated quantities and appears to have minimal effect in the normal regulation of vascular tone, i.e., there is no appreciable decrease in blood pressure when an endothelin antagonist is administered by injection in normal circulation. Further, at present there does not appear b be any evidence suggesting that ET plays a physiological role even in a small portion of the circulation under normal conditions in experimental models. However, it is likely that the circulation may appear normal when in fact a specific region of the circulation reveals pathophysiological changes, such as occurs with **erectile dysfunction.** Penile erection demands specific local vasodilation and/or inhibition of local vasoconstrictor mechanisms. It is not surprising that findings of elevated levels of endothelin in the blood are not widespread, as the regulation of ET action indicates a release preferentially towards the smooth muscle side, away from the circulation. In addition, it is highly improbable that there would be increased ET found in the circulation resulting from increased activity in a small portion of the circulation. ET is known to have a very short half-life.

Web site: http://www.delphion.com/details?pn=US06586391__

- **Methods and compositions for misoprostol compound treatment of erectile dysfunction**

Inventor(s): Kanakaris; Panagiotis (33 Koletti Street, GR-106, 77 Athens, GR), Karouzakis; Petros (9 Bakou Street, GR-115, 24 Athens, GR)

Assignee(s): none reported

Patent Number: 6,589,990

Date filed: February 2, 2000

Abstract: Therapeutic formulations and methods for treating **erectile dysfunction** with a misoprostol compound in a subject are provided, a method comprising: obtaining a therapeutic formulation having an effective dose of a misoprostol compound in an excipient carrier; and applying the therapeutic formulation topically to the subject.

Excerpt(s): The invention relates to the use of misoprostol, as well as its metabolites, misoprostol acid, for methods and compositions for topical use for the purpose of treating **erectile dysfunction** (ED). A current pharmaceutical treatment for ED comprises oral administration of sildenafil (Viagra.RTM.), a treatment counter indicated for subjects who are: allergic to this material; or are concurrently being treated with a nitrate medicine such as nitroglycerin; a transdermal nitrate; isosorbide nitrate (Imdur.RTM.); cimetidine (Tagamet.RTM.); mibefradil (Posicor.RTM.); or an anti-infective such as erythromycin, ketoconazole, itraconazole, or rifampin. Subjects suffering with ED due to hormonal insufficiency can be treated with suitable steroid hormone substitution therapy. Other current non-oral and non-steroid treatments include mainly the use of intracavernous injections consisting of direct injection of vasodilatory drugs (for example, injections Caverject.RTM.; and papaverine, phentolamine) into the corpora cavernosa of the penis (Campell's Urology, ed. W.B. Saunders Company, 6.sup.th Edition, Volume III, 3055-3057). Although in situ injection is efficient and scientifically approved, it has serious disadvantages of form (injection) as well as route of administration (introcarvernosal). Yohimbin, an indole alkaloid which is an a.sub.2 -adrenergic inhibitor, is administrated per os, however the efficiency of this method is questionable (Campell's Urology, ed. W. B. Saunders Company, 6.sup.th Edition, Volume III, 3053). Nitroglycerin paste has been proposed as a topical composition (Claes, H. et al., 1989 Urol. Int. 44(5): 309-312), however the method has not been developed as a therapeutic because of concerns regarding efficacy and potential serious side effects (Campell's Urology, 25.sup.th ed. W. B. Saunders Company, 6th Edition, Volume III, 3053). The topical application of prostaglandin E.sub.1 (or alprostadil) in the form of an endourethral gel or a stick was recently proposed as a therapeutic to treat male impotence of vascular etiology (International Journal of Impotence Research, Stockton ed. Vol. 7, September 1995, Supplement I, 5-6 however it is considered to be of limited efficacy.

Web site: http://www.delphion.com/details?pn=US06589990__

- **Methods and compositions for treating male erectile dysfunction**

  Inventor(s): Neal; Gary W. (Knoxville, TN)

  Assignee(s): Androsolutions, Inc. (Knoxville, TN)

  Patent Number: 6,410,595

  Date filed: October 12, 1999

  Abstract: Administration of a pharmaceutical composition comprising:(a) a vasodilator; and(b) a 15-hydroxyprostaglandindehydrogenase inhibitor is effective for the treatment of male **erectile dysfunction.**

  Excerpt(s): The present invention relates to methods of treating male **erectile dysfunction.** The present invention further relates to pharmaceutical compositions useful for treating male **erectile dysfunction.** Impotence, or lack of a man's ability to have sexual intercourse, is often the subject of jokes. However, millions of men suffer from this condition. Impotence is generally characterized by an inability to maintain a penile erection, and is often referred to as **erectile dysfunction. Erectile dysfunction** affects men, regardless of age, place of birth, or prior sexual experience. In the context of the present invention, the term "erectile dysfunction" refers to certain disorders of the cavernous tissue of the penis and the associated fascia which produce impotence, the inability to attain a sexually functional erection. Impotence is estimated to affect about 10 million men in the United States alone. Impotence results from disruption of any of numerous physiological or psychological factors which cause the blood flow to and from the penis to remain in balance thereby preventing retention of sufficient blood to cause rigid dilation of the corpus cavernosa and spongiosa. In the context of the present invention, the term "impotence" is used in its broadest sense as the inability to attain a sexually functional erection when desired.

  Web site: http://www.delphion.com/details?pn=US06410595__

- **Methods for the preparation of biphenyl isoxazole sulfonamides**

  Inventor(s): Chen; Chien-Kuang (Marlboro, NJ), Delaney; Edward J. (Princeton, NJ), Grosso; John A. (Princeton Jct, NJ), Polniaszek; Richard P. (Dayton, NJ), Singh; Ambarish (Bordentown, NJ), Thottathil; John K. (Princeton, NJ), Wang; Xuebao (East Brunswick, NJ)

  Assignee(s): Bristol-Myers Squibb Company (Princeton, NJ)

  Patent Number: 6,313,308

  Date filed: March 20, 2000

  Abstract: Methods for the preparation of biphenyl isoxazole sulfonamides and intermediates therof. The present invention also relates to the novel intermediates prepared by these methods. The biphenyl isoxazole sulfonamides prepared by the present methods are endothelin antagonists useful, inter alia, for the treatment of hypertension, congestive heart failure and male **erectile dysfunction.**

  Excerpt(s): The present invention relates to methods for the preparation of biphenyl isoxazole sulfonamides and intermediates thereof. The present invention also relates to the novel intermediates prepared by these methods. The biphenyl isoxazole sulfonamides prepared by the present methods are endothelin antagonists useful, inter alia, for the treatment of hypertension. in the 4'-position. p is 0 or an integer from 1 to 2.

Web site: http://www.delphion.com/details?pn=US06313308__

- **Nasal delivery of apomorphine**

Inventor(s): Achari; Raja G. (Millington, NJ), Ahmed; Shamim (Central Islip, NY), Behl; Charanjit R. (Hauppauge, NY), deMeireles; Jorge C. (Syosset, NY), Liu; Tianquing (Central Islip, NY), Romeo; Vincent D. (Massapequa Park, NY), Sileno; Anthony P. (Brookhaven Hamlet, NY)

Assignee(s): Nastech Pharmaceutical Company, Inc. (Hauppauge, NY)

Patent Number: 6,436,950

Date filed: June 16, 1999

Abstract: Intranasal delivery methods and compositions for the delivery of dopamine receptor agonists are provided which are effective for the amelioration of **erectile dysfunction** in a mammal without causing substantial intolerable adverse side effects to the mammal. Nasally administered compositions for treating male **erectile dysfunction** in a mammal are also provided which include a therapeutically effective amount of a dopamine receptor agonist which has been dispersed in a system to improve its solubility and/or stability.

Excerpt(s): The present invention relates generally to intranasal delivery methods and dosage forms. More particularly, methods and dosage forms for the safe and reliable intranasal delivery of apomorphine to ameliorate **erectile dysfunction** in a mammal are provided. Apomorphine is a potent dopamine receptor agonist which has a variety of uses. For example, it has been effectively used as an adjunctive medication in the treatment of Parkinson's disease which is complicated by motor fluctuations (T. van Laar et al., Arch. Neurol., 49: 482-484 (1992)). In particular, apomorphine has been used for relieving "off-period" symptoms in Parkinson patients with such response fluctuations. In the study by van Laar et al., the intranasally applied apomorphine used to achieve the results reportedly included an aqueous solution of apomorphine hydrochloride (HCL) at a concentration of 10 mg/ml. This formulation is also used for parenteral application and is published in different Pharmacopeia's. Also, U.S. Pat. No. 5,756,483 issued to Merkus (hereinafter "the '483 patent") which is hereby incorporated by reference, discloses the intranasal delivery of a variety of compositions, including apomorphine in combination with a cyclodextrin and/or a polysaccharide and/or a sugar alcohol for treating Parkinson's disease. The '483 patent, however, discloses very narrow dosage ranges of 0.1 to 2 mg of apomorphine per nostril which is specifically tailored for the amelioration of the "off-period" symptoms of Parkinson's disease.

Web site: http://www.delphion.com/details?pn=US06436950__

- **PDE III inhibitors for treating sexual dysfunction**

Inventor(s): Cutler; Neal R. (Los Angelos, CA)

Assignee(s): R.T. Alamo Ventures I, LLC (Beverly Hills, CA)

Patent Number: 6,541,487

Date filed: September 1, 2000

Abstract: Compositions that are selective PDE III inhibitors and that are effective to treat sexual dysfunction in males and females, including, but not limited to, **erectile**

dysfunction in males. The compositions comprise halogenated quinolines, isoquinolines, quinolones, thioquinolones and 2-oxoquinolones, including derivatives thereof. The compounds can be taken orally or by a number of different routes or can be used to coat the interior of a condom to induce erection.

Excerpt(s): The present invention relates to methods for the treatment of sexual dysfunction in males and females, including but not limited to **erectile dysfunction** in males. Impotence or erectile insufficiency is a widespread disorder that is thought to affect about twelve percent of adult men under age forty-five, about twenty percent of men at age sixty, and about fifty-five percent of men at age seventy-five. Similar to male sexual dysfunction, the prevalence of female sexual dysfunction has been shown to increase with age and be associated with the presence of vascular risk factors and the development of menopause. There is more than one cause of **erectile dysfunction.** For example, **erectile dysfunction** can be psychological, resulting from anxiety or depression, with no apparent somatic or organic impairment. Such **erectile dysfunction,** which is referred to as "psychogenic", is responsible for about fifteen to twenty percent of cases of impotence. In other cases, the **erectile dysfunction** is associated with atherosclerosis of the arteries supplying blood to the penis; such dysfunction is referred to as "arteriogenic" or "atherosclerotic." About forty to sixty percent of cases of impotence are arteriogenic in origin.

Web site: http://www.delphion.com/details?pn=US06541487__

- **Process for the treatment of erectile dysfunction and product therefor**

Inventor(s): Egerland; Ute (Radebeul, DE), Hofgen; Norbert (Medingen, DE), Kronbach; Thomas (Radebeul, DE), Marx; Degenhard (Radebeul, DE), Szelenyi; Stefan (Schwaig, DE)

Assignee(s): Arzneimittelwerk Dresden GmbH (Radebeul, DE)

Patent Number: 6,465,465

Date filed: February 8, 2001

Abstract: The invention relates to the use of pyrido[3,2-e]-pyrazinones of formula 1 as inhibitors of phosphodiesterase 5 for the treatment of **erectile dysfunction** (impotence).

Excerpt(s): Impotence in a man can be defined as the inability to engage in sexual intercourse because of the absence of an erection and/or because of the failure to ejaculate. One speaks of **erectile dysfunction,** if the erection, with respect to strength or duration, is insufficient for sexual intercourse. Erectile disorders affect about 10% of the male population. About 52% of men between the ages of 40 and 70 are affected. Several million men worldwide suffer from this disease (about 7.5 million in Germany alone), which in most cases is due to organic causes and less frequently due to mental causes. **Erectile dysfunction** is a widespread problem among older men, particularly if other chronic diseases are present, such as a high blood pressure, arteriosclerosis and diabetes. Although different active ingredients can induce an erection, these act only after an injection directly into the penis (intracavernous, i.c.) or instillation into the urethra (intraurethral). This form of pharmacological therapy has been available for more than 10 years and involves the i.c. injection of vasoactive substances, such as papaverin, phenoxybenzamine, phenotolamine, moxisylyte and prostaglandin El (PGEI). However, the i.c. use of these substances frequently is accompanied by serious side effects such as priapismus, pain or penile fibrosis. PGE, can be used intraurethrally and nitroglycerin and minoxidil transdermally (on the penis). However, this can cause side effect in the man as well as in the partner.

Web site: http://www.delphion.com/details?pn=US06465465__

- **Sildenafil citrate chewing gum formulations and methods of using the same**

Inventor(s): Gmunder; Charlean B. (Branchburg, NJ), Li; Weisheng (Bridgewater, NJ), Ream; Ronald L (Plano, IL)

Assignee(s): Wm. Wrigley Jr. Company (Chicago, IL)

Patent Number: 6,531,114

Date filed: November 16, 2000

Abstract: Methods and chewing gum formulations for delivering a medicament, namely sildenafil citrate, to an individual are provided. Further, an improved dosage form and method of treating **erectile dysfunction** are provided. Methods of treating esophageal spasms, dysphagia, and gastroparesis utilizing chewing gum formulations containing sildenafil citrate are also provided.

Excerpt(s): The present invention generally relates to medicaments and other agents. More specifically, the present invention relates to the delivery of medicaments or other agents. It is of course known to provide agents to individuals for various purposes. There are a great variety of such agents. These agents can be used to treat diseases and as such are typically referred to as drugs or medicaments. Likewise, the drugs or medicaments can be used for prophylactic purposes. In addition, some agents are taken on an as needed basis while others must be taken at regular intervals by the individual being treated. Still, it is known to provide such agents to an individual for a variety of indicated medicinal purposes such as sildenafil citrate for the treatment of male **erectile dysfunction.** Typically, drugs (medicaments) are administered parenterally or enterally. Of course, parenteral administration is the administration of the drug intravenously directly into the blood stream. Enteral refers to the administration of the drug into the gastrointestinal tract. In either case, the goal of the drug administration is to move the drug from the site of administration towards the systemic circulation. Except when given intravenously, a drug must traverse several semi-permeable cell membranes before reaching general circulation. These membranes act as a biological barrier that inhibits the passage of drug molecules. There are believed to be four processes by which drugs move across a biological barrier: passive diffusion; facilitated diffusion; active transport; and pinocytosis.

Web site: http://www.delphion.com/details?pn=US06531114__

- **Spiropiperidine derivatives as melanocortin receptor agonists**

Inventor(s): Bakshi; Raman K. (Edison, NJ), Nargund; Ravi P. (East Brunswick, NJ), Palucki; Brenda L. (Belle Mead, NJ), Patchett; Arthur A. (Westfield, NJ), Van Der Ploeg; Leonardus H. T. (Scotchplains, NJ), Ye; Zhixiong (Lawrenceville, NJ)

Assignee(s): Merck & Co., Inc. (Rahway, NJ)

Patent Number: 6,410,548

Date filed: February 12, 2001

Abstract: Certain novel spiropiperidine compounds are agonists of melanocortin receptor(s) and are useful for the treatment, control or prevention of diseases and disorders responsive to the activation of melanocortin receptors. The compounds of the present invention are therefore useful for treatment of diseases and disorders such as obesity, diabetes, sexual dysfunction including **erectile dysfunction** and female sexual dysfunction.

Excerpt(s): Spiropiperidine derivatives are melanocortin receptor agonists, and as such are useful in the treatment of disorders responsive to the activation of melanocortin receptors, such as obesity, diabetes as well as male and/or female sexual dysfunction. Pro-opiomelanocortin (POMC) derived peptides are known to affect food intake. Several lines of evidence support the notion that the G-protein coupled receptors (GPCRs) of the melanocortin receptor (MC-R) family, several of which are expressed in the brain, are the targets of POMC derived peptides involved in the control of food intake and metabolism. A specific single MC-R that may be targeted for the control of obesity has not yet been identified. Evidence for the involvement of MC-Rs in obesity includes: i) the agouti (A.sup.vy) mouse which ectopically expresses an antagonist of the MC-1R, MC-3R and -4R is obese, indicating that blocking the action of these three MC-Rs can lead to hyperphagia and metabolic disorders; ii) MC-4R knockout mice (Huszar et al., Cell, 88, 131-141, 1997) recapitulate the phenotype of the agouti mouse and these mice are obese; iii) the cyclic heptapeptide MT-II (MC-1R, -3R, -4R, -5R, agonist) injected intracerebroventricularly (ICV) in rodents, reduces food intake in several animal feeding models (NPY, ob/ob, agouti, fasted) while ICV injected SHU-9119 (MC-3R, -4R antagonist; MC-1R and -5R agonist) reverses this effect and can induce hyperphagia; iv) chronic intraperitoneal treatment of Zucker fatty rats with an.alpha.-NDP-MSH derivative (HP228) has been reported to activate MC-1R, -3R, -4R and -5R and to attenuate food intake and body weight gain over a 12 week period.

Web site: http://www.delphion.com/details?pn=US06410548__

- **Substituted piperidines as melanocortin-4 receptor agonists**

Inventor(s): Bakshi; Raman K. (Edison, NJ), Barakat; Khaled J. (Brooklyn, NY), Nargund; Ravi P. (East Brunswick, NJ), Palucki; Brenda L. (Belle Mead, NJ), Patchett; Arthur A. (Westfield, NJ), Sebhat; Iyassu (Hoboken, NJ), Van Der Ploeg; Leonardus H. T. (Scotch Plains, NJ), Ye; Zhixiong (Princeton, NJ)

Assignee(s): Merck & Co., Inc. (Rahway, NJ)

Patent Number: 6,350,760

Date filed: June 1, 2000

Abstract: Certain novel substituted piperidine compounds are agonists of the human melanocortin receptor(s) and, in particular, are selective agonists of the human melanocortin-4 receptor (MC-4R). They are therefore useful for the treatment, control, or prevention of diseases and disorders responsive to the activation of MC-4R, such as obesity, diabetes, sexual dysfunction, including **erectile dysfunction** and female sexual dysfunction. Also provided are methods of treating sexual dysfunction with a compound that is a selective agonist of MC-4R over any other human melanocortin receptor.

Excerpt(s): Pro-opiomelanocortin (POMC) derived peptides are known to affect food intake. Several lines of evidence support the notion that the G-protein coupled receptors (GPCRs) of the melanocortin receptor (MC-R) family, several of which are expressed in the brain, are the targets of POMC derived peptides involved in the control of food intake and metabolism. A specific single MC-R that may be targeted for the control of obesity has not yet been identified. Evidence for the involvement of MC-R's in obesity includes: i) the agouti (A.sup.vy) mouse which ectopically expresses an antagonist of the MC-1R, MC-3R and -4R is obese, indicating that blocking the action of these three MC-R's can lead to hyperphagia and metabolic disorders; ii) MC-4R knockout mice (Huszar et al., Cell, 88, 131-141, 1997) recapitulate the phenotype of the agouti mouse and these mice are obese; iii) the cyclic heptapeptide MT-II (a non-selective MC-1R, -3R, -4R, and -5R agonist) injected intracerebroventricularly (ICV) in rodents, reduces food intake in several animal feeding models (NPY, ob/ob, agouti, fasted) while ICV injected SHU-9119 (MC-3R and 4R antagonist; MC-1R and -5R agonist) reverses this effect and can induce hyperphagia; iv) chronic intraperitoneal treatment of Zucker fatty rats with an.alpha.-NDP-MSH derivative (HP228) has been reported to activate MC-1R, -3R, -4R, and -5R and to attenuate food intake and body weight gain over a 12-week period. Five distinct MC-R's have thus far been identified, and these are expressed in different tissues. MC-1R was initially characterized by dominant gain of function mutations at the Extension locus, affecting coat color by controlling phaeomelanin to eumelanin conversion through control of tyrosinase. MC-1R is mainly expressed in melanocytes. MC-2R is expressed in the adrenal gland and represents the ACTH receptor. MC-3R is expressed in the brain, gut, and placenta and may be involved in the control of food intake and thermogenesis. MC-4R is uniquely expressed in the brain, and its inactivation was shown to cause obesity. MC-5R is expressed in many tissues, including white fat, placenta, and exocrine glands. A low level of expression is also observed in the brain. MC-5R knockout mice reveal reduced sebaceous gland lipid production (Chen et al., Cell, 1997, 91, 789-798).

Web site: http://www.delphion.com/details?pn=US06350760__

- **Therapeutic vibrator for correcting erectile dysfunction**

Inventor(s): Lebecque; Maurice (7222 Durocher,.pi.9, Montreal, Quebec, CA)

Assignee(s): none reported

Patent Number: 6,338,721

Date filed: December 7, 1999

Abstract: The vibrator includes a selectively powered vibrating casing, on which an arch is mounted, the combination of the arch with the casing forming a closed loop. A resilient and flexible strap extends through the loop thus created, the strap being bored at its two end portions and being engaged by the two arms of the arcuate arch. The strap is slidable along the two arms of the arch, so that its position be adjustable relative to both the vibrating casing and the upper web of the arch itself.

Excerpt(s): The present invention relates to a vibrator, and more particularly to a vibrator for use in correcting **erectile dysfunction.** in the case of hollow cylindrical vibrators, they are often not provided with an open outer end, which results in the penis ejaculating inside the vibrator, which requires cleaning of the vibrator and which can bring about hygiene problems. It is further known to provide small vibrators for women which are destined to be inserted into the woman's vagina. However, these vibrators cannot be used by men.

Web site: http://www.delphion.com/details?pn=US06338721__

- **Thienopyrimidines**

  Inventor(s): Christadler; Maria (Darmstadt, DE), Jonas; Rochus (Darmstadt, DE), Kluxen; Franz-Werner (Darmstadt, DE), Schelling; Pierre (Darmstadt, DE)

  Assignee(s): Merck Patent Gesellschaft mit beschraenkter Haftung (DE)

  Patent Number: 6,420,368

  Date filed: May 26, 2000

  Abstract: The thienopyrimidines of the formula (I) and their physiologically compatible salts display a phosphodiesterase V inhibiting activity and can be used for treating diseases of the cardiovascular system and for treatment and/or therapy of **erectile dysfunction.**

  Excerpt(s): and their physiologically acceptable salts. Pyrimidine derivatives are disclosed, for example, in EP 201 188 or WO 93/06104. The invention is based on the object of finding novel compounds having valuable properties, in particular those which can be used for the production of medicaments.

  Web site: http://www.delphion.com/details?pn=US06420368__

- **Topical preparation of alprostadil for the treatment of erectile dysfunction**

  Inventor(s): Chi; Sang-Cheol (Suwon-si, KR), Lee; Dong Soo (Pyoungtaek-si, KR), Lee; Kye Kwan (Suwon-si, KR)

  Assignee(s): Whan In Pharm Co., Ltd. (Seoul, KR)

  Patent Number: 6,500,440

  Date filed: August 29, 2000

  Abstract: The present invention relates to a composition of topical preparation containing alprostadil, which has excellent skin permeation rate with little skin irritation, which is prepared by dissolving alprostadil or a solid dispersion thereof prepared using poloxamer, into a mixture of an oily vehicle, a pyrrolidone and an anti-irritant agent.

  Excerpt(s): This invention relates to a composition of topical preparation containing alprostadil for the treatment of **erectile dysfunction,** which has excellent skin permeation rate with little skin irritation. Particularly, the present invention relates to a composition of topical preparation containing alprostadil, which is prepared by dissolving alprostadil itself or a solid dispersion thereof prepared using poloxamer, into a mixture of an oily vehicle, a pyrrolidone and an anti-irritant agent. Erectile dysfunction refers to a condition of the inability to achieve and maintain penile erection sufficient to complete satisfactory sexual intercourse. There are two major causes for the erectile dysfunction: psychogenic and organic causes. Previously, **erectile dysfunction** was thought to be of psychogenic origin. In these days, however, it is believed that most of **erectile dysfunction** comes from organic causes resulting from damage in nerve, blood vessel or hormone system, surgery, or drug administration. Erectile dysfunction can be cured with surgical or pharmacological means. For the pharmacological treatment, some effective drugs are available, orally or locally. As oral drugs, yohimbine and trazodone have been used, but their clinical effect is not pronounced. Recently, sildenafil, a selective inhibitor of phosphodiesterase, has been introduced into the market as an oral drug. This new oral drug showed positive result in the treatment of **erectile dysfunction.** However, the oral administration of a drug accompanies systemic side effects inevitably, since the drug reaches the site of action after it is distributed throughout the whole body by the systemic circulation. Sildenafil also has some systemic side effects such as headache, flushing, indigestion and changes in vision, etc. Particularly, it may cause a serious side effect, if taken by patient medicated with organic nitrates, due to the possibility of dramatic drop in blood pressure. Therefore, a local treatment is the method of choice for the treatment of **erectile dysfunction,** since it is a local disorder. For this purpose, alprostadil (prostaglandin E1), papaverine, or phentolamine has been used. Among them, alprostadil is demonstrated to be the most effective drug for the local treatment of **erectile dysfunction.** Until now, intracavernous injection and transurethral pellet of alprostadil are commercially available in the market. However, the injection formulation needs a direct injection to the penis. Thus, patients may feel uncomfortable, and a pain or bleeding, or even infection on the injected site may occur. The transurethral pellet also has inconvenience in inserting into urethra, and burning sense on urethra or pain on penis may occur.

Web site: http://www.delphion.com/details?pn=US06500440__

- **Transmucosal administration of phosphodiesterase inhibitors for the treatment of erectile dysfunction**

Inventor(s): Doherty, Jr.; Paul C. (Cupertino, CA), Place; Virgil A. (Kawaihae, HI), Smith; William L. (Mahwah, NJ)

Assignee(s): Vivus, Inc. (Mountain View, CA)

Patent Number: 6,548,490

Date filed: December 10, 1999

Abstract: A method is provided for treating **erectile dysfunction** in a mammalian male individual. The method involves the transmucosal administration of a phosphodiesterase inhibitor or a pharmaceutically acceptable salt, ester, amide or derivative thereof, within the context of an effective dosing regimen. Preferred modes of administration include transbuccal, sublingual and transrectal routes. Pharmaceutical formulations and kits are provided as well.

Excerpt(s): This invention relates generally to methods and pharmaceutical compositions for treating **erectile dysfunction;** more particularly, the invention relates to transmucosal (e.g., buccal, sublingual and transrectal), administration of phosphodiesterase inhibitors to treat **erectile dysfunction.** Impotence is the consistent inability to achieve or sustain an erection of sufficient rigidity for sexual intercourse. It has recently been estimated that approximately 10 million American men are impotent (R. Shabsigh et al., "Evaluation of Erectile Impotence," Urology 32:83-90 (1988); W. L. Furlow, "Prevalence of Impotence in the United States," Med. Aspects Hum. Sex. 19:13-6 (1985)). Impotence is recognized to be an age-dependent disorder, with an incidence of 1.9 percent at 40 years of age and 25 percent at 65 years of age (A. C. Kinsey et al., "Age and Sexual Outlet," in Sexual Behavior in the Human Male; A. C. Kinsey et al., eds., Philadelphia, Pa.: W. B. Saunders, 218-262 (1948)). In 1985 in the United States, impotence accounted for more than several hundred thousand outpatient visits to physicians (National Center for Health Statistics, National Hospital Discharge Survey, 1985, Bethesda, Md., Department of Health and Human Services, 1989 DHHS publication no. 87-1751). Depending on the nature and cause of the problem, treatments include psychosexual therapy, hormonal therapy, administration of vasodilators such as nitroglycerin and.alpha.-adrenergic blocking agents (".alpha.-blockers"), oral administration of other pharmaceutical agents, vascular surgery, implanted penile prostheses, vacuum constriction devices and external aids such as penile splints to support the penis or penile constricting rings to alter the flow of blood through the penis. A number of causes of impotence have been identified, including vasculogenic, neurogenic, endocrinologic and psychogenic. Vasculogenic impotence, which is caused by alterations in the flow of blood to and from the penis, is thought to be the most frequent organic cause of impotence. Common risk factors for vasculogenic impotence include hypertension, diabetes, cigarette smoking, pelvic trauma, and the like. Neurogenic impotence is associated with spinal-cord injury, multiple sclerosis, peripheral neuropathy caused by diabetes or alcoholism and severance of the autonomic nerve supply to the penis consequent to prostate surgery. **Erectile dysfunction** is also associated with disturbances in endocrine function resulting in low circulating testosterone levels and elevated prolactin levels.

Web site: http://www.delphion.com/details?pn=US06548490__

- **Treatment of erectile dysfunction using isoquinoline compound melanocortin receptor ligands**

Inventor(s): Basu; Amaresh (San Diego, CA), Gahman; Timothy C. (Encinitas, CA), Girten; Beverly E. (Sunnyvale, CA), Griffith; Michael C. (San Diego, CA), Hecht; Curtis C. (San Diego, CA), Kiely; John S. (San Diego, CA), Slivka; Sandra R. (San Diego, CA)

Assignee(s): Lion Bioscience AG (Heidelberg, DE)

Patent Number: 6,608,082

Date filed: May 6, 1999

Abstract: Methods for treating **erectile dysfunction** using tetrahydroisoquinoline aromatic amines that function as melanocortin receptor ligands.

Excerpt(s): The present invention relates generally to the fields of medicinal chemistry and molecular pathology and, more specifically, to novel isoquinoline compounds and their use as melanocortin receptor ligands and as agents for controlling cytokine-regulated physiologic processes and pathologies, as well as combinatorial libraries comprising such compounds. The melanocortin (MC) receptors are a group of cell surface proteins that mediate a variety of physiological effects, including regulation of adrenal gland function such as production of the glucocorticoids cortisol and aldosterone; control of melanocyte growth and pigment production; thermoregulation; immunomodulation; and analgesia. Five distinct MC receptors have been cloned and are expressed in a variety of tissues, including melanocytes, adrenal cortex, brain, gut, placenta, skeletal muscle, lung, spleen, thymus, bone marrow, pituitary, gonads and adipose tissue (Tatro, Neuroimmunomodulation 3:259-284 (1996)). Three MC receptors, MCR-1, MCR-3 and MCR-4, are expressed in brain tissue (Xia et al., Neuroreport 6:2193-2196 (1995)). A variety of ligands termed melanocortins function as agonists that stimulate the activity of MC receptors. The melanocortins include melanocyte-stimulating hormones (MSH) such as.alpha.-MSH,.beta.-MSH and.gamma.-MSH, as well as adrenocorticotropic hormone (ACTH). Individual ligands can bind to multiple MC receptors with differing relative affinities. The variety of ligands and MC receptors with differential tissue-specific expression likely provides the molecular basis for the diverse physiological effects of melanocortins and MC receptors. For example,.alpha.-MSH antagonizes the actions of immunological substances such as cytokines and acts to modulate fever, inflammation and immune responses (Catania and Lipton, Annals N. Y. Acad. Sci. 680:412-423 (1993)).

Web site: http://www.delphion.com/details?pn=US06608082__

- **Treatments for obesity and methods for identifying compounds useful for treating obesity**

Inventor(s): Hadcock; John R. (East Lyme, CT), Swick; Andrew G. (East Lyme, CT)

Assignee(s): Pfizer Inc. (New York, NY)

Patent Number: 6,451,783

Date filed: January 16, 2001

Abstract: The present invention provides a method of treating obesity, sexual dysfunction (including erectile dysfunction), diabetes, insulin resistance, hyperinsulinemia, Syndrome X, adrenal dysfunction, hypertension, hypercholesterolemia, atherosclerosis, hyperlipoproteinemia, hypertriglyceridemia, or substance abuse, the method comprising the step of administering to a patent having or at risk of having one of the above-mentioned diseases a therapeutically effective amount of a compound that attenuates the binding of agouti-related protein to melanocortin receptors, but does not attenuate the binding of.alpha.-melanocyte stimulating hormone to melanocortin receptors. The present invention also provides a method of identifying a compound that is useful for the treatment or prevention of obesity, sexual dysfunction (including erectile dysfunction), diabetes, insulin resistance, hyperinsulinemia, Syndrome X, adrenal dysfunction, hypertension, hypercholesterolemia, atherosclerosis, hyperlipoproteinemia, hypertriglyceridemia, or substance abuse, the method comprising the steps of: 1) determining if a compound affects the binding of agouti-related protein to melanocortin receptors; 2) determining if a compound affects the binding of.alpha.-melanocyte stimulating hormone to melanocortin receptors; and 3) selecting a compound that attenuates the binding of agouti-related protein to melanocortin receptors, but does not affect the binding of.alpha.-melanocyte stimulating hormone to melanocortin receptors.

Excerpt(s): The present invention provides methods of treating obesity, sexual dysfunction (including erectile dysfunction), diabetes, insulin resistance, hyperinsulinemia, Syndrome X, adrenal dysfunction, hypertension, hypercholesterolemia, atherosclerosis, hyperlipoproteinemia, hypertriglyceridemia, or substance abuse, the methods comprising the step of administering to a patient having or at risk of having one of the above-mentioned diseases or conditions a therapeutically effective amount of a compound that attenuates the binding of agouti-related protein to melanocortin receptors, but does not attenuate the binding of.alpha.-melanocyte stimulating hormone to melanocortin receptors. The present invention also provides methods of identifying a compound that is useful for the treatment of obesity, sexual dysfunction (including erectile dysfunction), diabetes, insulin resistance, hyperinsulinemia, Syndrome X, adrenal dysfunction, hypertension, hypercholesterolemia, atherosclerosis, hyperlipoproteinemia, hypertriglyceridemia, or substance abuse, the methods comprising the steps of: 1) determining if a compound affects the binding of agouti-related protein to melanocortin receptors; 2) determining if a compound affects the binding of.alpha.-melanocyte stimulating hormone to melanocortin receptors; and 3) selecting a compound that attenuates the binding of agouti-related protein to melanocortin receptors, but does not attenuate the binding of cc-melanocyte stimulating hormone to melanocortin receptors. Obesity is a devastating disease. In addition to harming physical health, obesity can wreak havoc on mental health because obesity affects self-esteem, which ultimately can affect a person's ability to interact socially with others. Unfortunately, obesity is not well understood, and societal stereotypes and presumptions regarding obesity only tend to exacerbate the psychological effects of the disease. Because of the impact of obesity on individuals and society, much effort has been expended to find ways to treat obesity, but little success has been achieved in the long-term treatment and/or prevention of obesity.

Web site: http://www.delphion.com/details?pn=US06451783__

Patent Applications on Erectile Dysfunction

As of December 2000, U.S. patent applications are open to public viewing.[10] Applications are patent requests which have yet to be granted. (The process to achieve a patent can take several years.) The following patent applications have been filed since December 2000 relating to erectile dysfunction:

- **Acylated indanyl amines and their use as pharmaceuticals**

   Inventor(s): Dharanipragada, Ramalinga M.; (Belle Meade, NJ), Safarova, Alena; (Tucson, AZ), Schonafinger, Karl; (Alzenau, DE), Strobel, Hartmut; (Liederbach, DE), Suzuki, Teri; (Tucson, AZ), Walser, Armin; (Tucson, AZ), Wohlfart, Paulus; (Bensheim, DE)

   Correspondence: Finnegan, Henderson, Farabow,; Garrett & Dunner, L.L.P.; 1300 I Street, N.W.; Washington; DC; 20005-3315; US

   Patent Application Number: 20030055093

   Date filed: February 13, 2002

   Abstract: The present invention relates to acylated indanyl amines according to the general formula (I) 1wherein R.sup.1-R.sup.4 have the meanings given in the description, A is CH.sub.2, CHOH or CH--(C.sub.1-C.sub.3-alkyl), B is CH.sub.2 or CH--(C.sub.1-C.sub.3-alkyl), and R.sup.5 is an aryl or heteroaryl group, possibly substituted by the substituents listed in the description. These compounds are useful in the upregulation of endothelial nitric oxide synthase (eNOS), and may therefore be useful for the manufacture of medicaments for the treatment of cardiovascular diseases, stable or unstable angina pectoris, coronary heart disease, Prinzmetal angina, acute coronary syndrome, heart failure, myocardial infarction, stroke, thrombosis, peripheral artery occlusive disease, endothelial dysfunction, atherosclerosis, restenosis, endothelial damage after PTCA, hypertension, essential hypertension, pulmonary hypertension, secondary hypertension, renovascular hypertension, chronic glomerulonephritis, **erectile dysfunction,** ventricular arrhythmia, diabetes or diabetes complications, nephropathy or retinopathy, angiogenesis, asthma bronchiale, chronic renal failure, cirrhosis of the liver, osteoporosis, restricted memory performance, a restricted ability to learn, or for the lowering of cardiovascular risk of postmenopausal women or after intake of contraceptives.

   Excerpt(s): Endothelial NO synthase (eNOS, NOS-III) belongs to a group of three isoenzymes which produce nitric oxide (NO) by oxidation of arginine. Endothelially released NO is of central importance in a number of key cardiovascular mechanisms. It has a vasodilating effect and inhibits the aggregation of platelets, the adhesion of leukocytes to the endothelium and the proliferation of intimal smooth muscle cells.

---

[10] This has been a common practice outside the United States prior to December 2000.

Endothelial NO synthase is subject to physiological and pathophysiological regulation both at the transcriptional and at the post-transcriptional level. Enzyme already present in the endothelium may undergo calcium-dependent and calcium-independent activation through phosphorylation of specific amino acids, but also by direct interactions with specific proteins. Stimulators of this, usually transient, NO release are, extracellular arginine, 17.beta.-estrogen and the mechanical stimulus exerted on the luminal surface of the endothelium by the blood flow (shear stress). The latter additionally leads to regulation of eNOS at the transcriptional level. Thus, for example, Sessa et al. (Circ. Research 74 (1994) 349-353) were able by means of exercise training and the increase in shear stress associated therewith to obtain a marked increase in ecNOS. Whether regulation at the post-transcriptional level is relevant in vivo, is not unambiguously proved. Thus, for example, administration of a high arginine dose is followed by only a transient improvement in the endothelium-dependent vasorelaxation in patients with coronary heart disease.

Web site: http://appft1.uspto.gov/netahtml/PTO/search-bool.html

- **Apomorphine-containing dosage form for ameliorating male erectile dysfunction**

Inventor(s): El-Rashidy, Ragab; (Deerfield, IL), Ronsen, Bruce; (River Forest, IL)

Correspondence: OLSON & HIERL, LTD.; 36th Floor; 20 North Wacker Drive; Chicago; IL; 60606; US

Patent Application Number: 20030073715

Date filed: October 23, 2001

Abstract: Impotence can be ameliorated without substantial undesirable side effects by nasal administration of apomorphine, optionally with an antiemetic agent present in an amount sufficient to substantially reduce nausea symptoms that may be associated with the use of apomorphine.

Excerpt(s): This application is a continuation-in-part of our application U.S. Ser. No. 09/606,919, filed on Jun. 29, 2000 and now U.S. Pat. No. 6,306,437, which is a continuation of U.S. Ser. No. 09/102,406, filed on Jun. 22, 1998 and now U.S. Pat. No. 6,121,276, which is a continuation-in-part of U.S. Ser. No. 08/546,498 filed on Oct. 20, 1995 and now U.S. Pat. No. 5,770,606, which in turn is a continuation-in-part of U.S. Ser. No. 08/231,250, filed on Apr. 22, 1994, abandoned. This invention, in one aspect, relates to dosage forms and methods for ameliorating **erectile dysfunction** in psychogenic male patients. In another aspect this invention relates to diagnosis of **erectile dysfunction.** More particularly, this invention relates to the use of apomorphine-containing compositions for amelioration of **erectile dysfunction** in male patients and for diagnostic purposes. A normal erection occurs as a result of a coordinated vascular event in the penis. This is usually triggered neurally and consists of vasodilation and smooth muscle relaxation in the penis and its supplying arterial vessels. Arterial inflow causes enlargement of the substance of the corpora cavernosa. Venous outflow is trapped by this enlargement, permitting sustained high blood pressures in the penis sufficient to cause rigidity. Muscles in the perineum also assist in creating and maintaining penile rigidity. Erection may be induced centrally in the nervous system by sexual thoughts or fantasy, and is usually reinforced locally by reflex mechanisms. Erectile mechanics are substantially similar in the female for the clitoris.

Web site: http://appft1.uspto.gov/netahtml/PTO/search-bool.html

- **Aromatic nitrogen-containing 6-membered cyclic compounds**

Inventor(s): Kikkawa, Kohei; (Kawaguchi-shi, JP), Matsuki, Kenji; (Saitama-ken, JP), Omori, Kenji; (Saitama-shi, JP), Yamada, Koichiro; (Saitama-ken, JP)

Correspondence: Finnegan, Henderson, Farabow,; Garrett & Dunner, L.L.P.; 1300 I Street, N.W.; Washington; DC; 20005-3315; US

Patent Application Number: 20030032647

Date filed: August 10, 2001

Abstract: An aromatic nitrogen-containing 6-membered cyclic compound of the formula (I): 1wherein Ring A is a substituted or unsubstituted nitrogen-containing heterocyclic group; R.sup.1 is a substituted or unsubstituted lower alkyl group, --NH--Q--R.sup.3 (R.sup.3 is a substituted or unsubstituted nitrogen containing heterocyclic group, and Q is a lower alkylene group or a single bond), or --NH--R.sup.4 (R.sup.4 is a substituted or unsubstituted cycloalkyl group); R.sup.2 is a substituted or unsubstituted aryl group; one of Y and Z is.dbd.CH--, and the other is.dbd.N--, or a pharmaceutically acceptable salt thereof, these compounds exhibiting excellent selective PDE V inhibitory activities, and hence, being useful in the prophylaxis or treatment of penile **erectile dysfunction,** etc.

Excerpt(s): This application is a continuation application of PCT international application No. PCT/JP00/06258 which has an international filing date of Sep. 13, 2000 which designated the United States, the entire contents of which are incorporated by reference. The present invention relates to a novel aromatic nitrogen-containing 6-membered cyclic compound exhibiting a cGMP specific phosphodiesterase (PDE) inhibitory activity (PDE V inhibitory activity) and being useful as a medicament, and a process for preparing the same. In general, it is known that cGMP, which is an intracellular second messenger, is decomposed and inactivated by phosphodiesterase which widely distributes in many cell types and tissues of the living body, and when said PDE activity is inactivated, the level of cGMP in cells is increased, and as a result, various pharmacological activities, for example, relaxation of vascular smooth muscle, relaxation of bronchial smooth muscle, and inhibition of platelet aggregation are exhibited.

Web site: http://appft1.uspto.gov/netahtml/PTO/search-bool.html

- **Benzimidazole derivatives as therapeutic agents**

Inventor(s): Gopalaswamy, Ramesh; (Jamestown, NC), M. Mjalli, Adnan M.; (Jamestown, NC)

Correspondence: Cynthia B. Rothschild, Esq.; Kilpatrick Stockton LLP; 1001 West Fourth Street; Winston-Salem; NC; 27101-2400; US

Patent Application Number: 20030032663

Date filed: March 5, 2002

Abstract: This invention provides certain compounds, methods of their preparation, pharmaceutical compositions comprising the compounds, and their use in treating human or animal disorders. The compounds of the invention are useful as modulators of the interaction between the receptor for advanced glycated end products (RAGE) and its ligands, such as advanced glycated end products (AGEs), S100/calgranulin/EN-RAGE,.beta.-amyloid and amphoterin, and for the management, treatment, control, or as an adjunct treatment for diseases in humans caused by RAGE. Such diseases or disease states include acute and chronic inflammation, the development of diabetic late complications such as increased vascular permeability, nephropathy, atherosclerosis, and retinopathy, the development of Alzheimer's disease, **erectile dysfunction,** and tumor invasion and metastasis.

Excerpt(s): This invention relates to compounds which are modulators of the receptor for advanced glycated end products (RAGE) and interaction with its ligands such as advanced glycated end products (AGEs), S100/calgranulin/EN-RAGE,.beta.-amyloid and amphoterin, for the management, treatment, control, or as an adjunct treatment of diseases caused by RAGE. Incubation of proteins or lipids with aldose sugars results in nonenzymatic glycation and oxidation of amino groups on proteins to form Amadori adducts. Over time, the adducts undergo additional rearrangements, dehydrations, and cross-linking with other proteins to form complexes known as Advanced Glycosylation End Products (AGEs). Factors which promote formation of AGEs included delayed protein turnover (e.g. as in amyloidoses), accumulation of macromolecules having high lysine content, and high blood glucose levels (e.g. as in diabetes) (Hori et al., J. Biol. Chem. 270: 25752-761, (1995)). AGEs have implicated in a variety of disorders including complications associated with diabetes and normal aging. AGEs display specific and saturable binding to cell surface receptors on endothelial cells of the microvasculature, monocytes and macrophages, smooth muscle cells, mesengial cells, and neurons. The Receptor for Advanced Glycated Endproducts (RAGE) is a member of the immunoglobulin super family of cell surface molecules. The extracellular (N-terminal) domain of RAGE includes three immunoglobulin-type regions, one V (variable) type domain followed by two C-type (constant) domains (Neeper et al., J. Biol. Chem. 267:14998-15004 (1992). A single transmembrane spanning domain and a short, highly charged cytosolic tail follow the extracellular domain. The N-terminal, extracellular domain can be isolated by proteolysis of RAGE to generate soluble RAGE (sRAGE) comprised of the V and C domains.

Web site: http://appft1.uspto.gov/netahtml/PTO/search-bool.html

- **Combination effective for the treatment of impotence**

  Inventor(s): Wyllie, Michael G.; (Herne, GB)

  Correspondence: PFIZER INC.; PATENT DEPARTMENT, MS8260-1611; EASTERN POINT ROAD; GROTON; CT; 06340; US

  Patent Application Number: 20030040514

  Date filed: September 25, 2002

  Abstract: This invention relates to the treatment of **erectile dysfunction** with a combination of (1) a compound selected from.alpha.-adrenergic receptor antagonists, and (2) a compound selected from agents which elevate cGMP levels. Sildenafil or a pharmaceutically acceptable salt thereof is preferred as the cGMP PDE elevator. Also included are compositions and kits comprising such impotence treating compounds.

  Excerpt(s): This invention relates to the treatment of impotence comprising co-administering (1) an.alpha.-adrenergic receptor antagonist and (2) an agent which elevates cyclic guanosine 3',5'-monophosphate (cGMP) levels. The combination is particularly suitable for the treatment of patients suffering from impotence or **erectile dysfunction.** Impotence is the inability to obtain and/or sustain an erection sufficient for penetration of the vagina and/or intercourse. Thus, impotence is also referred to as "erectile insufficiency" or "erectile dysfunction". It has been estimated that 10-12 million American men between the ages of 18 and 75 suffer from chronic impotence, with the great majority being over age 55. The penis normally becomes erect when certain tissues, in particular the corpora cavernosa in the central portion of the penis, become engorged with blood, thereby causing them to become less flaccid, and in turn causing an erection. Impotence can result from psychologic disturbances (psychogenic), from physiologic abnormalities (organic) or from a combination of both. Thus, in some males **erectile dysfunction** may be due to anxiety or depression, with no apparent somatic or organic impairment In other cases, **erectile dysfunction** is associated with atherosclerosis of the arteries supplying blood to the penis. In still other cases, the dysfunction may be due to venous leakage or abnormal drainage in which there is leakage from veins in the penis such that sufficient pressure for an erection can be neither obtained nor maintained. In still other cases, the dysfunction is associated with a neuropathy or due to nerve damage arising from, for example, surgery or a pelvic injury. Typically, multiple factors are responsible for impotence.

Web site: http://appft1.uspto.gov/netahtml/PTO/search-bool.html

- **Combinations**

Inventor(s): Cohen, David Saul; (New Providence, NJ)

Correspondence: THOMAS HOXIE; NOVARTIS, PATENT AND TRADEMARK DEPARTMENT; ONE HEALTH PLAZA 430/2; EAST HANOVER; NJ; 07936-1080; US

Patent Application Number: 20030114469

Date filed: August 28, 2002

Abstract: The present invention relates to a pharmaceutical composition, comprising(a) a phosphodiesterase 5 inhibitor or a pharmaceutically acceptable salt thereof and(b) at least one of the active ingredients selected from the group consisting of(i) an anti-diabetic agent;(ii) HMG-Co-A reductase inhibitors;(iii) an anti-hypertensive agent; and(iv) a serotonin reuptake inhibitor (SSRI) or, in each case, or a pharmaceutically acceptable salt thereof; anda pharmaceutically acceptable carrier. The pharmaceutical composition may be employed for the treatment of sexual dysfunction, hyperglycemia, hyperinsulinaemia, hyperlipidaemia, hypertriglyceridemia, diabetes, insulin resistance, impaired glucose metabolism, conditions of impaired glucose tolerance (IGT), conditions of impaired fasting plasma glucose, obesity, diabetic retinopathy, diabetic nephropathy, glomerulosclerosis, diabetic neuropathy, syndrome X, **erectile dysfunction,** coronary heart disease, hypertension, especially ISH, angina pectoris, myocardial infarction, stroke, vascular restenosis, endothelial dysfunction, impaired vascular compliance, congestive heart failure.

Excerpt(s): a pharmaceutically acceptable carrier. Anti-diabetic agents include insulin secretion enhancers which are active ingredients that have the property to promote the secretion of insulin from pancreatic.beta.-cells. Examples of insulin secretion enhancers are a biguanide derivative, for example, metformin or, if appropriate, a pharmaceutically acceptable salt thereof, especially the hydrochloride thereof. Other insulin secretion enhancers include sulfonylureas (SU), especially those which promote the secretion of insulin from pancreatic.beta.-cells by transmitting signals of insulin secretion via SU receptors in the cell membrane including, but are not limited to, tolbutamide; chlorpropamide; tolazamide; acetohexamide; 4-chloro-N-[(1-pyrolidinylamino)carbonyl]-benzensulfonamide (glycopyramide); glibenclamide (glyburide); gliclazide; 1-butyl-3-metanilylurea; carbutamide; glibonuride; glipizide;

gliquidone; glisoxepid; glybuthiazole; glibuzole; glyhexamide; glymidine; glypinamide; phenbutamide; and tolylcyclamide, or pharmaceutically acceptable salts thereof. and repaglinide [(S)-2-ethoxy-4-{2-[[3-methyl-1-[2-(1-piperidinyl)p- henyl]butyl]amino]-2-oxoethyl}benzoic acid]. Repaglinide is disclosed in EP 589874, EP 147850 A2, in particular Example 11 on page 61, and EP 207331 A1. It can be administered in the form as it is marketed, e.g., under the trademark NovoNorm.TM.; calcium (2S)-2-benzyl-3-(cis-hexahydro-- 2-isoindolinlycarbonyl)-propionate dihydrate (mitiglinide--cf. EP 507534); furthermore representatives of the new generation of SUs such as glimepiride (cf. EP 31058); in free or pharmaceutically acceptable salt form. The term nateglinide likewise comprises crystal modifications such as disclosed in EP 0526171 B1 or U.S. Pat. No. 5,488,510, respectively, the subject matter of which, especially with respect to the identification, manufacture and characterization of crystal modifications, is herewith incorporated by reference to this application, especially the subject matter of claims 8-10 of said U.S. patent (referring to H-form crystal modification) as well as the corresponding references to the B-type crystal modification in EP 196222 B1 the subject matter of which, especially with respect to the identification, manufacture and characterization of the B-form crystal modification. Preferably, in the present invention, the B- or H-type, more preferably the H-type, is used. Nateglinide can be administered in the form as it is marketed, e.g., under the trademark STARLIX.TM.

Web site: http://appft1.uspto.gov/netahtml/PTO/search-bool.html

- **Compositions and methods for inhibiting arginase activity**

Inventor(s): Baggio, Ricky; (Waltham, MA), Christianson, David; (Media, PA), Elbaum, Daniel; (Newton, MA)

Correspondence: AKIN, GUMP, STRAUSS, HAUER & FELD, L.L.P.; ONE COMMERCE SQUARE; 2005 MARKET STREET, SUITE 2200; PHILADELPHIA; PA; 19103; US

Patent Application Number: 20030036529

Date filed: January 23, 2002

Abstract: Compositions and methods for inhibiting arginase activity, including arginase activity in a mammal, are provided. Methods of making the compositions of the invention are also provided as are methods of using the compositions therapeutically. The compositions described herein are useful for alleviating or inhibiting a variety of arinase- and NO synthase-related disorders, including heart diseae, gastrointestinal motility disorders, and penile **erectile dysfunction** in humans.

Excerpt(s): This application is a divisional of U.S. patent application Ser. No. 09/545,737 (allowed), which is itself a continuation-in-part of International Patent Application PCT/US98/21430, published in the English language on Oct. 9, 1998, and is entitled to priority pursuant to 35 U.S.C.sctn. 119(e) to U.S. provisional patent application No. 60/061,607, filed Oct. 10, 1997. The invention relates generally to enzyme inhibitors, more particularly to inhibitors of the enzyme designated arginase. Each individual excretes roughly ten kilograms of urea per year, as a result of the hydrolysis of arginine in the final cytosolic step of the urea cycle (Krebs et al., 1932, Hoppe-Seyler's Z. Physiol. Chem. 210:33-66). The activity of the liver enzyme, arginase, permits disposal of nitrogenous wastes which result from protein catabolism (Herzfeld et al., 1976, Biochem. J. 153:469-478). In tissues which lack a complete complement of the enzymes which catalyze the reactions of the urea cycle, arginase regulates cellular concentrations of arginine and ornithine, which are used for biosynthetic reactions (Yip et al., 1972, Biochem. J. 127:893-899). Arginine is used, by way of example, in the synthesis of nitric oxide. In macrophages, arginase activity is reciprocally coordinated with the activity of the enzyme, nitric oxide synthase. Reciprocal coordination of the activities of arginase and nitric oxide (NO) synthase modulates NO-dependent cytotoxicity (Corraliza et al., 1995, Biochem. Biophys. Res. Commun. 206:667-673; Daghigh et al., 1994, Biochem. Biophys. Res. Commun. 202:174-180; Chnais et al., 1993, Biochem. Biophys. Res. Commun. 196:1558-1565; Klatt et al., 1993, J. Biol. Chem. 268:14781-14787; Keller et al., 1991, Cell. Immunol. 134:249-256; Albina et al., 1995, J. Immunol. 155:4391-4396).

Web site: http://appft1.uspto.gov/netahtml/PTO/search-bool.html

- **Compositions and methods for the diagnosis and treatment of psychogenic erectile dysfunction**

  Inventor(s): Mann, Maria A.; (Glendale, AZ), Mann, Morris; (Glendale, AZ)

  Correspondence: The Halvorson Law Firm; Ste 1; 405 W. Southern Ave.; Tempe; AZ; 85282; US

  Patent Application Number: 20030036514

  Date filed: July 18, 2002

  Abstract: The present invention is directed to a group of linear and cyclic peptides having the structures:Ac-Nle-Asp-His-D-Phe-Cl-Arg-Trp-Lys-NH.sub.2;Ac-Nle-Asp-His-D-Phe-Cl-Arg-Trp-Lys-NH.sub.2;Ac-Nle-Asp-His-D-Phe-Cl-Arg-Trp-Lys-Gly-NH.sub.2;Ac-Nle-Asp-His-D-Phe-Cl-Arg-Trp-Lys-Gly-Pro-NH.sub.2;Ac-Ser-Tyr-Ser-Nle-Asp-His-D-Phe-Cl-Arg-Trp-Lys-NH.sub.2;Ac-Tyr-Ser-Nle-Asp-His-D-Phe-Cl-Arg-Trp-Lys-NH.sub.2;   andAc-Ser-Nle-Asp-His-D-Phe-Cl-Arg-Trp-Lys-NH.sub.2.These peptides, when systemically administered to animals, will bring about a sexual response and are thus useful for the diagnosis and treatment of psychogenic sexual dysfunction in the male.

  Excerpt(s): This application claims the benefit of U.S. Provisional Application No. 60/312,358, filed on Aug. 15, 2001. The present invention is related to the field erectogenic compositions. More specifically, the present invention is related to specific peptide compositions for the treatment of **erectile dysfunction.** Erectile dysfunction, or impotence, is probably the most common male sexual symptom encountered by the practicing physician, and an improved understanding of the problem and new approaches to diagnosis and treatment have greatly increased the chances of helping patients with this problem.

  Web site: http://appft1.uspto.gov/netahtml/PTO/search-bool.html

- **Cynomoriaceae extract and use in treating erectile dysfunction**

  Inventor(s): Huang, Yaoge; (Saskatoon, CA), Wang, Rui; (Saskatoon, CA), Zhao, Weimin; (Nepean, CA)

  Correspondence: GREENLEE WINNER AND SULLIVAN P C; 5370 MANHATTAN CIRCLE; SUITE 201; BOULDER; CO; 80303; US

  Patent Application Number: 20030157208

  Date filed: December 20, 2002

  Abstract: An extract from the herb of the family Cynomoriaceae, preferably Cynomorium songaricum Rupr, which is also commonly known as Suo Yang in Chinese

Medicine, has been prepared and found to have medicinal properties. The extract is preferably prepared from stems of the plant, and is most preferably extracted with an solvent including butanol, herein abbreviated as "BuSY". The extract is shown to have efficacy in the treatment of **erectile dysfunction** and the enhancement of male sexual health in vertebrates. A pharmaceutical preparation of this extract can be formulated with a pharmaceutically acceptable carrier to treat **erectile dysfunction** in host animals. The components of the nutraceutical extract can be combined in differing combinations to enhance and/or improve male sexual health.

Excerpt(s): This application claims priority from U.S. Provisional Patent Application No. 60/341,210, filed Dec. 20, 2001. To the extent that it is consistent herewith, the aforementioned application is incorporated herein by reference. The present invention relates to a plant extract prepared from the family of Cynomoriaceae such as Cynomorium songaricum Rupr. and its use in the treatment of **erectile dysfunction** or impotence in host animals. Erectile dysfunction or ED (also called impotence) affects over 30 million men, about half of all men aged between 40 to 70 years, to some degree in the United States, and much more in the world. ED is the inability for a man to get and/or keep an erection sufficient for sexual activity. When a man is sexually aroused, the arteries in the penis relax and widen, allowing more blood to flow into the penis. As the arteries in the penis expand and harden, the veins that normally carry blood away from the penis become compressed, restricting the blood flow out of the penis. With more blood flowing in and less flowing out, the penis enlarges, resulting in an erection. In men with ED, the chemical reactions responsible for erections do not take place as usual, so the arteries don't expand and the penis cannot fill with blood. The majority of cases of ED are associated with physical conditions, not just age. ED is a treatable condition in most men who have it.

Web site: http://appft1.uspto.gov/netahtml/PTO/search-bool.html

- **Daily treatment for erectile dysfunction using a PDE5 inhibitor**

Inventor(s): Ferguson, Kenneth M.; (Bothell, WA), Tejada, Inigo Saenz de; (Madrid, ES), Whitaker, John S.; (Woodinville, WA)

Correspondence: MARSHALL, GERSTEIN & BORUN; 6300 SEARS TOWER; 233 SOUTH WACKER; CHICAGO; IL; 60606-6357; US

Patent Application Number: 20030144296

Date filed: January 14, 2003

Abstract: The present invention relates to phosphodiesterase (PDE) enzyme inhibitors and to their use in pharmaceutical articles of manufacture. In particular, the present invention relates to potent inhibitors of cyclic guanosine 3',5'-monophosphate specific phosphodiesterase type 5 (PDE5) that when incorporated into a pharmaceutical product at about 1 to about 10 mg unit dosage are useful for the treatment of sexual dysfunction by daily administration of the PDE5 inhibitor. The articles of manufacture described herein are characterized by PDE5 inhibition, and accordingly, provide a benefit in therapeutic areas where inhibition of PDE5 is desired, especially **erectile dysfunction,** with minimization or elimination of adverse side effects resulting from inhibition of other phosphodiesterase enzymes and with an improvement of vascular conditioning.

Excerpt(s): This application is a continuation-in-part of U.S. application Ser. No. 09/558,911, filed Apr. 26, 2000, which claims the benefit of provisional patent application Serial No. 60/132,036, filed Apr. 30, 1999. The biochemical, physiological, and clinical effects of cyclic guanosine 3',5'-monophosphate specific phosphodiesterase (cGMP-specific PDE) inhibitors suggest their utility in a variety of disease states in which modulation of smooth muscle, renal, hemostatic, inflammatory, and/or endocrine function is desired. Type 5 cGMP-specific phosphodiesterase (PDE5) is the major cGMP hydrolyzing enzyme in vascular smooth muscle, and its expression in penile corpus cavernosum has been reported (Taher et al., J. Urol., 149:285A (1993)). Thus, PDE5 is an attractive target in the treatment of sexual dysfunction (Murray, DN&P 6(3):150-56 (1993)).

Web site: http://appft1.uspto.gov/netahtml/PTO/search-bool.html

- **Delivery of erectile dysfunction drugs through an inhalation route**

Inventor(s): Rabinowitz, Joshua D.; (Mountain View, CA), Zaffaroni, Alejandro C.; (Atherton, CA)

Correspondence: Richard R. Eckman; Morrison & Foerster LLP; 755 Page Mill Road; Palo Alto; CA; 94304-1018; US

Patent Application Number: 20030017120

Date filed: May 22, 2002

Abstract: The present invention relates to the delivery of **erectile dysfunction** drugs through an inhalation route. Specifically, it relates to aerosols containing **erectile dysfunction** drugs that are used in inhalation therapy. In a composition aspect of the present invention, the aerosol comprises particles comprising at least 5 percent by weight of an **erectile dysfunction** drug. In a method aspect of the present invention, an **erectile dysfunction** drug is delivered to a mammal through an inhalation route. The method comprises: a) heating a composition, wherein the composition comprises at least 5 percent by weight of an **erectile dysfunction** drug, to form a vapor; and, b) allowing the vapor to cool, thereby forming a condensation aerosol comprising particles, which is inhaled by the mammal. In a kit aspect of the present invention, a kit for delivering an **erectile dysfunction** drug through an inhalation route to a mammal is provided which comprises: a) a composition comprising at least 5 percent by weight of an **erectile dysfunction** drug; and, b) a device that forms an **erectile dysfunction** drug aerosol from the composition, for inhalation by the mammal.

Excerpt(s): This application claims priority to U.S. provisional application Ser. No. 60/294,203 entitled "Thermal Vapor Delivery of Drugs," filed May. 24, 2001, Rabinowitz and Zaffaroni, the entire disclosure of which is hereby incorporated by reference. This application further claims priority to U.S. provisional application Ser. No. 60/317,479 entitled "Aerosol Drug Delivery," filed Sept. 5, 2001, Rabinowitz and Zaffaroni, the entire disclosure of which is hereby incorporated by reference. The present invention relates to the delivery of **erectile dysfunction** drugs through an inhalation route. Specifically, it relates to aerosols containing **erectile dysfunction** drugs that are used in inhalation therapy. There are a number of compositions currently marketed for the treatment of **erectile dysfunction**. The compositions contain at least one active ingredient that provides for observed therapeutic effects. Among the active ingredients given in such **erectile dysfunction** compositions are sildenafil, tadalafil and vardenafil.

Web site: http://appft1.uspto.gov/netahtml/PTO/search-bool.html

- **High level insect expression of rage proteins**

Inventor(s): Harris, Robert B.; (Midlothian, VA), Shahbaz, Manouchehr; (Escondido, CA), Shen, Jane M.; (Winston-Salem, NC)

Correspondence: Cynthia B. Rothschild, Esq.; Kilpatrick Stockton LLP; 1001 West Fourth Street; Winston-Salem; NC; 27101; US

Patent Application Number: 20030166063

Date filed: March 5, 2002

Abstract: The present invention provides a method for high level expression of human sRAGE using insect cell culture. In an embodiment, the method comprises (a) subcloning a nucleotide sequence encoding RAGE or a fragment thereof into a virus; (b) preparing a high-titer stock of recombinant virus; and (c) infecting host cells with the high-titer recombinant virus under conditions such that pre-determined levels of RAGE or a fragment thereof is produced, wherein said pre-determined levels of RAGE are at least 25 mg recombinant protein per liter of culture. The invention comprises use of sRAGE prepared by the methods of the invention for treatment of AGE-related syndromes including complications associated with atherosclerosis, diabetes, kidney failure, systemic lupus nephritis or inflammatory lupus nephritis, amyloidoses, Alzheimer's disease, cancer, inflammation, and **erectile dysfunction.**

Excerpt(s): This application claims priority to U.S. Provisional Application Serial No. 60/273,418, filed Mar. 5, 2001. The disclosure of U.S. Provisional Application Serial No. 60/273,418 is hereby incorporated by reference in its entirety. The invention relates to methods for high level expression of recombinant forms of the Receptor for Advanced Glycated Endproducts (RAGE). More particularly, the present invention describes high level expression of sRAGE in insect cells. Incubation of proteins or lipids with aldose sugars results in nonenzymatic glycation and oxidation of amino groups on proteins to form Amadori adducts. Over time, the adducts undergo additional rearrangements, dehydrations, and cross-linking with other proteins to form complexes known as Advanced Glycosylation End Products (AGEs). Factors which promote formation of AGEs included delayed protein turnover (e.g. as in amyloidoses), accumulation of macromolecules having high lysine content, and high blood glucose levels (e.g. as in diabetes) (Hori et al., J. Biol. Chem. 270: 25752-761, (1995)). AGEs have been implicated in a variety of disorders including complications associated with diabetes and normal aging.

Web site: http://appft1.uspto.gov/netahtml/PTO/search-bool.html

- **Individualization of therapy with erectile dysfunction agents**

Inventor(s): Leyland-Jones, Brian; (Miami, FL)

Correspondence: HAMILTON, BROOK, SMITH & REYNOLDS, P.C.; 530 VIRGINIA ROAD; P.O. BOX 9133; CONCORD; MA; 01742-9133; US

Patent Application Number: 20030073133

Date filed: April 26, 2002

Abstract: The invention relates to the individualization of therapy on the basis of a phenotypic profile of an individual. More specifically, the present invention relates to the use of metabolic phenotyping for the individualization of treatment with ED agents.

Excerpt(s): This application is a new application which claims the benefit of U.S. Provisional Application No. 60/286,336, filed on Apr. 26, 2001. The entire teachings of the above application is incorporated herein by reference. The invention relates to a system and method for individualization of therapy with Erectile Disfunction (ED) agents. More specifically, the present invention relates to the use of metabolic phenotyping in individualizing treatment with ED agents. For the majority of drugs (or xenobiotics) administered to humans, their fate is to be metabolized in the liver, into a form less toxic and lipophilic with their subsequent excretion in the urine. Their metabolism involves two systems (Phase I and Phase II) which act consecutively: Phase I enzymes include the cytochrome P450 system which includes at least 20 enzymes catalyzing oxidation reactions as well as carboxylesterase, amindases, epoxide hydrolase, quinine reductase, alcohol and aldehyde dehydrogenase, xanthine oxidase and flavin-containing monooxygenase. These enzymes are localized in the microsomal fraction. Phase II enzymes include the conjugation system which involves at least 5 enzymes including, N-acetyltransferases (NAT), UDP-glucoronyltransferases (UGT), sulfotransferases (SUT), and glutathione-S-transferases (GST). A detailed description of the complex human drug metabolizing systems is provided in Kumar and Surapaneni (Medicinal Res. Rev. (2001) 21(5):397-411) and patent application WO 01/59127 A2.

Web site: http://appft1.uspto.gov/netahtml/PTO/search-bool.html

- **Intranasal formulations for treating sexual disorders**

  Inventor(s): Billotte, Anne; (Sandwich, GB), Dunn, Peter James; (Sandwich, GB), Henry, Brian Thomas; (Sandwich, GB), Marshall, Peter Vallance; (Sandwich, GB), Woods, Joanna Jayne; (Sandwich, GB)

  Correspondence: CONNOLLY BOVE LODGE & HUTZ, LLP; 1220 N MARKET STREET; P O BOX 2207; WILMINGTON; DE; 19899

  Patent Application Number: 20030158206

  Date filed: March 14, 2003

  Abstract: Intranasal formulations of sildenafil mesylate for the treatment of male **erectile dysfunction** or female sexual disorders.

  Excerpt(s): This invention relates to intranasal formulations of cyclic guanosine 3',5'-monophosphate phosphodiesterase type five (cGMP PDE5) inhibitors, including in particular the compound sildenafil, for the treatment of sexual disorders such as impotence. The invention also includes sildenafil mesylate and intranasal formulations thereof and its use in treating sexual disorders. According to the specification of our International patent application WO94/28902 we have discovered that compounds which are inhibitors of the cGMP PDE5 enzyme are potent and effective compounds for the treatment of male **erectile dysfunction** (MED, impotence) and for female sexual disorders. This discovery led to the development of the compound sildenafil (5-[2-ethoxy-5-(4-methylpiperazin-1-ylsulphonyl)pheny-   1]-1,6-dihydro-1-methyl-3-propylpyrazolo[4,3-d]pyrimidin-7-one) (VIAGRA.TM.) which has proved to be outstandingly successful as the first orally effective treatment for MED. WO98/53819 which was published on Dec. 3, 1998 (after the priority date of the present invention) claims intranasal compositions of cGMP phosphodiesterase inhibitors, including sildenafil, for treating **erectile dysfunction.** The intranasal route has previously been employed as a mode of administration for certain pharmaceutical products. The absorption rate of an agent from the nasal cavity is dependent on a number of variables; however two key factors are the surface area available for absorption and the local blood flow of the nasal cavity. The available surface area for absorption is dictated by the nasal cavity airflow resistance which is under the control of a dense capillary bed of erectile carvernous tissue in the nasal cavity. Vasodilation of these tissues leads to nasal congestion or rhinitis, for example, which increases resistance to air flow and reduces the available surface area for drug absorption. However, vasodilation can also increase bloodflow and enhance absorption by increasing the rate of remove of the drug from the site of absorption.

Web site: http://appft1.uspto.gov/netahtml/PTO/search-bool.html

- **L-arginine and phosphodiesterase (PDE) inhibitor synergism**

Inventor(s): Wallace, Arthur W.; (San Rafael, CA)

Correspondence: QUINE INTELLECTUAL PROPERTY LAW GROUP, P.C.; P O BOX 458; ALAMEDA; CA; 94501; US

Patent Application Number: 20030166661

Date filed: September 23, 2002

Abstract: This invention pertains to the discovery that L-arginine and type V phosphodiesterases act synergistically to inhibit vasospasm and/or to induce vasodilation. Methods are provided using combinations of L-arginine and type V phosphodiesterase inhibitors in the treatment of cardiac pathologies and/or the treatment of **erectile dysfunction.**

Excerpt(s): This invention was made with Government support by the Veteran's Administration. The Government of the United States of America may have certain rights in this invention. This invention relates the regulation of vascular hemodynamics in various pathologies. In particular this invention pertains to the discovery that L-arginine and type V phosphodiesterases act synergistically to inhibit vasospasm and/or to induce vasodilation. Impotence (erectile dysfunction) is the consistent inability to achieve or sustain an erection of sufficient rigidity for sexual intercourse. It has recently been estimated that approximately 10 million American men are impotent (Shabsigh et al. (1988) Urology 32: 83-90; Furlow (1985) Med Aspects Hum. Sex. 19:13-16). Impotence is recognized to be an age-dependent disorder, with an incidence of 1.9 percent at 40 years of age and 25 percent at 65 years of age (Kinsey et al. (1948) pages 218-262 in Sexual Behavior in the Human Male; A. C. Kinsey et al., eds., Philadelphia, Pa.: W. B. Saunders). In 1985 in the United States, impotence accounted for more than several hundred thousand outpatient visits to physicians Rational Center for Health Statistics (National Hospital Discharge Survey, 1985, Bethesda, Md., Department of Health and Human Services, 1989 DES publication no. 87-1751). Depending on the nature and cause of the problem, treatments include psychosexual therapy, hormonal therapy, administration of vasodilators such as nitroglycerin and.alpha.-adrenergic blocking agents (".alpha.-blockers-"), oral administration of other pharmaceutical agents, vascular surgery, implanted penile prostheses, vacuum constriction devices and external aids such as penile splints to support the penis or penile constricting rings to alter the flow of blood through the penis.

Web site: http://appft1.uspto.gov/netahtml/PTO/search-bool.html

- **Male sexual impotence treatment apparatus**

Inventor(s): Forsell, Peter; (Zug, SE)

Correspondence: NIXON & VANDERHYE, PC; 1100 N GLEBE ROAD; 8TH FLOOR; ARLINGTON; VA; 22201-4714; US

Patent Application Number: 20030135089

Date filed: November 25, 2002

Abstract: A **male sexual impotence** treatment apparatus comprises an adjustable restriction device (234) implanted in an impotent patient and engaging the corpora cavernosa or crura or the prolongation thereof (244). An implanted adjustment device is adapted to adjust the restriction device to temporarily contract the corpora cavernosa, in order to restrict the blood flow leaving the penis when the patient desires to achieve erection. An implanted powered hydraulic operation device (246) operates the adjustment device.

Excerpt(s): The present invention relates to a **male sexual impotence** treatment apparatus comprising an adjustable restriction device implantable in a male impotent patient for engaging the corpora cavernosa or crura or the prolongations thereof of the patient's penile tissue. An implantable adjustment device is provided for adjusting the restriction device to temporarily contract the corpora cavernosa or crura or the prolongations thereof to restrict the blood flow leaving the penis, and an implantable operation device is provided for operating the adjustment device. Male sexual impotence is a widespread problem. Many different solutions to this problem have been tried. A main solution currently practised and disclosed in for instance U.S. Pat. Nos. 5,437,605 and 4,841,461 is to implant a hydraulic inflatable/contractable silicon prosthesis in the cavities of the corpora cavernosa of the patient's penis. In fluid connection with this prosthesis is a reservoir implanted in the scrotum. By manual pumping action the prosthesis is filled with fluid from the reservoir to effect errect penile condition or is emptied of fluid, which returns to the reservoir, to effect flaccid penile condition. However, there are several more or less severe disadvantages of this main solution. Above all, the penis is more or less damaged by the operation and it is practically impossible to reverse the operation. Another disadvantage is that rather strong forces act against this implanted prosthesis resulting in a significant risk of the prosthesis being broken. Another solution to achieve erection is to restrict the blood flow leaving the penis. For example, U.S. Pat. No. 4,829,990 discloses two hydraulically operated inflatable cuffs wrapped around the respective crura. A disadvantage of such a solution is that it involves complicated surgery. Another example on this solution is U.S. Pat. No. 4,828,544, which discloses an artificial fistula system surgically implanted and providing a primary fistula between the femoral artery and the femoral vein and a secondary fistula for leading blood from the the primary fistula to the penis. An inflatable balloon engages the primary fistula between the secondary fistula and the vein. The balloon is in fluid connection with a manually compressible reservoir implanted in the scrotum. Again, implantation of this artifical fistula system requires delicate surgery.

Web site: http://appft1.uspto.gov/netahtml/PTO/search-bool.html

- **Method for treating nerve injury caused as a result of surgery**

Inventor(s): Burnett, Arthur L.; (Baltimore, MD), Snyder, Solomon; (Baltimore, MD), Steiner, Joseph P.; (Mount Airy, MD)

Correspondence: GUILFORD PHARMACEUTICALS C/O; FOLEY & LARDNER; 3000 K STREET, NW; WASHINGTON; DC; 20007-5143; US

Patent Application Number: 20030203890

Date filed: May 29, 2002

Abstract: The present invention relates generally to methods for treating or preventing nerve injury in a warm-blooded animal caused as a consequence of surgery by administering neurotrophic compounds described below. The invention relates more specifically to methods for treating or preventing nerve injury caused as a consequence of prostate surgery as well as **erectile dysfunction.**

Excerpt(s): The invention relates generally to methods for treating nerve injury caused as a consequence of surgery. The present invention relates more specifically to methods for treating nerve injury caused as a consequence of prostate surgery, or for methods of neuroprotection of penile innervation, by administering a neurotrophic compound to a patient in need thereof. The peptidyl-prolyl isomerases ("PPIases") are a family of ubiquitous enzymes which catalyze the interconversion of cis and trans amide bond rotamers adjacent to proline residues in peptide substrates. See, for example, Galat, A., Eur. J. Biochem. (1993) 216:689-707 and Kay, J. E., Biochem. J. (1996) 314:361-385. The PPIases have been referred to as "immunophilins" because of their interaction with certain immunosuppressant drugs. Schreiber, S. L., Science (1991) 251:283-287; Rosen, M. K. and Schreiber, S. L., Angew. Chem. Intl. Ed. Engi. (1992) 31:384-400. The PPIase, cyclophilin A, was found to be the intracellular protein target for the potent immunosuppressant drug cyclosporin A. Subsequently, the structurally unrelated macrolide immunosuppressant FK506 was discovered to bind to a different PPIase enzyme which was named FK506-binding protein, or FKBP. Rapamycin, another macrolide drug which is a structural analogue of FK506, also interacts with FKBP.

Web site: http://appft1.uspto.gov/netahtml/PTO/search-bool.html

- **Methods and compositions for preventing and treating male erectile dysfunction and female sexual arousal disorder**

Inventor(s): Carroll, Peter; (San Francisco, CA), Kan, Yuet W.; (San Francisco, CA), Lin, Ching-Shwun; (San Mateo, CA), Lue, Tom F.; (Hillsborough, CA)

Correspondence: Peng Chen; Morrison & Foerster LLP; Suite 500; 3811 Valley Centre Drive; San Diego; CA; 92130-2332; US

Patent Application Number: 20030096747

Date filed: May 23, 2002

Abstract: The invention provides a method for preventing or treating male **erectile dysfunction** or female sexual arousal disorder by administering an effective amount of one or more factors from a group of factors including vascular endothelial growth factor, brain-derived neurotrophic factor, basic fibroblast growth factor, neurotrophin-3, neurotrophin-4, or angiopoietin-1, wherein the factor is a full length protein or a nucleic acid encoding the factor, or a functional derivative or fragment thereof, or an agent that enhances production and/or male erection or female sexual arousal stimulating function of the factor(s). Combinations, kits, and combinatorial methods are also provided.

Excerpt(s): This invention relates generally to the field of urology. In particular, the invention provides a method for preventing or treating male **erectile dysfunction** or female sexual arousal disorder in a mammal in need of such treatment, comprising administering an effective amount of a factor from a group of factors including vascular endothelial growth factor (VEGF), brain-derived neurotrophic factor (BDNF), basic fibroblast growth factor (bFGF), platelet-derived growth factor (PDGF), neurotrophin-3 (NT-3), neurotrophin-4 (NT-4), or angiopoietin-1 (Ang-1), wherein the factor is a full length protein or a functional derivative or fragment thereof, or a nucleic acid encoding said factor or functional derivative or fragment thereof, or an agent that enhances production and/or male erection or female sexual arousal stimulating function of the factor, thereby preventing or treating male **erectile dysfunction** or female sexual arousal disorder in the mammal. Combinations, kits, and combinatorial methods for preventing or treating male **erectile dysfunction** or female sexual arousal disorder are also provided. VEGF is a family of proteins that were discovered on the basis of their ability to stimulate VEC (vascular endothelial cell) growth (angiogenesis). It now comprises five members, namely, VEGF-A, VEGF-B, VEGF-C, VEGF-D, and PLGF (placenta growth factor) that are encoded from distinct genes. Achen, et al., Proc. Nat'l. Acad. Sci. USA, 95: 548 (1998), Joukov, et al., EMBO J., 15: 1571 (1996), Maglione, et al., Oncogene, 8: 925 (1993), Olofsson, et al., Proc. Nat'l. Acad. Sci. USA, 93: 2576 (1996), Yamada, et al., Genomics, 42: 483 (1997). Each of the five members in turn comprises two or more isoforms that arise by the splicing of their respective pre-mRNAs. For example, the VEGF-A family includes VEGF.sub.206, VEGF.sub.189, VEGF.sub.83, VEGF.sub.165, VEGF.sub.145, VEGF.sub.121, and VEGF.sub.111. Anthony, et al., Placenta, 15: 557 (1994), Neufeld, et al., FASEB J., 13: 9 (1999), Lei, et al., Biochim. Biophys. Acta, 1443: 400 (1998), Jingjing, et al., Ophthamol. Vis. Sci., 40: 752 (1999), Cheung, et al., Am. J. Obstet. Gynecol., 173: 753 (1995), Burchardt, et al., Biol. Reprod., 60: 398 (1999). Among all VEGF proteins and isoforms, VEGF.sub.165 is by far the most frequently used form of VEGF both in basic and clinical studies. It has been shown that, among different vascular cell types (endothelial, smooth muscle cells (SMC), and fibroblasts), SMC is the principal source for the secreted VEGF. Pueyo, et al., Exp. Cell Res., 238: 354 (1998). Expression of VEGF in SMC is upregulated by multiple factors including phorbol esters (Tischer, et al., J. Biol. Chem., 266: 11947 (1991)), cAMP (Claffey, et al., J. Biol. Chem., 267: 16317 (1992)), and hypoxia (Goldberg, et al., J. Biol. Chem., 269: 4355 (1994), Shweiki, et al., Proc. Nat'l Acad. Sci. USA, 92: 768 (1995)). The secreted VEGF acts on VEC principally through two different cell surface receptors, VEGFR-1 and VEGFR-2. Activation of VEGFR-1 results in VEC migration, while activation of VEGFR-2 VEC migration and proliferation. Waltenberger, et al., J. Biol. Chem., 269: 26988 (1994), Neufeld, et al., FASEB J., 13: 9 (1999), Ortega, et al., Front. Biosci., 4: D141 (1999). Although VEGFR-1 and VEGFR-2 have long been considered endothelium-specific, they have both been detected in human uterine and bovine aorta SMC. Grosskreutz, et al., Microvasc. Res., 58: 128 (1999), Brown, et al., Lab. Invest., 76: 254 (1997). Cultured uterine SMC responded to VEGF in the form of cell proliferation and cultured aorta SMC cell migration. Cultured human colon SMC, however, did not express VEGF receptors, nor did they respond to VEGF treatment. Brown, et al., Lab. Invest., 76: 254 (1997).

Web site: http://appft1.uspto.gov/netahtml/PTO/search-bool.html

- **Methods and compositions for treatment of erectile dysfunction**

  Inventor(s): Ha, Quoc Huan; (Irvine, CA), Sallis, Ramsey; (St. Peters, AU)

  Correspondence: Gregory A. Nelson; AKERMAN SENTERFITT; P.O. BOX 3188; WEST PALM BEACH; FL; 33402-3188; US

  Patent Application Number: 20030144318

  Date filed: January 24, 2003

  Abstract: Disclosed are methods and compositions for treatment of male sexual dysfunction. A method of treating male sexual dysfunction includes administering a pharmaceutical composition effective to cause said male to sustain an erection. The composition is formulated based on diagnostic assessment and an individualized formulation test step. Also within the invention is a method of treating male sexual dysfunction in a population of subjects. The invention further provides kits for treatment of male **erectile dysfunction.**

  Excerpt(s): This application claims priority from U.S. Provisional Application Serial No. 60/351,634 filed Jan. 25, 2002. The foregoing is herein incorporated by reference. This invention relates generally to the fields of medicine and urology. More particularly, the invention relates to methods and compositions for treatment of male **erectile dysfunction.** Sexual dysfunction in both males and females has received a significant amount of popular attention with the greater concerns directed to the particular male problems of erectile capacity and penetration ability. Male sexual dysfunction associated with impotence is generally defined as the inability to attain or sustain an erection satisfactory for normal coitus. Prevalence of erectile problems, including premature ejaculation, has been estimated to be surprisingly high, perhaps as much as 45% worldwide. This is a particular concern among the over-50 male population in the United States, where estimates of impotency range from 18 to 75% for this age group.

  Web site: http://appft1.uspto.gov/netahtml/PTO/search-bool.html

- **Methods of treating or preventing erectile dysfunction**

  Inventor(s): Fang, Qun K.; (Wellesley, MA), Jerussi, Thomas P.; (Framingham, MA), Senanayake, Chrisantha H.; (Shrewsbury, MA)

  Correspondence: PENNIE & EDMONDS LLP; 1667 K STREET NW; SUITE 1000; WASHINGTON; DC; 20006

  Patent Application Number: 20030195261

  Date filed: March 25, 2003

  Abstract: Methods are disclosed for the treatment and prevention of disorders and conditions including, but are not limited to, **erectile dysfunction,** affective disorders, weight gain, cerebral functional disorders, pain, obsessive-compulsive disorder, substance abuse, chronic disorders, anxiety, eating disorders, migraines, and incontinence. The methods comprise the administration of a dopamine reuptake inhibitor and optionally an additional pharmacologically active compound. Pharmaceutical compositions and dosage forms are also disclosed that comprise a dopamine reuptake inhibitor and optionally an additional pharmacologically active compound. Preferred dopamine reuptake inhibitors are racemic or optically pure sibutrarnine metabolites and pharmaceutically acceptable salts, solvates, and clathrates thereof. Preferred additional pharmacologically active compounds include drugs that affect the central nervous system, such as 5-HT.sub.3 antagonists.

Excerpt(s): This application claims the benefit of U.S. Provisional Application No. 60/097,665, filed Aug. 24, 1998, and U.S. Provisional Application No. 60/099,306, filed Sep. 2, 1998, both of which are incorporated herein in their entireties by reference. The invention relates to methods of using, and compositions comprising, dopamine reuptake inhibitors and, in particular, racemic and optically pure metabolites of sibutramine. Sibutramine, chemically named [N-1-[1-(4-chlorophenyl)cyclobutyl]-3- -methylbutyl]-N,N-dimethylamine, is a neuronal monoamine reuptake inhibitor which was originally disclosed in U.S. Pat. Nos. 4,746,680 and 4,806,570. Sibutramine inhibits the reuptake of norepinephrine and, to a lesser extent, serotonin and dopamine. See, e.g., Buckett et al., Prog. Neuro-psychopharm. & Biol. Psychiat., 12:575-584, 1988; King et al., J. Clin. Pharm., 26:607-611 (1989).

Web site: http://appft1.uspto.gov/netahtml/PTO/search-bool.html

- **Nitric oxide-producing hydrogel materials**

Inventor(s): Masters, Kristyn Simcha; (Northglenn, CO), West, Jennifer L; (Pearland, TX)

Correspondence: JOHN S. PRATT, ESQ; KILPATRICK STOCKTON, LLP; 1100 PEACHTREE STREET; SUITE 2800; ATLANTA; GA; 30309; US

Patent Application Number: 20030012816

Date filed: May 17, 2002

Abstract: Hydrogels releasing or producing NO, most preferably polymerizable biodegradable hydrogels capable of releasing physiological amounts of NO for prolonged periods of time, are applied to sites on or in a patient in need of treatment thereof for disorders such as restenosis, thrombosis, asthma, wound healing, arthritis, penile **erectile dysfunction** or other conditions where NO plays a significant role. The polymeric materials can be formed into films, coatings, or microparticles for application to medical devices, such as stents, vascular grafts and catheters. The polymeric materials can also be applied directly to biological tissues and can be polymerized in situ. The hydrogels are formed of macromers, which preferably include biodegradable regions, and have bound thereto groups that are released in situ to elevate or otherwise modulate NO levels at the site where treatment is needed. The macromers can form a homo or hetero-dispersion or solution, which is polymerized to form a hydrogel material, that in the latter case can be a semi-interpenetrating network or interpenetrating network. Compounds to be released can be physically entrapped, covalently or ionically bound to macromer, or actually form a part of the polymeric material. The hydrogel can be formed by ionic and/or covalent crosslinking. Other active agents, including therapeutic, prophylactic, or diagnostic agents, can also be included within the polymeric material.

Excerpt(s): The present invention relates to polymerizable hydrogel materials that produce physiologically relevant amounts of nitric oxide (NO). Endothelial cells, normally present as a monolayer in the intimal layer of the arterial wall, are believed to play an important role in the regulation of smooth muscle cell (SMC) proliferation in vivo. Endothelial cells are seriously disrupted by most forms of vascular injury, including that caused by percutaneous transluminal coronary angioplasty and similar procedures. Approximately 35-50% of patients treated by percutaneous transluminal coronary angioplasty experience clinically significant renarrowing of the artery, or restenosis, within six months of the initial treatment. Restenosis is due, at least in part, to migration and proliferation of smooth muscle cells in the arterial wall along with increases in secretion of matrix proteins to form an obstructive neointimal layer within the arterial wall. Similar issues limit the performance of vascular grafts. The processes that regulate arterial wound healing following vascular injury, such as that caused by angioplasty, are as yet poorly understood, but are believed to involve a complex cascade of blood and vessel wall-derived factors. Numerous factors that stimulate intimal thickening and restenosis have been identified through administration of exogenous proteins, genetic alteration of cells, or through the blockade of certain signals using antibodies or other specific growth factor inhibitors. These smooth muscle cell mitogens and chemoattractants derive from both the blood or thrombus formation and from the vessel wall itself. Endothelial cells produce a number of substances known to down-regulate smooth muscle cell proliferation, including heparin sulfate, prostacyclin (PG12), and NO.

Web site: http://appft1.uspto.gov/netahtml/PTO/search-bool.html

- **Non-invasive erectile dysfunction aid**

Inventor(s): Lanton, Ralph H. JR.; (Ferguson, MO)

Correspondence: Gregory P. Gadson, Esq.; 19375 Amber Way; Noblesville; IN; 46060; US

Patent Application Number: 20030136415

Date filed: January 19, 2002

Abstract: A simple, non-invasive artificial erection apparatus for **erectile dysfunction** sufferers has a semi-rigid tube with an inflatable bladder coupled to its inside wall. The apparatus also contains a valve and a pump for inflating the bladder through the valve. When inflated, the bladder forms a contracting lumen that provides pressure around the penile shaft to provide the artificial erection. The valve allows the bladder to substantially deflate the bladder for removal of the apparatus, or incrementally deflate to adjust the pressure of the bladder for comfort during intercourse. Other aspects of the present invention include, inter alia, peristaltic inflation of the bladder to help congregate blood around the penile end, the ability to adjust the length of the apparatus by unrolling (or re-rolling) the distal end of the apparatus, which integrates the tube and bladder.

Excerpt(s): The present invention generally relates to non-pharmacological therapies for **erectile dysfunction,** which allow the artificial achievement or maintenance of erections. Erectile dysfunction can be broadly defined as the difficulty to, or the inability to, achieve or maintain a penile erection. While there is no age floor, **erectile dysfunction** is especially prevalent in older men who may still have an interest in sexual intercourse. Prior art remedies—both short-term and long-term-have met with only limited success, and have serious drawbacks.

Web site: http://appft1.uspto.gov/netahtml/PTO/search-bool.html

- **Non-invasive, quantitative somatosensory method for the evaluation of erectile dysfunction**

  Inventor(s): Arezzo, Joseph; (Mahwah, NJ), Bleustein, Clifford B.; (New York, NY), Melman, Arnold; (Ardsley, NY)

  Correspondence: DICKSTEIN SHAPIRO MORIN & OSHINSKY LLP; 1177 AVENUE OF THE AMERICAS; NEW YORK; NY; 10038-2714; US

  Patent Application Number: 20030105413

  Date filed: September 23, 2002

Abstract: A non-invasive quantitative somatosensory method is provided for evaluating erectile dysfunctions and involves the applications to the glans penis of different temperatures in increments of about 1.degree. C. until the patient can correctly identify which temperature starting at an ambient temperature was warmer for at least two consecutive times. The method of this invention provides a relatively simple procedure to assess a patient's neurological response to therapies. Incremental decreases in temperature can also be used to assess a patients's neurological response. The method of this invention can also be supplemented, if desired, by determination of the spatial perception threshold and/or the application of pressure, i.e., the sensitivity to touch determination to provide a two-point determination.

  Excerpt(s): This invention relates to a simple non-invasive method for the evaluation of **erectile dysfunction** (ED). The results obtained can be useful to assess a patient's neurological response to therapies. Erectile dysfunction (ED) is defined as the inability to achieve or maintain an erection sufficient for satisfactory sexual performance. The prevalence in United States is 10 to 20 million men. The male erectile response is a neurovascular event reliant on the complex interaction between neurological and vascular responses. **Erectile dysfunction** is multifactoral and has been typically classified by the primary presumed cause: vasculogenic, psychogenic, neurogenic, and endocrinologic disease. Any condition or injury that impairs the transmission of impulses along the psychogenic or reflexogenic neurological pathway, may be associated with neurogenic **erectile dysfunction.** The penis is innervated by the dorsal penile and perineal nerves. These nerves are a continuation of sympathetic and parasympathetic autonomic nerves as well as sensory and motor somatic nerves. The somatic sensory system is responsible for the specialize structures that transmit information about the external environment. There are four major classes of somatic sensation: pain, temperature, position sense, and touch-pressure sensation. These stimuli are transmitted in the autonomic nervous system through both large (.alpha. and.beta.) and small (.delta. and C) caliber nerves.

  Web site: http://appft1.uspto.gov/netahtml/PTO/search-bool.html

- **Novel alpha adrenergic agents**

  Inventor(s): Hong, Seoung-Soo; (Cheongju, KR), Miller, Duane D.; (Germantown, TN)

  Correspondence: Jeffrey J. Skelton; 10310 27th Ave. N.; Plymouth; MN; 55441; US

  Patent Application Number: 20030092741

  Date filed: August 9, 2002

Abstract: Aspects of the present invention are directed towards compounds of Formula I for the treatment of human erectile disorders including **erectile dysfunction** in men.

1wherein:R.sub.1 is hydrogen, halo, hydroxy, nitro, cyano, phenyl, trifluoromethyl, C.sub.1-C.sub.6 alkyl, C.sub.1-C.sub.6 alkoxy, carboxy, amino, cyclohexyl, C.sub.1-C.sub.6 alkylamino, or (C.sub.1-C.sub.6 alkyl).sub.2amino;R.sub.2 is hydrogen, halo, hydroxy, nitro, cyano, trifluoromethyl, C.sub.1-C.sub.6 alkyl, C.sub.1-C.sub.6 alkoxy, carboxy, amino, C.sub.1-C.sub.6 alkylamino, or (C.sub.1-C.sub.6 alkyl).sub.2amino;R.sub.3 is a group of the formula 2R.sub.4 is hydrogen or C.sub.1-C.sub.6 alkyl;R.sub.5 is hydrogen, halo, hydroxy, nitro, cyano, phenyl, trifluoromethyl, C.sub.1-C.sub.6 alkyl, C.sub.1-C.sub.6 alkoxy, carboxy, amino, C.sub.1-C.sub.6 alkylamino, or (C.sub.1-C.sub.6 alkyl).sub.2amino; andR.sub.6 is hydrogen, halo, hydroxy, nitro, cyano, trifluoromethyl, C.sub.1-C.sub.6 alkyl, C.sub.1-C.sub.6 alkoxy, carboxy, amino, C.sub.1-C.sub.6 alkylamino, or (C.sub.1-C.sub.6 alkyl).sub.2amino; or pharmaceutically acceptable salts thereof

Excerpt(s): This Application claims priority from and benefit of U.S. provision application No. 60/311,320 filed Aug. 10, 2001. Aspects of the current invention are directed towards the field of organic chemistry and more specifically toward the field of medicinal chemistry. The human sexual response in both males and females results from a complex interplay of psychological, hormonal, and other physiological influences. One important aspect of the human sexual response common to both men and women is the erectile response, which itself results from an interplay between the autonomic nervous system, the endocrine system, and the circulatory system.

Web site: http://appft1.uspto.gov/netahtml/PTO/search-bool.html

- **Phthalazine compounds and therapeutic agents for erectile dysfunction**

  Inventor(s): Adachi, Hideyuki; (Ibaraki, JP), Ishihara, Hiroki; (Ibaraki, JP), Kamada, Atsushi; (Ibaraki, JP), Kaneko, Toshihiko; (Ibaraki, JP), Karibe, Norio; (Saitama, JP), Kodama, Kohtarou; (Ibaraki, JP), Miyazaki, Kazuki; (Ibaraki, JP), Miyazawa, Shuhei; (Ibaraki, JP), Nagakura, Tadashi; (Ibaraki, JP), Naoe, Yoshimitsu; (Ibaraki, JP), Ozaki, Fumihiro; (Ibaraki, JP), Tsukada, Itaru; (Ibaraki, JP), Watanabe, Nobuhisa; (Ibaraki, JP)

  Correspondence: BIRCH STEWART KOLASCH & BIRCH; PO BOX 747; FALLS CHURCH; VA; 22040-0747; US

  Patent Application Number: 20030105074

  Date filed: October 28, 2002

Abstract: The present invention provides a phthalazine compound as a therapeutic agent for **erectile dysfunction** represented by the following formula, a pharmacologically acceptable salt thereof or a hydrate thereof: 1wherein R.sup.1 and R.sup.2 are the same as or different from each other and represent a halogen atom, a C1 to C4 alkyl group which may be substituted with a halogen atom, a C1 to C4 alkoxy group which may be substituted with a halogen atom or a cyano group; X represents a cyano group, a nitro group, a halogen atom, a hydroxyimino group which may be substituted or a heteroaryl group which may be substituted; Y represents a heteroaryl group, an aryl group which may be substituted, an alkynyl group which may substituted, an alkenyl group, an alkyl group, an optionally substituted saturated or unsaturated 4- to 8-membered amine ring, and the cyclic amine compound is a monocyclic compound, bicyclic compound or a spiro compound; l is an integer of 1 to 3; provided that the case where l is 1 or 2, X is a cyano group, a nitro group or a chlorine atom, R.sup.1 is a chlorine atom, R.sup.2 is a methoxy group and Y is a 5- or 6-memberred amine ring substituted with a hydroxyl group is excluded.

Excerpt(s): The present invention relates to phthalazine compounds. More specifically, it relates to prophylactic and therapeutic agents for male **erectile dysfunction,** and prophylactic and therapeutic agents for female sexual dysfunction or dysmenorrhea. It is said that the number of latent patients with **erectile dysfunction** amounts to about 3,000,000 in Japan. In U.S.A., it is reported that the number of patients with **erectile dysfunction** reaches 20,000,000 and 15% of males in the fifties and about 1/3 of those in the sixties suffer from this disease. In this aging society, sexual intercourse is regarded as a pleasant and emotional behavior. With the needs for the improved quality of life, it is anticipated that **erectile dysfunction** will raise not only a medical problem but also a social problem in future. This disease is classified into organic impotence caused by disorders in the nerves, blood vessels or muscles in the penis per se or sexual hormones and functional (psychic) impotence caused by mental or psychologic troubles. There are three factors necessary for erection, i.e., an increase in the penile arterial blood flow, the regulation of blood leakage from the penile veins, and the relaxation of the cavernous tissue. **Erectile dysfunction** arises when at least one of these conditions is inhibited. The urological treatments for **erectile dysfunction** effected today involve drug therapy and operative penile prosthesis with the use of penile prosthetic appliances.

Web site: http://appft1.uspto.gov/netahtml/PTO/search-bool.html

- **Preparations for oral administration**

Inventor(s): Murakami, Hideki; (Hyogo, JP), Takebe, Shoji; (Osaka-fu, JP)

Correspondence: BIRCH STEWART KOLASCH & BIRCH; PO BOX 747; FALLS CHURCH; VA; 22040-0747; US

Patent Application Number: 20030195220

Date filed: March 3, 2003

Abstract: The present invention provides a preparation for oral administration containing a medicinal substance having cGMP-specific phosphodiesterase inhibitory activity and showing decrease of solubility in the neutral and alkaline regions, wherein an acidic substance is compounded promote the dissolution of the medicinal substance in digestive tract and thus the efficacy can be expressed at the early stage after administration, and which preparation is useful in treatment of **erectile dysfunction.**

Excerpt(s): The present invention relates to a preparation for oral administration, which contains a cGMP-specific phosphodiesterase inhibitor and has an improved capacity of expressing the drug efficacy. More specifically, the present invention related to an oral preparation containing a medicinal substance having cGMP-specific phosphodiesterase inhibitory activity and showing decrease of solubility in the neutral and alkaline regions, which preparation is compounded with an acidic substance and thereby being capable of expressing the drug efficacy rapidly after oral administration. Latent patients with **erectile dysfunction** increases as the population ages and, considering the advent of an aging society in near future, attention has been concentrated on the significance of improving the quality of life (QOL) of patients by treatment. As a therapeutic agent, a cyclic GMP (cGMP)-specific phosphodiesterase (PDE) inhibitor, especially PDE-V inhibitor is used. A therapeutic agent for **erectile dysfunction** preferably exerts the drug efficacy immediately after taking the agent so that the sexual response can be regulated on demand. However, some PDE-V inhibitors are known to show marked decrease in solubility in the neutral and alkaline regions compared to the acidic region. For example, the solubility of sildenafil citrate is 2.52 mg/ml at pH 1.2, while it is only 0.11 mg/ml at pH 6.8 (WO00/20033, page 4).

Web site: http://appft1.uspto.gov/netahtml/PTO/search-bool.html

- **Prostaglandin compositions and methods of treatment for male erectile dysfunction**

  Inventor(s): Buyuktimkin, Nadir; (Robbinsville, NJ), Buyuktimkin, Servet; (Robbinsville, NJ), Yeager, James L.; (Lake Forest, IL)

  Correspondence: ROGER P. ZIMMERMAN, ESQ.; BOWDITCH & DEWEY, LLP; 161 Worcester Road; P.O. Box 9320; Framingham; MA; 01701-9320; US

  Patent Application Number: 20030134903

  Date filed: September 6, 2002

  Abstract: The invention provides methods and compositions for treating **erectile dysfunction.** The methods include the step of placing within the fossa navicularis of the patient an effective erection-inducing amount of a vasoactive prostaglandin composition of a semi-solid consistency. The composition comprises a vasoactive prostaglandin, a penetration enhancer, a shear-thinning polysaccharide, a lipophilic compound, and an acidic buffer system. The penetration enhancer is an alkyl-2-(N-substituted amino)-alkanoate ester, a (N-substituted amino)-alkanol alkanoate, or a mixture of these enhancers. The lipophilic compound may be an aliphatic C_1 to C_8 alcohol, aliphatic C_2 to C_{30} ester, an aliphatic C_8 to C_{30} ester, or a mixture of these. The composition includes a buffer system providing a buffered pH value for said composition in the range of about 3 to about 7.4.

  Excerpt(s): This application is a continuation-in-part of co-pending application Ser. No. 09/947,617, filed Sep. 6, 2001, that is a continuation-in-part of application Ser. No. 09/480,738, now U.S. Pat. No. 6,323,241 and a continuation-in-part of International Application Serial No. PCT/US01/00852, filed Jan. 10, 2001. This invention relates to the compositions and methods for treatment of **erectile dysfunction,** and more particularly to methods and pharmaceutical compositions for intranavicular administration of vasodilator medicaments to the fossa naviscularis of a patient. The term "impotence" has been used to signify the inability of the male to attain and maintain erection of the penis sufficient to permit satisfactory sexual intercourse. The term "erectile dysfunction" has been suggested as a more precise term "to signify an inability of the male to achieve an erect penis as part of the overall multifaceted process of male sexual function." Droller, M. J. et al. Impotence. Consensus Development Conference Statement, National Institutes of Health (1993).

  Web site: http://appft1.uspto.gov/netahtml/PTO/search-bool.html

- **Pyrazolopyrimidinones for the treatment of female sexual dysfunction**

  Inventor(s): Ellis, Peter; (Sandwich, GB), Terrett, Nicholas Kenneth; (Sandwich, GB)

  Correspondence: PFIZER INC.; PATENT DEPARTMENT, MS8260-1611; EASTERN POINT ROAD; GROTON; CT; 06340; US

  Patent Application Number: 20030027824

  Date filed: July 24, 2002

  Abstract: The use of a compound of formula (I) wherein R^1 is H; C_1-C_3 alkyl; C_1-C_3 perfluomalkyl; or C_3-C_5 cycloalkyl; R^2 is H; optionally substituted C_1-C_6 alkyl; C_1-C_3 pefluoroalkyl; or C_3-

C.sub.6 cycloalkyl; R.sup.3 is optionally substituted C.sub.1-C.sub.6 alkyl; C.sub.1-C.sub.6 perfluoroalkyl; C.sub.3-C.sub.5 cycloalkyl; C.sub.3-C.sub.6 alkenyl; or C.sub.3-C.sub.6 alkynyl; R.sup.4 is optionally substituted C.sub.1-C.sub.4 alkyl, C.sub.2-C.sub.4 alkenyl, C.sub.2-C.sub.4 alkanoyl, (hydroxy)C.sub.2-C.sub.4 alkyl or (C.sub.2-C.sub.3 alkoxy)C.sub.1-C.sub.2 alkyl; CONR.sup.5R.sup.6; CO.sub.2R.sup.7; halo; NR.sup.5R.sup.6; NHSO.sub.2NR.sup.5R.sup.6; NHSO.sub.2R.sup.8; SO.sub.2NR.sup.9R.sup.10; or phenyl, pyridyl, pyrimidinyl, imidazolyl, oxazolyl, thiazolyl, thienyl or triazolyl any of which is optionally substituted with methyl; R.sup.5 and R.sup.6 are each independently H or C.sub.1-C.sub.4 alkyl, or together with the nitrogen atom to which they are attached form an optionally substituted pyrrolidinyl, piperidino, morpholino, 4-N(R.sup.11)-piperazinyl or imidazolyl group; R.sup.7 is H or C.sub.1-C.sub.4 alkyl; R.sup.8 is optionally substituted C.sub.1-C.sub.3 alkyl; R.sup.9 and R.sup.10 together with the nitrogen atom to which they are attached form an optionally substituted pyrrolidinyl, piperidino, morpholino or 4-N(R.sup.12)-piperazinyl group; R.sup.11 is H; optionally substituted C.sub.1-C.sub.3 alkyl; (hydroxy)C.sub.2-C.sub.3 alkyl; or C.sub.1-C.sub.4 alkanoyl; R.sup.12 is H; optionally substituted C.sub.1-C.sub.6 alkyl; CONR.sup.13R.sup.14. CSNR.sup.13R.sup.14; or C(NH)NR.sup.13R.sup.14; and R?13? and R.sup.14 are each independently H; C.sub.1-C.sub.4 alkyl; or substituted C.sub.2-C.sub.4 alkyl; or a pharmaceutically acceptable salt thereof, or a pharmaceutical composition containing either entity, for the manufacture of a medicament for the curative or prophylactic treatment of **erectile dysfunction** in a male animal, including man; a pharmaceutical composition for said treatment; and a method of said treatment of said male animal with said pharmaceutical composition or with said either entity.

Excerpt(s): This invention relates to the use of a series of pyrazolo[4,3-d]pyrimidin-7-ones for the treatment of impotence. Impotence can be defined literally as a lack of power, in the male, to copulate and may involve an inability to achieve penile erection or ejaculation, or both. More specifically, erectile impotence or dysfunction may be defined as an inability to obtain or sustain an erection adequate for intercourse. Its prevalence is claimed to be between 2 and 7% of the human male population, increasing with age, up to 50 years, and between 18 and 75% between 55 and 80 years of age. In the USA alone, for example, it has been estimated that there are up to 10 million impotent males, with the majority suffering from problems of organic rather than of psychogenic origin. Reports of well-controlled clinical trials in man are few and the efficacy of orally administered drugs is low. Although many different drugs have been shown to induce penile erection, they are only effective after direct injection into the penis, e.g. intraurethrally or intracavernosally (i.c.), and are not approved for **erectile dysfunction.** Current medical treatment is based on the i.c injection of vasoactive substances and good results have been claimed with phenoxybenzamine, phentolamine, papaverine and prostaglandin E.sub.1, either alone or in combination; however, pain, priapism and fibrosis of the penis are associated with the i.c. administration of some of these agents. Potassium channel openers (KCO) and vasoactive intestinal polypeptide (VIP) have also been shown to be active i.c., but cost and stability issues could limit development of the latter. An alternative to the i.c. route is the use of glyceryl trinitrate (GTN) patches applied to the penis, which has been shown to be effective but produces side-effects in both patient and partner.

Web site: http://appft1.uspto.gov/netahtml/PTO/search-bool.html

- **Relieving symptoms of erectile dysfunction with proanthocyanidins**

  Inventor(s): Ferrari, Victor; (Feutersoey, CH), Rohdewald, Peter; (Munster, DE)

  Correspondence: GIBBONS, DEL DEO, DOLAN, GRIFFINGER & VECCHIONE; 1 RIVERFRONT PLAZA; NEWARK; NJ; 07102-5497; US

  Patent Application Number: 20030104077

  Date filed: January 13, 2003

  Abstract: Use of proanthocyanidins as an active ingredient of a stimulator and L-arginine or its salts as a source of nitric oxide in the treatment of **erectile dysfunction.** The active ingredient stimulates the endothelial NO-synthase enzyme, which acts as a catalyst for the synthesis of nitric oxide from its substrate L-arginine or its salts. The nitric oxide in turn activates the guanylyl cyclase, which leads to an increased development of cyclic guanosine monophosphate, which causes relaxation of smooth muscles. Blood vessel diameter may increase. The stimulator may also have Sildenafil or enzymes that inhibit an enzyme phosphodiesterase type from reducing an amount of the cyclic guanosine monophosphate.

  Excerpt(s): This is a continuation patent application of utility patent application Ser. No. 09/865,189, filed May 24, 2001, which claims priority from U.S. Provisional Patent Application Serial No. 60/207,520 filed May 26, 2000. The invention relates to the use of proanthocyanidins to stimulate the enzyme NO-synthase, which acts as a catalyst to release nitric oxide from L-arginine (or its salts). Such is advantageous in relieving symptoms of **erectile dysfunction.** As a result of sexual stimuli, the enzyme NO-synthase (NOS) gets activated in endothelial cells of the erectile tissue. This enzyme acts as a catalyst for the synthesis of nitric oxide (NO) from its substrate, amino acid L-arginine. The NO in turn activates the guanylyl cyclase which leads to an increased development of cyclic guanosine monophosphate (cGMP).

  Web site: http://appft1.uspto.gov/netahtml/PTO/search-bool.html

- **Rho-kinase inhibitors**

  Inventor(s): Nagarathnam, Dhanaphalan; (Bethany, CT), Wang, Chunguang; (Hamden, CT)

  Correspondence: MILLEN, WHITE, ZELANO & BRANIGAN, P.C.; 2200 CLARENDON BLVD.; SUITE 1400; ARLINGTON; VA; 22201; US

  Patent Application Number: 20030087919

  Date filed: March 22, 2002

  Abstract: Disclosed are compounds and derivatives thereof, their synthesis, and their use as Rho-kinase inhibitors. These compounds of the present invention are useful for inhibiting tumor growth, treating **erectile dysfunction,** and treating other indications mediated by Rho-kinase, e.g., coronary heart disease.

  Excerpt(s): This application claims the benefit of the filing date of U.S. Provisional Application Serial No. 60/277,974, filed Mar. 23, 2001 and U.S. Provisional Application Serial No.: 60/315,338, filed Aug. 29, 2001. The present invention relates to compounds and derivatives thereof, their synthesis, and their use as Rho-kinase inhibitors. These compounds of the present invention are useful for inhibiting tumor growth, treating **erectile dysfunction,** and treating other indications mediated by Rho-kinase, e.g., coronary heart disease. The pathology of a number of human and animal diseases including hypertension, erectile dysfunction, coronary cerebral circulatory impairments, neurodegenerative disorders and cancer can be linked directly to changes in the actin cytoskeleton. These diseases pose a serious unmet medical need. The actin cytoskeleton is composed of a meshwork of actin filaments and actin-binding proteins found in all eukaryotic cells. In smooth muscle cells the assembly and disassembly of the actin cytoskeleton is the primary motor force responsible for smooth muscle contraction and relaxation. In non-muscle cells, dynamic rearrangements of the actin cytoskeleton are responsible for regulating cell morphology, cell motility, actin stress fiber formation, cell adhesion and specialized cellular functions such as neurite retraction, phagocytosis or cytokinesis (Van Aelst, et al. Genes Dev 1997, 11, 2295).

Web site: http://appft1.uspto.gov/netahtml/PTO/search-bool.html

- **Therapeutic combinations for the treatment of hormone deficiencies**

Inventor(s): van der Hoop, Roland Gerritsen; (Marietta, GA)

Correspondence: Joseph A. Mahoney; Mayer, Brown & PlaTT; P.O. Box 2828; Chicago; IL; 60690; US

Patent Application Number: 20030027804

Date filed: June 27, 2001

Abstract: The present invention relates to methods of treating, preventing, or reducing the risk of developing a male or female menopause disorder or symptom in a mammal by administering to the mammal a sex hormone binding globulin synthesis inhibiting agent and one or more steroids, including, for example, an androgen or an estrogen; to combinations for treating, preventing or reducing the risk of developing a male or female menopause disorder or symptom in a mammal; and to compositions for treating, preventing, or reducing the risk of developing a male or female menopause disorder or symptom in a mammal, where the composition comprises a sex binding globulin synthesis inhibiting agent and one or more steroids, including, for example, an androgen or an estrogen. In addition, the methods, combinations and compositions may be used in conjunction with other pharmaceutical agents aimed at improving sexual performance or impotence, increasing libido, or treating erectile dysfunction, such as VIAGRA.RTM., to enhance their effectiveness.

Excerpt(s): The present invention relates to methods, combinations, and compositions for treating, preventing, or reducing the risk of developing an androgenic or estrogenic hormone deficiency in a male or female subject, or for treating, preventing, or reducing the risk of developing the symptoms associated with, or related to, an androgenic or estrogenic deficiency in a male or female subject. Research into "male menopause" or "andropause" shows that there is a drastic drop of serum levels of free testosterone of about 1.5% per year after puberty. While the total testosterone of a male does not drop drastically, the free testosterone, which is the biologically active part of the testosterone, does drop precipitously with aging. In fact, a significant drop of free testosterone can occur as early as the early forties. Studies have shown that men with high testosterone levels live longer, healthier lives and maintain sexual potency. Studies have also shown that testosterone has the ability to stop the spread of breast cancer in females. Additionally, research has shown that testosterone has a protective effect against autoimmune diseases. The female hormones, estrogen and progesterone, are known to drop drastically to very low levels after menopause. The American College of Physicians and the American College of Obstetricians and Gynecologists has released position papers saying post-menopausal women should seriously consider preventive estrogen/progesterone hormone replacement therapy for their benefit in reducing osteoporosis and heart disease. Maintaining estrogen and progesterone levels has also been shown to improve a number of key risk factors for heart disease in post-menopausal women. The benefits of estrogen/progesterone hormone replenishment therapy include prevention of osteoporosis and heart disease, prevention of vaginal dryness and thinning of the vaginal wall, relief from menopausal symptoms and hot flashes, and the possible benefit of reducing the onset of Alzheimer's disease, dementia, and cataracts. Studies have shown that when estrogen is replenished in conjunction with progesterone, the risks of uterine or breast cancer is nullified.

Web site: http://appft1.uspto.gov/netahtml/PTO/search-bool.html

- **Thiophenyl triazol-3-one derivatives as smooth muscle relaxants**

Inventor(s): Hewawasam, Piyasena; (Middletown, CT), King, Dalton; (Hamden, CT), Lodge, Nicholas J.; (Madison, CT), Starrett, John E.; (Middletown, CT), Sun, Li-Quang; (Glastonbury, CT)

Correspondence: STEPHEN B. DAVIS; BRISTOL-MYERS SQUIBB COMPANY; PATENT DEPARTMENT; P O BOX 4000; PRINCETON; NJ; 08543-4000; US

Patent Application Number: 20030144333

Date filed: October 8, 2002

Abstract: The present invention provides novel [1,2,4]triazole-3-one derivatives having the general formula (I) 1wherein:Q is 2and R.sup.1, R.sup.2, R.sup.3, R.sup.4, R.sup.5 and R.sup.6 are as defined herein or a nontoxic pharmaceutically acceptable salt or solvate thereof which are smooth muscle relaxants and useful in treating disorders responsive to relaxation of smooth muscle such as asthma, irritable bowel syndrome, male **erectile dysfunction** and urinary incontinence.

Excerpt(s): This is a non-provisional application which claims the benefit of U.S. Provisional Application No. 60/336,865 filed Nov. 2, 2001. The present invention is directed to novel 2phenyl-5thiophenyl-2,4-- dihydro-[1,2,4]-triazol-3-one derivatives which are smooth muscle relaxants and therefore are useful in treating disorders responsive to relaxation of smooth muscle such as asthma, irritable bowel syndrome, male **erectile dysfunction** and particularly urinary incontinence. The present invention is also directed to a method of treatment with the novel compounds and to pharmaceutical compositions containing them. Urinary incontinence is a common condition that is the frequent cause of confinement to nursing homes among the elderly. It afflicts significant numbers among both men and women and all ages. In addition studies show some degree of daily incontinence reported among as many as 17% of young apparently healthy women. Safe and reliable methods for treating incontinence are clearly needed. Urinary incontinence is a manifestation of the failure to control the muscles of the bladder or urinary sphincter. Incontinence results when the pressure within the bladder is too great as a result of excessive force exerted by the bladder muscles, or when the sphincter muscles are too weak. Urinary incontinence can be a manifestation of other diseases such as Parkinsonism, multiple sclerosis, lesions of the central nervous system, or bladder infections. Interstitial cysts can result in instability of the bladder detusor muscles and a particularly unpleasant form of urge incontinence. Urinary incontinence is believed to currently affect over 12 million people in the United States alone, and to occur in between 15 and 30% of the population over 60. The current standard of care is quite unsatisfactory. All of the current drugs now utilized to treat urinary incontinence suffer from polypharmacology and unwanted side effects.

Web site: http://appft1.uspto.gov/netahtml/PTO/search-bool.html

- **Transmucosal phosphodiesterase inhibitors for the treatment of erectile dysfunction**

Inventor(s): Doherty, Paul C. JR.; (Cupertino, CA), Place, Virgil A.; (Kawaihae, HI), Smith, William L.; (Mahwah, NJ)

Correspondence: REED & EBERLE LLP; 800 MENLO AVENUE, SUITE 210; MENLO PARK; CA; 94025; US

Patent Application Number: 20030134861

Date filed: January 24, 2003

Abstract: A pharmaceutical formulation is provided for treating **erectile dysfunction** in a mammalian male individual. The pharmaceutical formulation includes a phosphodiesterase inhibitor or a pharmaceutically acceptable salt, ester, amide or derivative thereof, that is administered transmucosally within the context of an effective dosing regimen. Preferred modes of administration include transbuccal, sublingual and transrectal routes. A kit for the administration of the pharmaceutical formulation is also provided.

Excerpt(s): This application is a divisional application of U.S. Ser. No. 09/467,094, filed Dec. 10, 1999, which is a continuation-in-part of U.S. Ser. No. 09/181,070, filed Oct. 27, 1998, which is a continuation-in-part of U.S. Ser. No. 08/958,816, filed Oct. 28, 1997, the disclosures of which are hereby incorporated by reference. This invention relates generally to methods and pharmaceutical compositions for treating **erectile dysfunction;** more particularly, the invention relates to transmucosal (e.g., buccal, sublingual and transrectal), phosphodiesterase inhibitors that are used to treat **erectile dysfunction.** Impotence is the consistent inability to achieve or sustain an erection of sufficient rigidity for sexual intercourse. It has recently been estimated that approximately 10 million American men are impotent (R. Shabsigh et al., "Evaluation of Erectile Impotence," Urology 32:83-90 (1988); W. L. Furlow, "Prevalence of Impotence in the United States," Med. Aspects Hum. Sex. 19:13-6 (1985)). Impotence is recognized to be an age-dependent disorder, with an incidence of 1.9 percent at 40 years of age and 25 percent at 65 years of age (A. C. Kinsey et al., "Age and Sexual Outlet," in Sexual Behavior in the Human Male; A. C. Kinsey et al., eds., Philadelphia, Pa.: W. B. Saunders, 218-262 (1948)). In 1985 in the United States, impotence accounted for more than several hundred thousand outpatient visits to physicians (National Center for Health Statistics, National Hospital Discharge Survey, 1985, Bethesda, Md., Department of Health and Human Services, 1989 DHHS publication no. 87-1751). Depending on the nature and cause of the problem, treatments include psychosexual therapy, hormonal therapy, administration of vasodilators such as nitroglycerin and -adrenergic blocking agents ("-blockers"), oral administration of other pharmaceutical agents, vascular surgery, implanted penile prostheses, vacuum constriction devices and external aids such as penile splints to support the penis or penile constricting rings to alter the flow of blood through the penis.

Web site: http://appft1.uspto.gov/netahtml/PTO/search-bool.html

- **Treatment of erectile dysfunction**

  Inventor(s): Buyuktimkin, Nadir; (Robbinsville, NJ), Buyuktimkin, Servet; (Robbinsville, NJ), Okada, Koichi; (Saitama, JP), Yeager, James L.; (Lake Forest, IL)

  Correspondence: ROGER P. ZIMMERMAN, ESQ.; BOWDITCH & DEWEY, LLP; 161 Worcester Road; P.O. Box 9320; Farmingham; MA; 01701-9320; US

  Patent Application Number: 20030220292

  Date filed: February 14, 2003

  Abstract: Methods for the treatment of **erectile dysfunction** are provided comprising placing in the fossa navicularis an amount of a semi-solid vasoactive prostaglandin composition sufficient to increase blood flow in the glans penis and resulting in increased tumescence of the penis. In preferred embodiments, the method further comprises providing erotic stimuli. Another embodiment, the invention provides a method for increasing the tumescence of the glans penis. In another aspect, the invention provides compositions and articles of manufacture for the practice of the methods of the invention.

  Excerpt(s): The present application claims the benefit of U.S. Provisional Application No. 60/357,282, filed Feb. 15, 2002. The entire contents of the above application are incorporated herein by reference in entirety. This invention relates to the compositions and methods for treatment of **erectile dysfunction,** and more particularly to methods and pharmaceutical compositions for increasing the microcirculation of the glans penis and increasing the tumescence of the glans penis by the administration of medicaments to the fossa navicularis of a patient. Prior treatments for impotence and **erectile dysfunction** (ED) have focussed on the task of achieving an erection adequate for intercourse, and specifically for vaginal penetration. While progress has been made in this area, there remains the problem that an erection that is adequate may not be satisfactory to either the patient or his sexual partner.

  Web site: http://appft1.uspto.gov/netahtml/PTO/search-bool.html

- **Treatment of male sexual dysfunction**

  Inventor(s): Naylor, Alasdair Mark; (Sandwich, GB), Van Der Graaf, Pieter Hadewijn; (Sandwich, GB), Wayman, Christopher Peter; (Sandwich, GB)

  Correspondence: Gregg C. Benson; Pfizer Inc.; Patent Department, MS4159; Eastern Point Road; Groton; CT; 06340; US

  Patent Application Number: 20030119714

  Date filed: December 12, 2001

  Abstract: The use of an inhibitor of a neuropeptide Y (NPY), preferably of a NPY Y1 receptor, which inhibitor is selective for an NPY or NPY Y1 receptor associated with male genitalia, in the preparation/manufacture of a medicament for the treatment or prevention of male **erectile dysfunction** (MED).

  Excerpt(s): The present invention relates to a compound and a pharmaceutical that is useful for the treatment and/or prevention of male sexual dysfunction (MSD), in particular male **erectile dysfunction** (MED). The present invention also relates to a method of prevention and/or treatment of MSD, in particular MED. The present invention also relates to assays to screen for the compounds useful in the treatment of MSD, in particular MED.

Web site: http://appft1.uspto.gov/netahtml/PTO/search-bool.html

- **Use of PDE V inhibitors**

  Inventor(s): Brandle, Marian; (Rottenburg, DE), Ehring, Thomas; (Remscheid, DE), Wilm, Claudia; (Darmstadt, DE)

  Correspondence: MILLEN, WHITE, ZELANO & BRANIGAN, P.C.; 2200 CLARENDON BLVD.; SUITE 1400; ARLINGTON; VA; 22201; US

  Patent Application Number: 20030022906

  Date filed: September 3, 2002

  Abstract: The invention relates to the use of a highly penis-specific PDE V inhibitor, or a physiologically acceptable salt or solvate thereof, for the production of a medicament for the treatment of **erectile dysfunction** in males, without the previous circulatory side effects caused by PDE V inhibitors, in particular, with concomitant administration of vasodilators, whose mode of action is by means of the NO/cGMP system.

  Excerpt(s): The invention relates to the use of a highly penis-specific PDE V inhibitor, or a physiologically acceptable salt and/or solvate thereof, for the preparation of a medicament for the treatment of **erectile dysfunction** in men without circulatory side effects caused by PDE V inhibitors. The use of PDE V inhibitors is described, for example, in WO 94/28902. Pyrimidine derivatives are known, for example, from EP 201 188 and WO 93/06104. The use of PDE (phosphodiesterase) V inhibitors for the treatment of **erectile dysfunction** is known, for example, from EP 702 555 and WO 99/55708.

  Web site: http://appft1.uspto.gov/netahtml/PTO/search-bool.html

- **USES OF VASCULAR ENDOTHELIAL GROWTH FACTOR IN THE TREATMENT OF ERECTILE DYSFUNCTION**

  Inventor(s): SHABSIGH, RIDWAN; (WAYNE, NJ)

  Correspondence: JOHN P WHITE; ALBERT WAI-KIT CHAN; COOPER & DUNHAM; 1185 AVENUE OF THE AMERICAS; NEW YORK; NY; 10063

  Patent Application Number: 20030124094

  Date filed: January 21, 1999

  Abstract: This invention provides a method of increasing or maintaining the blood supply in the penis of a male subject which comprises administering to the subject an amount of vascular endothelial growth factor effective to increase or maintain the blood supply in the subject's penis. This invention provides a method of treating **erectile dysfunction** in a subject which comprises administering to the subject an amount of vascular endothelial growth factor effective to increase the blood supply in the subject's penis and thereby treat the subject's **erectile dysfunction.** This invention provides a method of increasing or maintaining the blood supply in the penis of a subject which comprises introducing a nucleic acid comprising a gene encoding a vascular endothelial growth factor into a suitable cell under conditions such that the nucleic acid expresses vascular endothelial growth factor so as to thereby increase or maintain the blood supply in the subject's penis. This invention provides a method of increasing or maintaining the blood supply in the genital area of a female subject which comprises administering to the subject an amount of vascular endothelial growth factor effective to increase or maintain the blood supply in the subject's genital area.

Excerpt(s): Throughout this application, various publications are referenced by Arabic numerals. Full citations for these publications may be found at the end of the specification immediately preceding the claims. The disclosure of these publications is hereby incorporated by reference into this application to describe more fully the art to which this invention pertains. Mammalian reproduction requires a physiological stimulation of male erectile tissues in the penis to mechanistically support the transfer of sperm from the male to the female. Obviously then, defects that prevent an appropriate erectile tissue response can drastically interfere with reproductive capability. In humans, **erectile dysfunction** is considered to be a disease state and is referred to as the condition of "impotence". This condition impacts on the quality of life both of the male patients, as well as their wives/partners (1). Erection is a hemodynamic phenomenon involving the tissue of the corpora cavernosa as well as the corpus spongiosum in the penis. This tissue is a complex admixture of smooth muscle, endothelial cells, fibroblasts and nerves interacting under stimulatory conditions to drastically enhance and maintain an accessory blood supply that imparts rigidity to the penis. Given the need for stringent control of blood flow during this response, it is no surprise that vascular insufficiency has the ability to drastically suppress erectile capability. In fact, penile vascular insufficiency is believed to be a very common pathomechanism of **erectile dysfunction** (2). This is associated with substantial pathologic changes in the erectile tissue leading to reduction in vascular smooth muscle cells and increases in collagen and fibrosis (3-6).

Web site: http://appft1.uspto.gov/netahtml/PTO/search-bool.html

Keeping Current

In order to stay informed about patents and patent applications dealing with erectile dysfunction, you can access the U.S. Patent Office archive via the Internet at the following Web address: **http://www.uspto.gov/patft/index.html**. You will see two broad options: (1) Issued Patent, and (2) Published Applications. To see a list of issued patents, perform the following steps: Under "Issued Patents," click "Quick Search." Then, type "erectile dysfunction" (or synonyms) into the "Term 1" box. After clicking on the search button, scroll down to see the various patents which have been granted to date on erectile dysfunction.

You can also use this procedure to view pending patent applications concerning erectile dysfunction. Simply go back to **http://www.uspto.gov/patft/index.html** Select "Quick Search" under "Published Applications." Then proceed with the steps listed above.

CHAPTER 7. BOOKS ON ERECTILE DYSFUNCTION

Overview

This chapter provides bibliographic book references relating to erectile dysfunction. In addition to online booksellers such as **www.amazon.com** and **www.bn.com**, excellent sources for book titles on erectile dysfunction include the Combined Health Information Database and the National Library of Medicine. Your local medical library also may have these titles available for loan.

Book Summaries: Federal Agencies

The Combined Health Information Database collects various book abstracts from a variety of healthcare institutions and federal agencies. To access these summaries, go directly to the following hyperlink: **http://chid.nih.gov/detail/detail.html**. You will need to use the "Detailed Search" option. To find book summaries, use the drop boxes at the bottom of the search page where "You may refine your search by." Select the dates and language you prefer. For the format option, select "Monograph/Book." Now type "erectile dysfunction" (or synonyms) into the "For these words:" box. You should check back periodically with this database which is updated every three months. The following is a typical result when searching for books on erectile dysfunction:

- **It's Not All In Your Head: A Couple's Guide to Overcoming Impotence**

  Source: Louisville, TN: Byron's Graphic Arts. 1988. 192 p.

  Contact: Available from Impotence Institute of America. P.O. Box 410, Bowie, MD 20718-0410. (800) 669-1603 or (301) 262-2400. Fax (301) 262-6825. E-mail: iwabowie@aol.com. Website: www.impotenceworld.org. PRICE: $16.95.

  Summary: Chronic impotence affects at least 30 million American couples. In this book, the founders of Impotents Anonymous (IA) and IAnon reveal that as many as 80 percent of men who suffer from **erectile dysfunction** (ED, or impotence) do so because of physical, not psychological, problems. The authors, who for years struggled with ED themselves, first explode the many myths surrounding impotence, then offer updated information on the treatment options available. Treatments discussed include medication, sex therapy, vascular surgery, penile implants, external management (such as vacuum erection devices), and injection programs (drug therapy which is either administered via injection to the penis or administered intraurethrally). The authors also discuss new developments in the treatment of ED that has a psychogenic cause. The authors emphasize that there are treatment options available for all situations where ED is problematic. However, they stress that reaching a successful resolution requires the active participation of both partners. The book includes actual stories and letters from some of the many individuals who have been in contact with the authors through their national organizations: Impotence Institute of America, Impotence Institute International, Impotence World Services, Impotents Anonymous, and I-Anon. A glossary of terms and a subject index conclude the book.

- **Beyond Viagra: Plain Talk About Treating Male and Female Sexual Dysfunction**

Source: Montgomery, AL: Starrhill Press. 1999. 196 p.

Contact: Available from Black Belt Press. P.O. Box 551, Montgomery, AL 36101. (800) 959-3245 or (334) 265-6753. Fax (334) 265-8880. PRICE: $13.95 plus shipping and handling. ISBN: 1573590142.

Summary: This book discusses the drug sildenafil (Viagra) in the context of a larger discussion about sexuality and sexual dysfunction. Twenty-four chapters cover normal male sexual function, an overview of male sexual dysfunction, the causes of male **erectile dysfunction,** evaluating the male with **erectile dysfunction,** treatment strategies for metabolic disorders (including diabetes and prolactinoma), hormone replacement therapy, penile injections with vasoactive drugs, urethral suppository with vasoactive drugs, vacuum erection devices, vascular surgery for impotence, an overview of penile implants, treatment of Peyronie's disease, treatment of psychological impotence, the role of impotence support groups, herbal medicine for males, Viagra for male **erectile dysfunction,** Viagra in combination with injections or vacuum erection devices, Viagra in combination with penile implants, future treatments for **erectile dysfunction,** normal female sexual function, the causes and treatment of female sexual dysfunction, Viagra and apomorphine for females, herbal medicine for females, and healthy relationships and sexual function. The chapters are written in nontechnical language but include enough medical information to be of use to medical professionals wishing to learn more about sexual dysfunction. The book concludes with a list of resources and a subject index. 10 figures. 5 tables. 237 references.

- **Difficult Diabetes**

Source: Malden, MA: Blackwell Science, Inc. 2001. 308 p.

Contact: Available from Blackwell Science, Inc. 350 Main Street, Commerce Place, Malden, MA 02148. (800) 215-1000 or (617) 388-8250. Fax (617) 388-8270. E-mail: books@blacksci.com. Website: www.blackwell-science.com. PRICE: $154.95. ISBN: 0632053240.

Summary: This book is intended for diabetes specialists and endocrinologists who want to keep abreast of the most topical and controversial aspects of diabetes management. Four sections cover diagnostic and screening issues; management issues in type 2 diabetes; management issues in type 1 diabetes; and general diabetes issues such as managing coexisting disease and employment and driving restrictions. Specific topics including screening for diabetes, patient selection, impaired glucose tolerance, gestational diabetes, microalbuminuria (microscopic protein in the urine), obesity, oral hypoglycemic agents, the use of insulin in type 2 diabetes, foot ulcers, management in adolescents, brittle diabetes, hypoglycemia unawareness, intensive diabetes management, insulin pumps, transplantation of the pancreas, **erectile dysfunction,** and hypertension (high blood pressure). Each chapter concludes with a list of references and the text concludes with a subject index.

- **Live Now, Age Later: Proven Ways to Slow Down the Clock**

  Source: New York, NY: Warner Books. 1999. 398 p.

  Contact: Available from Warner Books. 1271 Avenue of the Americas, New York, NY 10020. (800) 759-0190. E-mail: cust.service@littlebrown.com. Website: www.twbookmark.com. PRICE: $7.99 plus shipping and handling.

  Summary: This book offers practical strategies and healthy living advice for people who want to slow down their own aging process. The book is written in casual language with an emphasis on explaining medical and health issues for the general public. Twenty chapters cover Alzheimer's disease, cancer, constipation, depression, hearing loss, heart attacks, **erectile dysfunction** (impotence), insomnia, libido, menopause, osteoarthritis, osteoporosis, prostate enlargement, aging skin, stroke, diminished taste and smell, tinnitus, tooth loss, and loss of vision (macular degeneration, cataracts, glaucoma). Each chapter reviews the topic in question, risk factors, the type of symptoms that can be expected, diagnostic tests that are used to confirm the problem, treatment options, and prognosis. A final section offers general health guidelines that focus on the importance of positive thinking and healthy lifestyle choices. A subject index concludes the book.

- **101 Tips for Staying Healthy with Diabetes (and Avoiding Complications). 2nd ed**

  Source: Alexandria, VA: American Diabetes Association. 1999. 127 p.

  Contact: Available from American Diabetes Association (ADA). Order Fulfillment Department, P.O. Box 930850, Atlanta, GA 31193-0850. (800) 232-6733. Fax (770) 442-9742. Website: www.diabetes.org. PRICE: $14.95 plus shipping and handling. ISBN: 1580400078.

  Summary: This book presents a collection of tips, techniques, and strategies for preventing and treating diabetes complications. One question appears on each page, with the answer immediately below. Questions in chapter one provide general information about diabetes and diabetes complications. Chapter two focuses on glucose control. The third chapter answers questions about various foods and nutrients, including chromium, fiber, fructose, ginseng, folic acid, magnesium, and melatonin. Questions in chapter four provide general information about nutrition, meal planning, and weight management. This is followed by a chapter that describes small blood vessel complications, including eye and kidney disease, diabetic gastroparesis, and foot problems. Chapter six answers questions about large blood vessel complications, including heart disease, **erectile dysfunction,** and bladder problems. The next two chapters answer miscellaneous questions and offer new tips. The final chapter lists the name, address, and telephone number of helpful organizations. The book also includes an index.

- **Shy Bladder Syndrome: Your Step-by-Step Guide to Overcoming Paruresis**

  Source: Oakland, CA: New Harbinger Publications, Inc. 2001. 147 p.

  Contact: Available from New Harbinger Publications, Inc. 5674 Shattuck Avenue, Oakland, CA 94609. (800) 748-6273 or (510) 652-2002. Fax (510) 652-5472. Website: www.newharbinger.com. PRICE: $13.95 plus shipping and handling. ISBN: 1572242272.

Summary: This book provides a comprehensive overview of paruresis (shy bladder) and explains what it is, how the condition is diagnosed, and how it can be treated. The author notes that other than **erectile dysfunction** (impotence) and incontinence (involuntary loss of urine), shy bladder syndrome is perhaps the most embarrassing bodily dysfunction to discuss. The book includes eight chapters that cover a description of the condition and its symptoms; the physiology of the brain, bladder, and urination; determining the causes of bashful bladder syndrome; self treatment for paruresis; adjunct therapies, support groups and workshops; the medical community and paruresis; how family members, intimate partners, and friends can support the patient's recovery; and evolving legal ramifications, including those related to mandatory drug testing and the Americans with Disabilities Act (ADA). The book includes many personal stories from people who have shy bladder; these stories are taken from anonymous postings on the hternational Paruresis Association's (IPA) talk board or from personal communications with the authors. The authors recommend that readers use a journal when reading the book, to help identify and keep track of those issues that are important. Three appendices offer a literature review, a historical overview of the evolution of the bathroom, and resources for additional help. The book concludes with a list of references. 2 figures. 93 references.

- **Diabetes Sourcebook. 3rd ed**

  Source: Detroit, MI: Omnigraphics. 2003. 621 p.

  Contact: Available from Omnigraphics. 615 Griswold Street, Detroit, MI 48226. (800) 234-1340. Fax (800) 875-1340. Website: www.omnigraphics.com. ISBN: 780806298.

  Summary: This book provides information for people seeking to understand the risk factors, complications, and management of type 1 diabetes, type 2 diabetes, and gestational diabetes. The book offers 67 chapters in seven sections: diabetes types and diagnosis; lifestyle and related diabetes management concerns; exercise and nutrition for diabetes management; medication management of diabetes; complications of diabetes; treatment of end stage renal disease (ESRD); and diabetes-related research and statistics. Specific topics include risk factors, impaired glucose tolerance (IGT), insulin resistance, HbA1c (glycosylated hemoglobin) testing, blood glucose testing, urine testing, SMBG (self monitoring of blood glucose), non-invasive blood glucose monitors, preventing complications, how stress affect diabetes, alternative therapies for diabetes, exercise, exchange lists, carbohydrate counting, eating at restaurants, insulin administration and dosage, oral medications, amputation, kidney disease (diabetic nephropathy), diabetic retinopathy (eye disease), diabetic neuropathy (nerve disease), gastroparesis (reduced motility of stomach contents), hypoglycemia (low blood glucose levels), hyperglycemia (high blood glucose levels), **erectile dysfunction** (ED formerly called impotence), research advances in diabetes, and diabetes in ethnic and racial groups. The book includes a glossary of related terms, information about locating financial help for diabetes care, and a list of resources, including organizations, recipes and cookbooks.

- **Making Love Again: Hope for Couples Facing Loss of Sexual Intimacy**

  Source: Sandwich, MA: North Star Publications. 2002. 250 p.

  Contact: Available from North Star Publications Ant Hill Press. 7 Lantern Lane, Sandwich, MA 02563. (800) 949-4416. Fax (631) 979-5989. E-mail: ibmarket@optonline.net. ISBN: 0965506789. PRICE: 24.94, plus shipping and handling.

Summary: This book was written by a couple who faced a lack of sexual intimacy after the husband's treatment for prostate cancer resulted in **erectile dysfunction.** While the radical prostatectomy had saved the husband's life, it had also taken away his ability to get an erection. This real-life couple offers the true and incredibly candid story of how they regained physical intimacy after sexual dysfunction. The authors stress that it is not erections that allow men and women to be intimate, it is an understanding of the need for a safe and nonjudgmental place where mutual physical pleasure and emotional care can flourish. Topics include postoperative recovery, the physiology of erection and male orgasm, oral sex, the use of self-injection for erection, the importance of attitude, libido versus arousal, drug therapy (Viagra, sildenafil), and Peyronie's disease. Throughout the book, the authors share their own thoughts and journals, as well as describe their experiences. The book concludes with a list of resources, a bibliography, and a subject index.

- **AAKP Patient Plan. Phase Three: Stabilization**

  Source: Tampa, FL: American Association of Kidney Patients. 2000. 43 p.

  Contact: Available from American Association of Kidney Patients (AAKP). 100 South Ashley Drive, Suite 280, Tampa, FL 33602. (800) 749-AAKP or (813) 223-7099. E-mail: AAKPnat@aol.com. Website: www.aakp.org. PRICE: Single copy free. Also available for free at http://www.aakp.org/ppbk3.pdf.

  Summary: This booklet is the third in a four phase series of instructional materials for kidney patients. Published by the American Association of Kidney Patients (AAKP), the booklets are designed to address questions and concerns at various phases of the disease process. The four phases covered are diagnosis and treatment options, access and initiation, stabilization, and ongoing treatment. During each of these phases, the patient can keep control of his or her life by staying active and learning as much as possible about kidney disease and treatment. This third booklet introduces the reader to the idea of stabilization and the importance of continuing to learn about kidney disease. During this phase, the patient has settled into the routine of treatments and medications. The booklet covers optimal dialysis (dialysis adequacy); optimal transplant; family, friends, and social life; work, employment and volunteering; and legal responsibilities. Specific topics include hemodialysis adequacy, peritoneal dialysis adequacy, the importance of nutrition, anemia and how to treat it, the use of erythropoietin (EPO), the role of exercise, the symptoms of transplant rejection, the physical changes that may accompany transplant, how to handle stress, **erectile dysfunction** (impotence) and its treatment, how to talk about end stage renal disease (ESRD) in a new relationship, strategies to help the ongoing adjustment to ESRD, the Americans With Disabilities Act (ADA), the ESRD Networks and how they can help, and how to report a grievance to the Network. The booklet concludes with a glossary of terms and an appendix that lists information resources, ESRD networks, questions to ask the health care team, and forms to record important medical information. The booklet encourages readers to educate themselves and become active members of their own health care team. There are quotes and suggestions from other kidney patients sprinkled throughout the text. When readers are finished with the book, there is a postage paid card to send in to receive the fourth booklet. The booklet is illustrated with black and white photographs and tables. 3 figures. 8 tables.

- **Before and After Your Radical Retropubic Prostatectomy: Information and Resources to Help You Cope**

  Source: Quebec, Canada: Canadian Continence Foundation. 2000. 29 p.

Contact: Canadian Continence Foundation. B.P/P.O. 30, Succ. Victoria Branch, Westmount, Quebec, Canada, H3Z 2V4. (514) 488-8379. Email: help@continence-fdn.ca. Website: www.continence-fdn.ca. PRICE: $4.95; discounts with bulk orders.

Summary: This booklet provides general information and tips about how to manage before and after a radical retropubic prostatectomy (removal of the prostate gland), both in the hospital and at home. Information was gathered from men who have undergone this surgery from their spouses, and from health professionals involved in their care. Written mostly in a question and answer format, the booklet addresses the decision to have surgery, a checklist of questions to ask before surgery, feelings and emotions, waiting for the date of surgery, the use of pelvic floor muscle exercises to help prevent and treat urinary incontinence, what to expect during the admission to the hospital, immediate postoperative concerns, nursing care, recovering at home, coping with the urinary catheter, the symptoms and treatment of a bladder infection, identifying and treating urinary incontinence, incontinence products, postoperative **erectile dysfunction** (problems with erections), followup visits to the health care provider, and returning to regular work and family relations. The booklet concludes with a list of resources, including a blank space for noting telephone numbers, and support groups, books, videos, and reliable web sites for more information. 5 figures. 6 tables.

- **Therapy for Diabetes Mellitus and Related Disorders. 3rd ed**

Source: Alexandria, VA: American Diabetes Association. 1998. 487 p.

Contact: Available from American Diabetes Association (ADA). Order Fulfillment Department, P.O. Box 930850, Atlanta, GA 31193-0850. (800) 232-6733. Fax (770) 442-9742. Website: www.diabetes.org. PRICE: $39.95 plus shipping and handling. ISBN: 0945448945.

Summary: This handbook focuses on the treatment of problems that are of importance in the management of people with diabetes mellitus. The book attempts to help health professionals apply major advances in health care to their patients. Topics include the diagnosis and classification of diabetes mellitus, genetic counseling for type 1 diabetes, gestational diabetes mellitus, the management of pregnant women who have diabetes, antepartum and intrapartum obstetric care, neonatal problems and their management, type 1 diabetes and diabetic ketoacidosis in children, psychosocial adjustment in children who have type 1 diabetes, psychosocial aspects in adults, diabetic ketoacidosis and hyperosmolar hyperglycemic nonketotic syndrome in adults, and lactic acidosis. Other topics include the role of diabetes education in patient management; self monitoring of blood glucose; the rationale for management of hyperglycemia; medical nutrition therapy; pharmacological treatment of obesity; exercise; oral hypoglycemic agents such as sulfonylureas, repaglinide, metformin, alpha glucosidase inhibitors, and thiazolidinediones; insulin treatment; insulin pump therapy; combination therapy for hyperglycemia; and diabetes complications. In addition, the book discusses surgery and anesthesia in people with diabetes, geriatric patient care, hypoglycemia in patients who have type 1 diabetes, insulin allergy and insulin resistance, drugs and hormones that increase blood glucose levels, diabetic dyslipidemia, antihypertensive therapy, cutaneous disorders associated with diabetes mellitus, infections, visual loss, ocular complications, drug induced renal dysfunction, diabetic nephropathy, chronic kidney disease, painful or insensitive lower extremity, mononeuropathy and amyoradiculopathy, gastrointestinal disturbances, and bladder dysfunction. Final topics include **erectile dysfunction,** female sexual disorders, postural hypotension, sudomotor dysfunction and dark vision, cardiac denervation syndrome, noninvasive cardiac testing, angina and congestive heart failure, myocardial infarction, peripheral vascular disease, and foot ulcers and infections. The book includes an index. Numerous figures. Numerous tables. Numerous references.

- **Getting Help: A Patient's Guide for Men With Impotence**

  Source: Lenexa, KS: Integrated Medical Resources, Inc. 1995. 48 p.

  Contact: Available from Integrated Medical Resources, Inc. 8326 Melrose Drive, Lenexa, KS 66214. (913) 894-0591. PRICE: $6.95.

  Summary: This handbook provides basic information about the diagnosis and treatment of male **erectile dysfunction,** or impotence. After introductory chapters defining impotence and discussing its causes, the author considers diagnostic issues, including the patient history and physical, specialized blood tests, erection monitoring during sleep, in-office impotence testing, and other specialized tests. The next chapter outlines treatment options, including sexual counseling, oral medications, testosterone hormone replacement, penile injections, vacuum constriction devices, penile implant surgery, and corrective surgeries. Also included is a chapter on penile curvature and Peyronie's disease. The handbook concludes with two brief sections to help readers determine if they really have a problem and to encourage them to consult a health care provider. A brief index concludes the book. Simple line drawings illustrate many of the concepts.

- **Manual of Urology: Diagnosis and Therapy. 2nd ed**

  Source: Hagerstown, MD: Lippincott Williams and Wilkins. 1999. 362 p.

  Contact: Available from Lippincott Williams and Wilkins. P.O. Box 1600, Hagerstown, MD 21741. (800) 638-3030 or (301) 714-2300. Fax (301) 824-7390. Website: www.lww.com. PRICE: $37.95 plus shipping and handling. ISBN: 078171785X.

  Summary: This manual is designed to be used by the house officer and medical student responsible for urology patients. The related endoscopic, medical, and diagnostic procedures are well described. Twenty two chapters cover imaging of the genitourinary tract, radionuclide imaging, endoscopic instruments and surgery, nontraumatic genitourinary emergencies, fluid and electrolyte disorders, lower urinary tract symptoms, hematuria (blood in the urine) and other urine abnormalities, evaluation of renal mass lesions, surgical disorders of the adrenal gland, urinary calculi (stones) and endourology, the management of urinary incontinence, male **erectile dysfunction** (impotence), male reproductive dysfunction, neoplasms (cancerous and benign) of the genitourinary tract, the medical management of genitourinary malignancy (cancer), radiation therapy of genitourinary malignancy, genitourinary infection, management of genitourinary trauma, pediatric urology, neurourology and urodynamic testing, and renal (kidney) transplantation. Each chapter presents information in outline form, with numerous tables and diagrams, as necessary. Each chapter concludes with a list of suggested reading. The handbook concludes with two appendices, presenting the American Urological Association Symptom Score (for benign prostatic hyperplasia) and the staging of genitourinary tumors, as well as a subject index.

- **20 Common Problems in Urology**

  Source: New York, NY: McGraw-Hill, Inc. 2001. 335 p.

  Contact: Available from McGraw-Hill, Inc. 1221 Avenue of the Americas, New York, NY 10020. (612) 832-7869. Website: www.bookstore.mcgraw-hill.com. PRICE: $45.00; plus shipping and handling. ISBN: 0070634130.

Summary: This text on common problems in urology is designed for the primary care provider. The text covers both pediatric and adult conditions and features quick reference algorithms, charts and tables that organize presenting signs and symptoms, diagnostic tests, and treatments. Twenty chapters cover fetal and postnatal hydronephrosis (fluid accumulation in the kidneys), urinary tract infections (UTIs) in children, cryptorchidism (undescended testicles), circumcision, nocturnal enuresis (bedwetting), UTIs in adults, urethritis, urinary incontinence, interstitial cystitis, geriatric urology, hematuria (blood in the urine), prostate cancer screening, benign prostatic hyperplasia (BPH), scrotal mass and pain, genital skin rash, urinary calculi (stones), **erectile dysfunction** (impotence), male infertility, vasectomy, male menopause, and imaging studies (diagnostic tests). Most chapters define the condition and then discuss the differential diagnosis, the physical examination, recommended diagnostic tests, special considerations, treatment options, and patient care strategies. The text also offers practice advice on when to refer to a specialist and what to expect post-referral. The text concludes with a subject index and is illustrated with black and white photographs and diagrams.

- **Comprehensive Urology**

  Source: Orlando, FL: Mosby, Inc. 2001. 704 p.

  Contact: Available from Mosby, Inc. Order Fulfillment Department, 6277 Sea Harbor Drive, Orlando FL 32887. (800) 321-5068. Fax (800)874-6418. E-mail: custserv.ehs@elsevier.com Website: www.elsevierhealth.com. PRICE: $249.00. ISBN: 723429499.

Summary: This textbook offers a comprehensive overview of urology in one volume incorporating clinical information concerning all aspects of urology. The internationally renowned contributors present detailed clinical information in a format which is not encyclopedic but contains carefully selected and nonbiased practical information backed by specific, relevant references. The first section concisely reviews basic anatomy, physiology, and molecular biology, which have relevance for the entire text. The remaining 42 chapters are presented in seven sections: investigative urology, pediatric urology, benign conditions of the upper urinary tract, urologic oncology, benign conditions of the lower urinary tract, andrology, and miscellaneous. Specific topics include diagnostic tests, interventional uroradiology, congenital diseases, vesicoureteral reflux, renal (kidney) transplantation, urinary tract infections, urinary tract stones, bladder cancer, prostate cancer, benign prostatic hyperplasia, female urology and incontinence, interstitial cystitis, the neuropathic bladder, urinary diversion and augmentations, urethral stricture disease, male infertility, **erectile dysfunction**, benign and malignant disorders of the penis, extracorporeal shock wave lithotripsy (ESWL), genitourinary trauma, radiation therapy, and chemotherapy. Each chapter concludes with lengthy references, and a subject index concludes the volume. The text is illustrated with full-color photographs and drawings.

- **Handbook of Diagnostic Endocrinology**

  Source: Totowa, NJ: The Humana Press, Inc. 2003. 360 p.

  Contact: Humana Press, Inc. 999 Riverview Dr., Suite 208 Totowa, NJ 07512. (973) 256-1699. Fax (973) 256-8341. E-mail: humana@humanapr.com PRICE: $99.50 plus shipping and handling. ISBN: 0896037576.

Summary: With the rapid development of new and more reliable diagnostic tests, and aided by the molecular and genetic approaches that continue to deepen the understanding of these diseases, the ability to diagnose patients with endocrine disease has dramatically increased. In this book, physicians concisely explain the pathophysiology and clinical manifestations of these disorders and survey all the latest laboratory tests used in their diagnosis. Topics range widely from an overview of the diagnosis of diabetes and the long-term monitoring of its complications to the evaluation of menstrual dysfunction. Other topics include the diagnosis of pituitary tumors, Cushing's syndrome, thyroid disease, and hypoglycemia; the evaluation of endocrine-induced hypertension; the assessment of dyslipidemia and obesity; new approaches to diagnosing hypercalcemia and hypocalcemia, osteoporosis, hypogonadism and **erectile dysfunction,** and hyperandrogenism in women. The authors review the complex physiological basis of the relevant endocrine processes and provide recommendations for the follow up and long term management of patients. Each chapter concludes with references and the text concludes with a subject index.

Book Summaries: Online Booksellers

Commercial Internet-based booksellers, such as Amazon.com and Barnes&Noble.com, offer summaries which have been supplied by each title's publisher. Some summaries also include customer reviews. Your local bookseller may have access to in-house and commercial databases that index all published books (e.g. Books in Print®). **IMPORTANT NOTE:** Online booksellers typically produce search results for medical and non-medical books. When searching for "erectile dysfunction" at online booksellers' Web sites, you may discover non-medical books that use the generic term "erectile dysfunction" (or a synonym) in their titles. The following is indicative of the results you might find when searching for "erectile dysfunction" (sorted alphabetically by title; follow the hyperlink to view more details at Amazon.com):

- **"Your Legs Are Too Long": Getting Beyond Excuses for Erectile Dysfunction** by Deborah Kathryn Hargis (2003); ISBN: 0971954100;
  http://www.amazon.com/exec/obidos/ASIN/0971954100/icongroupinterna

- **100 Questions & Answers About Erectile Dysfunction** by Pamela Ellsworth, Bob Stanley (2002); ISBN: 0763705896;
  http://www.amazon.com/exec/obidos/ASIN/0763705896/icongroupinterna

- **An Atlas of Erectile Dysfunction** by Roger S. Kirby; ISBN: 1850700427;
  http://www.amazon.com/exec/obidos/ASIN/1850700427/icongroupinterna

- **Conservative Treatment of Male Urinary Incontinence and Erectile Dysfunction** by Grace Dorey; ISBN: 1861563027;
  http://www.amazon.com/exec/obidos/ASIN/1861563027/icongroupinterna

- **Contemporary Diagnosis and Management of Male Erectile Dysfunction** by Tom F. Lue; ISBN: 1884065279;
  http://www.amazon.com/exec/obidos/ASIN/1884065279/icongroupinterna

- **Erectile Dysfunction** by W.F. Thon, et al; ISBN: 0387527486;
  http://www.amazon.com/exec/obidos/ASIN/0387527486/icongroupinterna

- **Erectile Dysfunction** by A. Rane; ISBN: 1873413696;
  http://www.amazon.com/exec/obidos/ASIN/1873413696/icongroupinterna

- **Erectile Dysfunction -- Current Investigation and Management** by Ian Eardley, et al; ISBN: 0723433658;
  http://www.amazon.com/exec/obidos/ASIN/0723433658/icongroupinterna

- **Erectile Dysfunction (Patient Pictures)** by Philip Kell, et al (2000); ISBN: 189954111X;
  http://www.amazon.com/exec/obidos/ASIN/189954111X/icongroupinterna

- **Erectile Dysfunction and Vascular Disease** by Michael Kirby (2003); ISBN: 1405107537;
  http://www.amazon.com/exec/obidos/ASIN/1405107537/icongroupinterna

- **Erectile Dysfunction: A Clinical Guide** by Roger S. Kirby (Editor), et al (1999); ISBN: 190186524X;
  http://www.amazon.com/exec/obidos/ASIN/190186524X/icongroupinterna

- **Erectile Dysfunction: Integrating Couple Therapy, Sex Therapy, and Medical Treatment** by Gerald R. Weeks, Nancy Gambescia; ISBN: 0393703304;
  http://www.amazon.com/exec/obidos/ASIN/0393703304/icongroupinterna

- **Erectile Dysfunction: issues in current pharmacotherapy** by Alvaro Morales (1998); ISBN: 1853175773;
  http://www.amazon.com/exec/obidos/ASIN/1853175773/icongroupinterna

- **Fast Facts: Erectile Dysfunction (Fast Facts)** by Roger Kirby, et al; ISBN: 1899541470;
  http://www.amazon.com/exec/obidos/ASIN/1899541470/icongroupinterna

- **Fast Facts: Male Erectile Dysfunction (Fast Facts)** by Simon Holmes, et al; ISBN: 1899541551;
  http://www.amazon.com/exec/obidos/ASIN/1899541551/icongroupinterna

- **Heart Disease and Erectile Dysfunction (Contemporary Cardiology)** by Robert A. Kloner (Editor) (2004); ISBN: 1588292169;
  http://www.amazon.com/exec/obidos/ASIN/1588292169/icongroupinterna

- **Impotence: Diagnosis and Management of Erectile Dysfunction** by Alan H. Bennett (Editor) (1997); ISBN: 072163768X;
  http://www.amazon.com/exec/obidos/ASIN/072163768X/icongroupinterna

- **Impotence: Diagnosis and Management of Male Erectile Dysfunction** by Culley C. Carson, et al (1991); ISBN: 0750613629;
  http://www.amazon.com/exec/obidos/ASIN/0750613629/icongroupinterna

- **Key Trials in Erectile Dysfunction** by Carson, Wagner (2002); ISBN: 1904218040;
  http://www.amazon.com/exec/obidos/ASIN/1904218040/icongroupinterna

- **Management of Erectile Dysfunction in Primary Care** by John Dean, et al (2002); ISBN: 1904218113;
  http://www.amazon.com/exec/obidos/ASIN/1904218113/icongroupinterna

- **Medical Biology of Yohimbine & Its Easy Use in Male Sex Erectile Dysfunction: Index of New Information With Authors, Subjects, Research Categories & References** by Henry Z. Poche (1997); ISBN: 0788315919;
  http://www.amazon.com/exec/obidos/ASIN/0788315919/icongroupinterna

- **Medical Management of Erectile Dysfunction : A Primary-Care Manual** by Harin Padma-Nathan (1999); ISBN: 1884735401;
  http://www.amazon.com/exec/obidos/ASIN/1884735401/icongroupinterna

- **Natural Penis Enlargement: New methods of avoiding and curing impotence, premature ejaculation, and erectile dysfunction safely and inexpensively. NEW Secrets that your doctor won¿t tell you, No Pumps, No Pills and No Gadgets!** by Platinum Millennium, Platinum Millennium Publishing; ISBN: 0972261311;
  http://www.amazon.com/exec/obidos/ASIN/0972261311/icongroupinterna

- **Pelvic Floor Exercises for Erectile Dysfunction** by Grace Dorey (2004); ISBN: 1861563655;
  http://www.amazon.com/exec/obidos/ASIN/1861563655/icongroupinterna

- **Pharmacotherapy for Erectile Dysfunction** by Harin Padma-Nathan (Editor), et al; ISBN: 1853177091;
  http://www.amazon.com/exec/obidos/ASIN/1853177091/icongroupinterna

- **Prostate and Renal Cancer, Benign Prostatic Hyperplasia, Erectile Dysfunction and Basic Research: An Update** by Ch. H. Bangma (Editor), et al; ISBN: 1842141961;
  http://www.amazon.com/exec/obidos/ASIN/1842141961/icongroupinterna

- **Report on the treatment of organic erectile dysfunction**; ISBN: 096497021X;
  http://www.amazon.com/exec/obidos/ASIN/096497021X/icongroupinterna

- **Research on Venous Outflow Reduction in Erectile Dysfunction (Acta Biomedica Lovaniensia , No 108)** by Hubert Claes; ISBN: 9061866782;
  http://www.amazon.com/exec/obidos/ASIN/9061866782/icongroupinterna

- **Textbook of Erectile Dysfunction** by Culley C. Carson MD (Editor), et al; ISBN: 1899066969;
  http://www.amazon.com/exec/obidos/ASIN/1899066969/icongroupinterna

- **Textbook of Erectile Dysfunction** by Bernard Levinson (Editor); ISBN: 1919713425;
  http://www.amazon.com/exec/obidos/ASIN/1919713425/icongroupinterna

- **The role of alprostadil in the diagnosis amd treatment of erectile dysfunction : proceedings of a symposium, August 3-4, 1993, Brook Lodge, Kalamazoo, Michigan**; ISBN: 0444019022;
  http://www.amazon.com/exec/obidos/ASIN/0444019022/icongroupinterna

- **The Viagra Alternative: The Complete Guide to Overcoming Erectile Dysfunction Naturally** by Marc Bonnard, Marc, M.D. Bonnard; ISBN: 0892817895;
  http://www.amazon.com/exec/obidos/ASIN/0892817895/icongroupinterna

- **UK Management Guidelines for Erectile Dysfunction: May 1999**; ISBN: 1853154245;
  http://www.amazon.com/exec/obidos/ASIN/1853154245/icongroupinterna

- **Understanding Erectile Dysfunction Chart** by Anatomical Chart (2003); ISBN: 1587795477;
  http://www.amazon.com/exec/obidos/ASIN/1587795477/icongroupinterna

- **Vascular Andrology: Erectile Dysfunction/Priapism Varicocele** by A. Ledda (Editor) (1996); ISBN: 3540594728;
  http://www.amazon.com/exec/obidos/ASIN/3540594728/icongroupinterna

The National Library of Medicine Book Index

The National Library of Medicine at the National Institutes of Health has a massive database of books published on healthcare and biomedicine. Go to the following Internet site, **http://locatorplus.gov/**, and then select "Search LOCATORplus." Once you are in the search area, simply type "erectile dysfunction" (or synonyms) into the search box, and select "books only." From there, results can be sorted by publication date, author, or relevance. The following was recently catalogued by the National Library of Medicine:[11]

---

[11] In addition to LOCATORPlus, in collaboration with authors and publishers, he National Center for Biotechnology Information (NCBI) is currently adapting biomedical books for the Web. The books may be accessed

- **Cardiovascular implications of PDE5 inhibition in men with erectile dysfunction.** Author: Jackson, Graham,; Year: 2002; London, U.K.: W.B. Saunders, c2002

- **Erectile dysfunction** Author: Jonas, Udo.; Year: 1991; Berlin; New York: Springer-Verlag, c1991; ISBN: 3540527486
  http://www.amazon.com/exec/obidos/ASIN/3540527486/icongroupinterna

- **Treatment options for male erectile dysfunction: a systematic review of published studies of effectiveness** Author: Wilt, Timothy J.; Year: 1999; Boston, MA: MDRC, HSR;D, [1999]

Chapters on Erectile Dysfunction

In order to find chapters that specifically relate to erectile dysfunction, an excellent source of abstracts is the Combined Health Information Database. You will need to limit your search to book chapters and erectile dysfunction using the "Detailed Search" option. Go to the following hyperlink: **http://chid.nih.gov/detail/detail.html**. To find book chapters, use the drop boxes at the bottom of the search page where "You may refine your search by." Select the dates and language you prefer, and the format option "Book Chapter." Type "erectile dysfunction" (or synonyms) into the "For these words:" box. The following is a typical result when searching for book chapters on erectile dysfunction:

- **Doc, I've Got a Problem: Evaluating the Male with Erectile Dysfunction**

  Source: in Newman, A.J. Beyond Viagra: Plain Talk About Treating Male and Female Sexual Dysfunction. Montgomery, AL: Starrhill Press. 1999. p. 45-57.

  Contact: Available from Black Belt Press. P.O. Box 551, Montgomery, AL 36101. (800) 959-3245 or (334) 265-6753. Fax (334) 265-8880. PRICE: $13.95 plus shipping and handling. ISBN: 1573590142.

  Summary: As with any other medical problem, evaluation of the patient who has complaints of erectile dysfunction begins with a comprehensive medical and psychosexual history, physical examination, and focused laboratory testing. This chapter on the evaluation of male erectile dysfunction is from a book that discusses the drug sildenafil (Viagra) in the context of a larger discussion about sexuality and sexual dysfunction. The author stresses that the psychosexual history is probably the most important part of the diagnostic process. While the medical history helps identify risk factors that contribute to an underlying physical etiology (for example, smoking, history of elevated cholesterol, history of hypertension, or history of previous radical prostate cancer surgery), the psychosexual history helps in determining whether the patient's problem is primarily physical or psychological. It is also very helpful to involve the patient's partner early in the evaluation process. This allows for a very accurate psychosexual history along with good communication and a better therapeutic alliance with the patient. The author reviews the common diagnostic tests used, including the nocturnal penile tumescence (NPT) testing, other sleep lab studies, ultrasound, cavernosometry, cavernosography, and urinalysis. The author concludes that today,

---

in two ways: (1) by searching directly using any search term or phrase (in the same way as the bibliographic database PubMed), or (2) by following the links to PubMed abstracts. Each PubMed abstract has a "Books" button that displays a facsimile of the abstract in which some phrases are hypertext links. These phrases are also found in the books available at NCBI. Click on hyperlinked results in the list of books in which the phrase is found. Currently, the majority of the links are between the books and PubMed. In the future, more links will be created between the books and other types of information, such as gene and protein sequences and macromolecular structures. See **http://www.ncbi.nlm.nih.gov/entrez/query.fcgi?db=Books**.

with the availability of Viagra, the first step after the history and physical exam is to start the patient on Viagra. After a 4 to 6 week trial with Viagra the patient is not having a successful response, the assessment can be conducted in greater depth. The chapter is written in nontechnical language but includes enough medical information to be of use to medical professionals wishing to learn more about sexuality and sexual dysfunction.

- **Enter Viagra!: Viagra for Male Erectile Dysfunction**

Source: in Newman, A.J. Beyond Viagra: Plain Talk About Treating Male and Female Sexual Dysfunction. Montgomery, AL: Starrhill Press. 1999. p. 118-129.

Contact: Available from Black Belt Press. P.O. Box 551, Montgomery, AL 36101. (800) 959-3245 or (334) 265-6753. Fax (334) 265-8880. PRICE: $13.95 plus shipping and handling. ISBN: 1573590142.

Summary: This chapter is from a book that discusses the drug sildenafil (Viagra) in the context of a larger discussion about sexuality and sexual dysfunction. The author offers a question and answer format that introduces sildenafil, its use, advantages and disadvantages, how it works, patient selection (and contraindications), age factors, costs, and insurance coverage for the drug. Readers are reminded that Viagra has no effect in the absence of sexual stimulation. The beneficial effect can be seen as late as 8 hours after taking the tablet, but the average time for maximum blood level is about 60 minutes. Adverse effects with Viagra can include mild headache, flushing, indigestion, runny nose, transient visual disturbance (blue haze), urinary tract infection, diarrhea, dizziness, and a rash. The only contraindication to Viagra therapy is the concurrent use of nitrates, including sublingual nitroglycerine, long acting oral nitrates, and nitrate paste. Viagra's cost is about the same as some of the newer, very potent antibiotics that are taken for severe prostate infections; it ranges from about $8 to $11 per tablet. The chapter is written in nontechnical language but includes enough medical information to be of use to medical professionals wishing to learn more about sexuality and sexual dysfunction.

- **What Next?: Future Treatment Developments for Male Erectile Dysfunction**

Source: in Newman, A.J. Beyond Viagra: Plain Talk About Treating Male and Female Sexual Dysfunction. Montgomery, AL: Starrhill Press. 1999. p. 134-137.

Contact: Available from Black Belt Press. P.O. Box 551, Montgomery, AL 36101. (800) 959-3245 or (334) 265-6753. Fax (334) 265-8880. PRICE: $13.95 plus shipping and handling. ISBN: 1573590142.

Summary: This chapter on future treatment developments for male erectile dysfunction is from a book that discusses the drug sildenafil (Viagra) in the context of a larger discussion about sexuality and sexual dysfunction. The author discusses new oral drugs, including oral phentolamine (Vasomax) and apomorphine, and other treatments, including several new topical agents and combinations of oral agents or oral and injectable agents. On the molecular level, several laboratories are making progress in the understanding of the biochemistry of the smooth muscle in the corpus cavernosum tissue. The chapter concludes with a brief discussion of a new surgical technique that can treat men with Peyronie's disease. Written in nontechnical language, the chapter includes enough medical information to be of use to medical professionals wishing to learn more about sexuality and sexual dysfunction.

- **Why Me?: Causes of Male Erectile Dysfunction**

Source: in Newman, A.J. Beyond Viagra: Plain Talk About Treating Male and Female Sexual Dysfunction. Montgomery, AL: Starrhill Press. 1999. p. 26-44.

Contact: Available from Black Belt Press. P.O. Box 551, Montgomery, AL 36101. (800) 959-3245 or (334) 265-6753. Fax (334) 265-8880. PRICE: $13.95 plus shipping and handling. ISBN: 1573590142.

Summary: This chapter on the causes of male erectile dysfunction is from a book that discusses the drug sildenafil (Viagra) in the context of a larger discussion about sexuality and sexual dysfunction. The author discusses the causes of male erectile dysfunction in two general categories: physical (or organic) and psychological. Factors prevent initiation of an erection usually involve the nerve supply, but can also be psychological. Factors that prevent the erectile tissue from fully filling with blood usually have to do with problems of arterial blood flow to the penis. Factors that lead to loss of the erection before orgasm and ejaculation tend to involve failure of the venous occlusive mechanism that traps blood in the penis and thus maintains the erection. Most men complaining of erectile dysfunction have at least one, and sometimes several, of the following problem areas: blood flow problems, nerve problems, diabetes, prior surgery, drugs, pelvic trauma or pelvic radiation, Peyronie's disease, and psychological problems. Psychological problems can include anxiety and fear of failure, depression, marital conflict, misinformation or lack of information about normal male sexual function and changes with aging, and psychiatric problems (including psychotic disorders and obsessive compulsive personality disorders). The chapter is written in nontechnical language but includes enough medical information to be of use to medical professionals wishing to learn more about sexuality and sexual dysfunction. One table reviews the drugs that may produce erectile dysfunction. 1 table.

- **Matter Over Mind: Treatment of Psychological Erectile Dysfunction**

Source: in Newman, A.J. Beyond Viagra: Plain Talk About Treating Male and Female Sexual Dysfunction. Montgomery, AL: Starrhill Press. 1999. p. 100-105.

Contact: Available from Black Belt Press. P.O. Box 551, Montgomery, AL 36101. (800) 959-3245 or (334) 265-6753. Fax (334) 265-8880. PRICE: $13.95 plus shipping and handling. ISBN: 1573590142.

Summary: This chapter on the treatment of psychological erectile dysfunction is from a book that discusses the drug sildenafil (Viagra) in the context of a larger discussion about sexuality and sexual dysfunction. The author stresses that purely psychogenic causes account for no more than 15 percent of the men with erectile dysfunction. However, it is rare indeed to see a man with a physical cause of erectile dysfunction who does not also complain of a marked psychological impact. Therefore, psychosexual therapy for impotence divides into two groups of patients: those whose underlying problem is primarily psychological and those whose underlying problem is primarily physical. Topics include psychotherapy for these two different groups and the use of sex therapy. Many patients with primarily psychological effects from a recent life event, such as the death of a family member or personal stresses at work or in their marriage, will see a return to normal erectile function once the relationship or work problems resolve, or an adequate amount of time has passed since the traumatic loss of a family member. The key to treating psychogenic erectile dysfunction is to involve the patient's partner in the treatment. The author notes that those people whose erectile dysfunction is primarily psychological in origin usually find minimally invasive treatments (vacuum erection devices, oral drugs like Viagra, or intracavernosal injections) effective. The chapter is written in nontechnical language but includes enough medical information to be of use to medical professionals wishing to learn more about sexuality and sexual dysfunction.

- **Kindest Cut: Vascular Surgery for Erectile Dysfunction**

  Source: in Newman, A.J. Beyond Viagra: Plain Talk About Treating Male and Female Sexual Dysfunction. Montgomery, AL: Starrhill Press. 1999. p. 80-83.

  Contact: Available from Black Belt Press. P.O. Box 551, Montgomery, AL 36101. (800) 959-3245 or (334) 265-6753. Fax (334) 265-8880. PRICE: $13.95 plus shipping and handling. ISBN: 1573590142.

  Summary: This chapter on vascular surgery for erectile dysfunction is from a book that discusses the drug sildenafil (Viagra) in the context of a larger discussion about sexuality and sexual dysfunction. Vascular surgery is a rarely needed treatment for erectile dysfunction. It can be divided into two major areas: arterial revascularization of the penis, namely, repairing damaged vessels bringing blood into the penis; and surgery for veno occlusive disorder, essentially correcting problems with the mechanics that clamp down on blood outflow. The author briefly reviews the criteria for evaluation for penile revascularization, and the criteria for surgery for veno occlusive disorder. The conclusion is that, in spite of great strides in surgical technique and results, long term results have been less than satisfactory; therefore, this type of surgery is only recommended in rare, specific situations. The chapter is written in nontechnical language but includes enough medical information to be of use to medical professionals wishing to learn more about sexuality and sexual dysfunction.

Directories

In addition to the references and resources discussed earlier in this chapter, a number of directories relating to erectile dysfunction have been published that consolidate information across various sources. The Combined Health Information Database lists the following, which you may wish to consult in your local medical library:[12]

- **Resource Guide: Products and Services for Incontinence**

  Source: Spartanburg, SC: National Association for Continence. 199x. [104 p.].

  Contact: Available from National Association for Continence (NAFC). (formerly Help For Incontinent People). P.O. Box 8310, Spartanburg, SC 29305-8310. (800) BLADDER or (864) 579-7900. Fax (864) 579-7902. PRICE: $10.00 plus $3.00 shipping and handling; free with membership.

  Summary: This directory, compiled by the National Association for Continence (formerly Help for Incontinent People, or HIP), lists products and services for incontinence. The resource guide was developed to assist people who are awaiting professional treatment for incontinence, people whose incontinence is presently being treated by a health professional, and for people whose incontinence cannot be cured.

---

[12] You will need to limit your search to "Directory" and "diseasex" using the "Detailed Search" option. Go directly to the following hyperlink: **http://chid.nih.gov/detail/detail.html**. To find directories, use the drop boxes at the bottom of the search page where "You may refine your search by." For publication date, select "All Years." Select your preferred language and the format option "Directory." Type "diseasex" (or synonyms) into the "For these words:" box. You should check back periodically with this database as it is updated every three months.

The guide is divided into five sections: product listings, manufacturers' index, distributors' index, mail and phone order index, and organizations and services index. The product listings section is divided into sixteen categories: disposable products, reusable products, external urinary devices and accessories, intermittent self-catheterization, fecal incontinence, skin care products, deodorizing products, nocturnal enuresis (bedwetting), pelvic muscle re-education equipment, pelvic organ support devices, implanted devices, treatments for **erectile dysfunction,** medications, support surface equipment, miscellaneous, and educational materials. Each product description is illustrated with a simple line drawing. The directory is revised each year.

CHAPTER 8. MULTIMEDIA ON ERECTILE DYSFUNCTION

Overview

In this chapter, we show you how to keep current on multimedia sources of information on erectile dysfunction. We start with sources that have been summarized by federal agencies, and then show you how to find bibliographic information catalogued by the National Library of Medicine.

Video Recordings

An excellent source of multimedia information on erectile dysfunction is the Combined Health Information Database. You will need to limit your search to "Videorecording" and "erectile dysfunction" using the "Detailed Search" option. Go directly to the following hyperlink: **http://chid.nih.gov/detail/detail.html**. To find video productions, use the drop boxes at the bottom of the search page where "You may refine your search by." Select the dates and language you prefer, and the format option "Videorecording (videotape, videocassette, etc.)." Type "erectile dysfunction" (or synonyms) into the "For these words:" box. The following is a typical result when searching for video recordings on erectile dysfunction:

- **Current Approaches to Erectile Dysfunction**

  Source: Madison, WI: University of Wisconsin Hospitals and Clinics, Department of Outreach Education. 1999. (videocassette).

  Contact: Available from University of Wisconsin Hospital and Clinics. Picture of Health, 702 North Blackhawk Avenue, Suite 215, Madison, WI 53705-3357. (800) 757-4354 or (608) 263-6510. Fax (608) 262-7172. PRICE: $19.95 plus shipping and handling; bulk copies available. Order number 060699A.

  Summary: Erectile dysfunction (impotence) is a common, treatable condition experienced by 10 to 20 million men in the United States. This videotape program, moderated by Carol Koby, discusses the current approaches to the diagnosis and treatment of erectile dysfunction (ED). The program features Dr. Wolfram Nolten, an endocrinologist, who first defines ED as the inability to achieve or maintain erection satisfactory for intercourse at least 50 percent of the time. Dr. Nolten stresses that effective treatments are available. Focusing primarily on Viagra (sildenafil), Dr. Nolten discusses the history of the drug's development, how Viagra works, cost considerations, side effects, patient selection issues, and the use of Viagra in women (an 'off label' use that is not recommended). Other topics covered include the role of depression and stress, hormones, systemic diseases (such as diabetes mellitus or cardiovascular diseases), and drug effects on the development of ED. Dr. Nolten then covers diagnostic issues, the appropriate use of primary care providers to treat most men with ED, other drugs used to treat ED (self injection and urethral administration of vasoactive drugs), penile implants, vacuum erection devices, and the implications of the presence of noctural erections. Dr. Nolten concludes by reminding viewers that 'erection is good for erection'; in other words, frequent erections oxygenate the penis and keep the physiology in good working condition. As the population ages, there is an accompanying change in awareness of sexuality and general health. The program concludes with a reference to a physician's guide to ED information and resources (www.pslgroup.com).

- **Recognizing and Managing Erectile Dysfunction**

  Source: Kansas City, MO: American Academy of Family Physicians. 2000. (videocassette).

  Contact: Available from American Academy of Family Physicians. 8880 Ward Parkway, Kansas City, MO 64114-2797. (800) 274-2237. PRICE: $17.95 for members; $25.00 for non-members, plus shipping and handling.

  Summary: Sexual dysfunction affects about 31 percent of men in the United States. The most common of these problems are erectile dysfunction (ED, formerly called impotence), premature ejaculation, inability to achieve orgasm or ejaculation, and decreased libido. This continuing education program focuses on ED, which is defined as the inability to achieve or maintain penile erection sufficient for sexual intercourse. The program includes a videotape program and study guide and covers the causes of ED, including vascular, neurologic, endocrine, anatomical, and medications and substance abuse; the evaluation of ED, including patient history, a focused physical examination, the indications for laboratory tests, and the role of referral; therapeutic options, including medical (drug) therapy, vacuum constriction devices, psychotherapy or sex therapy, intraurethral therapy, intracavernosal injection, and surgery; and patient education. The program stresses that any patient with a complaint of erectile problems should be thoroughly evaluated before treatment recommendations are made. The first step in treatment is addressing modifiable causes or exacerbating factors. If further treatment is necessary, a number of safe and effective options are available. Patients can be assured that ED is treatable. Men and their partners may also benefit from counseling to address related emotional and relationship issues. The program comes with a patient information fact sheet (which can be photocopied and distributed), and a form with which readers can qualify for continuing education credits. 11 tables. 13 references.

Bibliography: Multimedia on Erectile Dysfunction

The National Library of Medicine is a rich source of information on healthcare-related multimedia productions including slides, computer software, and databases. To access the multimedia database, go to the following Web site: **http://locatorplus.gov/**. Select "Search LOCATORplus." Once in the search area, simply type in erectile dysfunction (or synonyms).

Then, in the option box provided below the search box, select "Audiovisuals and Computer Files." From there, you can choose to sort results by publication date, author, or relevance. The following multimedia has been indexed on erectile dysfunction:

- **Current concepts of erectile dysfunction [videorecording]: diagnosis & treatment** Source: sponsored by Mayo Clinic; CME Information Services, Inc., CMEVideo; Year: 1998; Format: Videorecording; Mt. Laurel, NJ: CMEVideo, 1998

- **Erectile dysfunction [videorecording]: oral therapy: current treatment and future therapies** Source: Marshfield Clinic, Saint Joseph's Hospital; a presentation of the Marshfield Video Network; Year: 1998; Format: Videorecording; Marshfield, WI: The Network, c1998

- **Erectile dysfunction [videorecording]: recognition, diagnosis, and treatment** Source: Ridwan Shabsigh; Year: 1997; Format: Videorecording; Secaucus, N.J.: Network for Continuing Medical Education, 1997

- **Erectile dysfunction in primary care [videorecording]: broaching the subject, treating the problem** Source: Andre T. Guay, Louis Kurtizky, Jacob Rajfer; guest commentary, Louis Ignarro; Year: 2000; Format: Videorecording; Secaucus, N.J.: Network for Continuing Medical Education, c2000

- **Recognizing and managing erectile dysfunction [videorecording]** Source: American Academy of Family Physicians; Year: 2000; Format: Videorecording; Leawood, KS: American Academy of Family Physicians, c2000

- **The erectile dysfunction decision support system [electronic resource]** Source: [Bruce Block]; Year: 1995; Format: Electronic resource; Chapel Hill, NC: Health Sciences Consortium, c1995

- **The erectile dysfunction decision support system [electronic resource]** Source: Bruce Block; Year: 1993; Format: Electronic resource; Chapel Hill, NC: Health Sciences Consortium, c1993

CHAPTER 9. PERIODICALS AND NEWS ON ERECTILE DYSFUNCTION

Overview

In this chapter, we suggest a number of news sources and present various periodicals that cover erectile dysfunction.

News Services and Press Releases

One of the simplest ways of tracking press releases on erectile dysfunction is to search the news wires. In the following sample of sources, we will briefly describe how to access each service. These services only post recent news intended for public viewing.

PR Newswire

To access the PR Newswire archive, simply go to **http://www.prnewswire.com/**. Select your country. Type "erectile dysfunction" (or synonyms) into the search box. You will automatically receive information on relevant news releases posted within the last 30 days. The search results are shown by order of relevance.

Reuters Health

The Reuters' Medical News and Health eLine databases can be very useful in exploring news archives relating to erectile dysfunction. While some of the listed articles are free to view, others are available for purchase for a nominal fee. To access this archive, go to **http://www.reutershealth.com/en/index.html** and search by "erectile dysfunction" (or synonyms). The following was recently listed in this archive for erectile dysfunction:

- **One third of older men report erectile dysfunction**
  Source: Reuters Medical News
  Date: August 04, 2003

- **Lilly, ICOS yet to provide data to FDA on Cialis for erectile dysfunction**
  Source: Reuters Medical News
  Date: May 02, 2003

- **UK company trials inhaled drug for erectile dysfunction**
  Source: Reuters Industry Breifing
  Date: March 25, 2003

- **Sildenafil safe, effective for type 1 diabetic men with erectile dysfunction**
  Source: Reuters Industry Breifing
  Date: March 12, 2003

- **FDA lifts clinical hold on NexMed erectile dysfunction study**
  Source: Reuters Industry Breifing
  Date: February 27, 2003

- **Novel erectile dysfunction drug superior to sildenafil**
  Source: Reuters Medical News
  Date: January 22, 2003

- **Vardenafil for erectile dysfunction safe for men with exertional angina due to CAD**
  Source: Reuters Industry Breifing
  Date: December 27, 2002

- **Erectile dysfunction responds to treatment with Korean red ginseng**
  Source: Reuters Industry Breifing
  Date: November 22, 2002

- **Nexmed halts erectile dysfunction study at FDA's request**
  Source: Reuters Industry Breifing
  Date: November 13, 2002

- **TAP files in US for fast-acting erectile dysfunction pill**
  Source: Reuters Industry Breifing
  Date: October 29, 2002

- **Vardenafil shows encouraging results for treatment of erectile dysfunction**
  Source: Reuters Medical News
  Date: September 23, 2002

- **Bayer, Glaxo erectile dysfunction drug performs well in phase III studies**
  Source: Reuters Industry Breifing
  Date: September 23, 2002

- **Beta-blocker-related erectile dysfunction often psychogenic**
  Source: Reuters Industry Breifing
  Date: September 05, 2002

- **Diabetes duration influences risk of erectile dysfunction**
  Source: Reuters Medical News
  Date: August 22, 2002

- **Hepatitis C may cause erectile dysfunction**
  Source: Reuters Health eLine
  Date: August 13, 2002

- **Sildenafil effective for erectile dysfunction in CHF patients**
  Source: Reuters Industry Breifing
  Date: August 06, 2002

- **Sales in India of erectile dysfunction pills triple -- newspaper**
  Source: Reuters Industry Breifing
  Date: July 10, 2002

- **NexMed raises $6 million to fund completion of phase III erectile dysfunction trials**
  Source: Reuters Industry Breifing
  Date: July 02, 2002

- **Palatin erectile dysfunction drug effective in phase IIa trial**
  Source: Reuters Industry Breifing
  Date: May 30, 2002

The NIH

Within MEDLINEplus, the NIH has made an agreement with the New York Times Syndicate, the AP News Service, and Reuters to deliver news that can be browsed by the public. Search news releases at **http://www.nlm.nih.gov/medlineplus/alphanews_a.html**. MEDLINEplus allows you to browse across an alphabetical index. Or you can search by date at the following Web page: **http://www.nlm.nih.gov/medlineplus/newsbydate.html**. Often, news items are indexed by MEDLINEplus within its search engine.

Business Wire

Business Wire is similar to PR Newswire. To access this archive, simply go to **http://www.businesswire.com/**. You can scan the news by industry category or company name.

Market Wire

Market Wire is more focused on technology than the other wires. To browse the latest press releases by topic, such as alternative medicine, biotechnology, fitness, healthcare, legal, nutrition, and pharmaceuticals, access Market Wire's Medical/Health channel at **http://www.marketwire.com/mw/release_index?channel=MedicalHealth**. Or simply go to Market Wire's home page at **http://www.marketwire.com/mw/home**, type "erectile dysfunction" (or synonyms) into the search box, and click on "Search News." As this service is technology oriented, you may wish to use it when searching for press releases covering diagnostic procedures or tests.

Search Engines

Medical news is also available in the news sections of commercial Internet search engines. See the health news page at Yahoo (**http://dir.yahoo.com/Health/News_and_Media/**), or you can use this Web site's general news search page at **http://news.yahoo.com/**. Type in "erectile dysfunction" (or synonyms). If you know the name of a company that is relevant to erectile dysfunction, you can go to any stock trading Web site (such as **http://www.etrade.com/**) and search for the company name there. News items across various news sources are reported on indicated hyperlinks. Google offers a similar service at **http://news.google.com/**.

BBC

Covering news from a more European perspective, the British Broadcasting Corporation (BBC) allows the public free access to their news archive located at **http://www.bbc.co.uk/**. Search by "erectile dysfunction" (or synonyms).

Newsletter Articles

Use the Combined Health Information Database, and limit your search criteria to "newsletter articles." Again, you will need to use the "Detailed Search" option. Go directly to the following hyperlink: **http://chid.nih.gov/detail/detail.html** Go to the bottom of the search page where "You may refine your search by." Select the dates and language that you prefer. For the format option, select "Newsletter Article." Type "erectile dysfunction" (or synonyms) into the "For these words:" box. You should check back periodically with this database as it is updated every three months. The following is a typical result when searching for newsletter articles on erectile dysfunction:

- **Cautions in the Use of Oral Agents for the Management of Erectile Dysfunction**

  Source: AUA News. 3(4): 20. July-August 1998.

  Contact: Available from AUA News. Williams and Wilkins, 351 West Camden Street, Baltimore, MD 21201-2436.

  Summary: Few if any pharmaceutical agents have experienced more heralded releases or had more public media coverage than Viagra (sildenafil citrate), a new oral therapy for erectile dysfunction. This selective inhibitor of cyclic guanosine monophosphate specific phosphodiesterase type 5 acts on corpus cavernosal smooth muscle (in the penis) and has been extensively evaluated in studies of men with erectile dysfunction (ED) of organic, psychogenic, and mixed etiologies. This brief article reviews the cautions in the use of this drug for the management of ED. In clinical trials, adverse events were reported as mild, including headache, flushing, and dyspepsia occurring in 6 to 18 percent of men. Mild and transient visual effects have also been reported (approximately 3 percent of men). The author reports that as of June 8, 1998, the Food and Drug Administration had received 16 unduplicated reports of deaths of men taking Viagra. At least 3 of the 16 reported deaths occurred in men who were treated with nitroglycerin. The package insert for Viagra clearly states that an absolute contraindication for this drug is the concomitant use of organic nitrates. Because of sildenafil's vasodilatory effects, it acts synergistically with nitrates. During nitrate therapy, high levels of nitric oxide (NO) are present in the circulation. Sildenafil increases the vasodilatory effect of circulating NO, causing precipitous and potentially serious hypotension (low blood pressure). Although most if not all urologists are aware of the contraindication of combining sildenafil and nitrates, this may not be well known to emergency room physicians or technicians. 1 table. 1 reference.

Academic Periodicals covering Erectile Dysfunction

Numerous periodicals are currently indexed within the National Library of Medicine's PubMed database that are known to publish articles relating to erectile dysfunction. In addition to these sources, you can search for articles covering erectile dysfunction that have been published by any of the periodicals listed in previous chapters. To find the latest studies published, go to **http://www.ncbi.nlm.nih.gov/pubmed**, type the name of the periodical into the search box, and click "Go."

If you want complete details about the historical contents of a journal, you can also visit the following Web site: **http://www.ncbi.nlm.nih.gov/entrez/jrbrowser.cgi**. Here, type in the name of the journal or its abbreviation, and you will receive an index of published articles. At **http://locatorplus.gov/**, you can retrieve more indexing information on medical periodicals (e.g. the name of the publisher). Select the button "Search LOCATORplus." Then type in the name of the journal and select the advanced search option "Journal Title Search."

CHAPTER 10. RESEARCHING MEDICATIONS

Overview

While a number of hard copy or CD-ROM resources are available for researching medications, a more flexible method is to use Internet-based databases. Broadly speaking, there are two sources of information on approved medications: public sources and private sources. We will emphasize free-to-use public sources.

U.S. Pharmacopeia

Because of historical investments by various organizations and the emergence of the Internet, it has become rather simple to learn about the medications recommended for erectile dysfunction. One such source is the United States Pharmacopeia. In 1820, eleven physicians met in Washington, D.C. to establish the first compendium of standard drugs for the United States. They called this compendium the U.S. Pharmacopeia (USP). Today, the USP is a non-profit organization consisting of 800 volunteer scientists, eleven elected officials, and 400 representatives of state associations and colleges of medicine and pharmacy. The USP is located in Rockville, Maryland, and its home page is located at **http://www.usp.org/**. The USP currently provides standards for over 3,700 medications. The resulting USP DI® Advice for the Patient® can be accessed through the National Library of Medicine of the National Institutes of Health. The database is partially derived from lists of federally approved medications in the Food and Drug Administration's (FDA) Drug Approvals database, located at **http://www.fda.gov/cder/da/da.htm**.

While the FDA database is rather large and difficult to navigate, the Phamacopeia is both user-friendly and free to use. It covers more than 9,000 prescription and over-the-counter medications. To access this database, simply type the following hyperlink into your Web browser: **http://www.nlm.nih.gov/medlineplus/druginformation.html** To view examples of a given medication (brand names, category, description, preparation, proper use, precautions, side effects, etc.), simply follow the hyperlinks indicated within the United States Pharmacopeia (USP).

Below, we have compiled a list of medications associated with erectile dysfunction. If you would like more information on a particular medication, the provided hyperlinks will direct you to ample documentation (e.g. typical dosage, side effects, drug-interaction risks, etc.).

The following drugs have been mentioned in the Pharmacopeia and other sources as being potentially applicable to erectile dysfunction:

Albumin Microspheres Sonicated

- **Systemic - U.S. Brands:** Optison
  http://www.nlm.nih.gov/medlineplus/druginfo/uspdi/203714.html

Alprostadil

- **Local - U.S. Brands:** Caverject; Edex; Muse
  http://www.nlm.nih.gov/medlineplus/druginfo/uspdi/202023.html

Bromocriptine

- **Systemic - U.S. Brands:** Parlodel
  http://www.nlm.nih.gov/medlineplus/druginfo/uspdi/202094.html

Nicotine

- **Systemic - U.S. Brands:** Habitrol; Nicorette; Nicotrol; Prostep
  http://www.nlm.nih.gov/medlineplus/druginfo/uspdi/202407.html

Orlistat

- **Oral–Local - U.S.** Brands: Xenical
  http://www.nlm.nih.gov/medlineplus/druginfo/uspdi/500006.html

Orphenadrine

- **Systemic - U.S. Brands:** Antiflex; Banflex; Flexoject; Mio-Rel; Myolin; Myotrol; Norflex; Orfro; Orphenate
  http://www.nlm.nih.gov/medlineplus/druginfo/uspdi/202426.html

Orphenadrine and Aspirin

- **Systemic - U.S. Brands:** Norgesic; Norphadrine; Orphenagesic
  http://www.nlm.nih.gov/medlineplus/druginfo/uspdi/202427.html

Papaverine

- **Systemic - U.S. Brands:** Cerespan; Genabid; Pavabid; Pavacels; Pavacot; Pavagen; Pavarine; Pavased; Pavatine; Pavatym; Paverolan
  http://www.nlm.nih.gov/medlineplus/druginfo/uspdi/202439.html

Sildenafil

- **Systemic - U.S. Brands:** Viagra
  http://www.nlm.nih.gov/medlineplus/druginfo/uspdi/203533.html

Yohimbine

- **Systemic - U.S. Brands:** Actibine; Aphrodyne; Baron-X; Prohim; Thybine; Yocon; Yohimar; Yohimex; Yoman; Yovital
  http://www.nlm.nih.gov/medlineplus/druginfo/uspdi/202639.html

Commercial Databases

In addition to the medications listed in the USP above, a number of commercial sites are available by subscription to physicians and their institutions. Or, you may be able to access these sources from your local medical library.

Mosby's Drug Consult™

Mosby's Drug Consult™ database (also available on CD-ROM and book format) covers 45,000 drug products including generics and international brands. It provides prescribing information, drug interactions, and patient information. Subscription information is available at the following hyperlink: **http://www.mosbysdrugconsult.com/**.

PDR*health*

The PDR*health* database is a free-to-use, drug information search engine that has been written for the public in layman's terms. It contains FDA-approved drug information adapted from the Physicians' Desk Reference (PDR) database. PDR*health* can be searched by brand name, generic name, or indication. It features multiple drug interactions reports. Search PDR*health* at **http://www.pdrhealth.com/drug_info/index.html**

Other Web Sites

Drugs.com (**www.drugs.com**) reproduces the information in the Pharmacopeia as well as commercial information. You may also want to consider the Web site of the Medical Letter, Inc. (**http://www.medletter.com/**) which allows users to download articles on various drugs and therapeutics for a nominal fee.

If you have any questions about a medical treatment, the FDA may have an office near you. Look for their number in the blue pages of the phone book. You can also contact the FDA through its toll-free number, 1-888-INFO-FDA (1-888-463-6332), or on the World Wide Web at **www.fda.gov**.

APPENDICES

APPENDIX A. PHYSICIAN RESOURCES

Overview

In this chapter, we focus on databases and Internet-based guidelines and information resources created or written for a professional audience.

NIH Guidelines

Commonly referred to as "clinical" or "professional" guidelines, the National Institutes of Health publish physician guidelines for the most common diseases. Publications are available at the following by relevant Institute[13]:

- Office of the Director (OD); guidelines consolidated across agencies available at **http://www.nih.gov/health/consumer/conkey.htm**

- National Institute of General Medical Sciences (NIGMS); fact sheets available at **http://www.nigms.nih.gov/news/facts/**

- National Library of Medicine (NLM); extensive encyclopedia (A.D.A.M., Inc.) with guidelines: **http://www.nlm.nih.gov/medlineplus/healthtopics.html**

- National Cancer Institute (NCI); guidelines available at **http://www.cancer.gov/cancerinfo/list.aspx?viewid=5f35036e-5497-4d86-8c2c-714a9f7c8d25**

- National Eye Institute (NEI); guidelines available at **http://www.nei.nih.gov/order/index.htm**

- National Heart, Lung, and Blood Institute (NHLBI); guidelines available at **http://www.nhlbi.nih.gov/guidelines/index.htm**

- National Human Genome Research Institute (NHGRI); research available at **http://www.genome.gov/page.cfm?pageID=10000375**

- National Institute on Aging (NIA); guidelines available at **http://www.nia.nih.gov/health/**

---

[13] These publications are typically written by one or more of the various NIH Institutes.

- National Institute on Alcohol Abuse and Alcoholism (NIAAA); guidelines available at http://www.niaaa.nih.gov/publications/publications.htm

- National Institute of Allergy and Infectious Diseases (NIAID); guidelines available at http://www.niaid.nih.gov/publications/

- National Institute of Arthritis and Musculoskeletal and Skin Diseases (NIAMS); fact sheets and guidelines available at http://www.niams.nih.gov/hi/index.htm

- National Institute of Child Health and Human Development (NICHD); guidelines available at http://www.nichd.nih.gov/publications/pubskey.cfm

- National Institute on Deafness and Other Communication Disorders (NIDCD); fact sheets and guidelines at http://www.nidcd.nih.gov/health/

- National Institute of Dental and Craniofacial Research (NIDCR); guidelines available at http://www.nidr.nih.gov/health/

- National Institute of Diabetes and Digestive and Kidney Diseases (NIDDK); guidelines available at http://www.niddk.nih.gov/health/health.htm

- National Institute on Drug Abuse (NIDA); guidelines available at http://www.nida.nih.gov/DrugAbuse.html

- National Institute of Environmental Health Sciences (NIEHS); environmental health information available at http://www.niehs.nih.gov/external/facts.htm

- National Institute of Mental Health (NIMH); guidelines available at http://www.nimh.nih.gov/practitioners/index.cfm

- National Institute of Neurological Disorders and Stroke (NINDS); neurological disorder information pages available at http://www.ninds.nih.gov/health_and_medical/disorder_index.htm

- National Institute of Nursing Research (NINR); publications on selected illnesses at http://www.nih.gov/ninr/news-info/publications.html

- National Institute of Biomedical Imaging and Bioengineering; general information at http://grants.nih.gov/grants/becon/becon_info.htm

- Center for Information Technology (CIT); referrals to other agencies based on keyword searches available at http://kb.nih.gov/www_query_main.asp

- National Center for Complementary and Alternative Medicine (NCCAM); health information available at http://nccam.nih.gov/health/

- National Center for Research Resources (NCRR); various information directories available at http://www.ncrr.nih.gov/publications.asp

- Office of Rare Diseases; various fact sheets available at http://rarediseases.info.nih.gov/html/resources/rep_pubs.html

- Centers for Disease Control and Prevention; various fact sheets on infectious diseases available at http://www.cdc.gov/publications.htm

NIH Databases

In addition to the various Institutes of Health that publish professional guidelines, the NIH has designed a number of databases for professionals.[14] Physician-oriented resources provide a wide variety of information related to the biomedical and health sciences, both past and present. The format of these resources varies. Searchable databases, bibliographic citations, full-text articles (when available), archival collections, and images are all available. The following are referenced by the National Library of Medicine:[15]

- **Bioethics:** Access to published literature on the ethical, legal, and public policy issues surrounding healthcare and biomedical research. This information is provided in conjunction with the Kennedy Institute of Ethics located at Georgetown University, Washington, D.C.: **http://www.nlm.nih.gov/databases/databases_bioethics.html**

- **HIV/AIDS Resources:** Describes various links and databases dedicated to HIV/AIDS research: **http://www.nlm.nih.gov/pubs/factsheets/aidsinfs.html**

- **NLM Online Exhibitions:** Describes "Exhibitions in the History of Medicine": **http://www.nlm.nih.gov/exhibition/exhibition.html**. Additional resources for historical scholarship in medicine: **http://www.nlm.nih.gov/hmd/hmd.html**

- **Biotechnology Information:** Access to public databases. The National Center for Biotechnology Information conducts research in computational biology, develops software tools for analyzing genome data, and disseminates biomedical information for the better understanding of molecular processes affecting human health and disease: **http://www.ncbi.nlm.nih.gov/**

- **Population Information:** The National Library of Medicine provides access to worldwide coverage of population, family planning, and related health issues, including family planning technology and programs, fertility, and population law and policy: **http://www.nlm.nih.gov/databases/databases_population.html**

- **Cancer Information:** Access to cancer-oriented databases: **http://www.nlm.nih.gov/databases/databases_cancer.html**

- **Profiles in Science:** Offering the archival collections of prominent twentieth-century biomedical scientists to the public through modern digital technology: **http://www.profiles.nlm.nih.gov/**

- **Chemical Information:** Provides links to various chemical databases and references: **http://sis.nlm.nih.gov/Chem/ChemMain.html**

- **Clinical Alerts:** Reports the release of findings from the NIH-funded clinical trials where such release could significantly affect morbidity and mortality: **http://www.nlm.nih.gov/databases/alerts/clinical_alerts.html**

- **Space Life Sciences:** Provides links and information to space-based research (including NASA): **http://www.nlm.nih.gov/databases/databases_space.html**

- **MEDLINE:** Bibliographic database covering the fields of medicine, nursing, dentistry, veterinary medicine, the healthcare system, and the pre-clinical sciences: **http://www.nlm.nih.gov/databases/databases_medline.html**

---

[14] Remember, for the general public, the National Library of Medicine recommends the databases referenced in MEDLINE*plus* (http://medlineplus.gov/ or http://www.nlm.nih.gov/medlineplus/databases.html).

[15] See http://www.nlm.nih.gov/databases/databases.html.

- **Toxicology and Environmental Health Information (TOXNET):** Databases covering toxicology and environmental health: **http://sis.nlm.nih.gov/Tox/ToxMain.html**

- **Visible Human Interface:** Anatomically detailed, three-dimensional representations of normal male and female human bodies: **http://www.nlm.nih.gov/research/visible/visible_human.html**

The NLM Gateway[16]

The NLM (National Library of Medicine) Gateway is a Web-based system that lets users search simultaneously in multiple retrieval systems at the U.S. National Library of Medicine (NLM). It allows users of NLM services to initiate searches from one Web interface, providing one-stop searching for many of NLM's information resources or databases.[17] To use the NLM Gateway, simply go to the search site at **http://gateway.nlm.nih.gov/gw/Cmd**. Type "erectile dysfunction" (or synonyms) into the search box and click "Search." The results will be presented in a tabular form, indicating the number of references in each database category.

Results Summary

Category	Items Found
Journal Articles	9431
Books / Periodicals / Audio Visual	270
Consumer Health	284
Meeting Abstracts	24
Other Collections	0
Total	10009

HSTAT[18]

HSTAT is a free, Web-based resource that provides access to full-text documents used in healthcare decision-making.[19] These documents include clinical practice guidelines, quick-reference guides for clinicians, consumer health brochures, evidence reports and technology assessments from the Agency for Healthcare Research and Quality (AHRQ), as well as AHRQ's Put Prevention Into Practice.[20] Simply search by "erectile dysfunction" (or synonyms) at the following Web site: **http://text.nlm.nih.gov**.

---

[16] Adapted from NLM: **http://gateway.nlm.nih.gov/gw/Cmd?Overview.x**.

[17] The NLM Gateway is currently being developed by the Lister Hill National Center for Biomedical Communications (LHNCBC) at the National Library of Medicine (NLM) of the National Institutes of Health (NIH).

[18] Adapted from HSTAT: **http://www.nlm.nih.gov/pubs/factsheets/hstat.html**.

[19] The HSTAT URL is **http://hstat.nlm.nih.gov/**.

[20] Other important documents in HSTAT include: the National Institutes of Health (NIH) Consensus Conference Reports and Technology Assessment Reports; the HIV/AIDS Treatment Information Service (ATIS) resource documents; the Substance Abuse and Mental Health Services Administration's Center for Substance Abuse Treatment (SAMHSA/CSAT) Treatment Improvement Protocols (TIP) and Center for Substance Abuse Prevention (SAMHSA/CSAP) Prevention Enhancement Protocols System (PEPS); the Public Health Service (PHS) Preventive Services Task Force's *Guide to Clinical Preventive Services*; the independent, nonfederal Task Force on Community Services' *Guide to Community Preventive Services*; and the Health Technology Advisory Committee (HTAC) of the Minnesota Health Care Commission (MHCC) health technology evaluations.

Coffee Break: Tutorials for Biologists [21]

Coffee Break is a general healthcare site that takes a scientific view of the news and covers recent breakthroughs in biology that may one day assist physicians in developing treatments. Here you will find a collection of short reports on recent biological discoveries. Each report incorporates interactive tutorials that demonstrate how bioinformatics tools are used as a part of the research process. Currently, all Coffee Breaks are written by NCBI staff.[22] Each report is about 400 words and is usually based on a discovery reported in one or more articles from recently published, peer-reviewed literature.[23] This site has new articles every few weeks, so it can be considered an online magazine of sorts. It is intended for general background information. You can access the Coffee Break Web site at the following hyperlink: **http://www.ncbi.nlm.nih.gov/Coffeebreak/**.

Other Commercial Databases

In addition to resources maintained by official agencies, other databases exist that are commercial ventures addressing medical professionals. Here are some examples that may interest you:

- **CliniWeb International:** Index and table of contents to selected clinical information on the Internet; see **http://www.ohsu.edu/cliniweb/**.

- **Medical World Search:** Searches full text from thousands of selected medical sites on the Internet; see **http://www.mwsearch.com/**.

---

[21] Adapted from **http://www.ncbi.nlm.nih.gov/Coffeebreak/Archive/FAQ.html**.

[22] The figure that accompanies each article is frequently supplied by an expert external to NCBI, in which case the source of the figure is cited. The result is an interactive tutorial that tells a biological story.

[23] After a brief introduction that sets the work described into a broader context, the report focuses on how a molecular understanding can provide explanations of observed biology and lead to therapies for diseases. Each vignette is accompanied by a figure and hypertext links that lead to a series of pages that interactively show how NCBI tools and resources are used in the research process.

APPENDIX B. PATIENT RESOURCES

Overview

Official agencies, as well as federally funded institutions supported by national grants, frequently publish a variety of guidelines written with the patient in mind. These are typically called "Fact Sheets" or "Guidelines." They can take the form of a brochure, information kit, pamphlet, or flyer. Often they are only a few pages in length. Since new guidelines on erectile dysfunction can appear at any moment and be published by a number of sources, the best approach to finding guidelines is to systematically scan the Internet-based services that post them.

Patient Guideline Sources

The remainder of this chapter directs you to sources which either publish or can help you find additional guidelines on topics related to erectile dysfunction. Due to space limitations, these sources are listed in a concise manner. Do not hesitate to consult the following sources by either using the Internet hyperlink provided, or, in cases where the contact information is provided, contacting the publisher or author directly.

The National Institutes of Health

The NIH gateway to patients is located at **http://health.nih.gov/**. From this site, you can search across various sources and institutes, a number of which are summarized below.

Topic Pages: MEDLINEplus

The National Library of Medicine has created a vast and patient-oriented healthcare information portal called MEDLINEplus. Within this Internet-based system are "health topic pages" which list links to available materials relevant to erectile dysfunction. To access this system, log on to **http://www.nlm.nih.gov/medlineplus/healthtopics.html**. From there you can either search using the alphabetical index or browse by broad topic areas. Recently, MEDLINEplus listed the following when searched for "erectile dysfunction":

- Guides on erectile dysfunction

  Erectile Dysfunction - Viagra
  http://www.nlm.nih.gov/medlineplus/tutorials/erectiledysfunctionviagraloader.t
  ml

- Other guides

  Diabetes
  http://www.nlm.nih.gov/medlineplus/diabetes.html

  Infertility
  http://www.nlm.nih.gov/medlineplus/infertility.html

  Male Genital Disorders
  http://www.nlm.nih.gov/medlineplus/malegenitaldisorders.html

  Men's Health Issues
  http://www.nlm.nih.gov/medlineplus/menshealthissues.html

  Prostate Cancer
  http://www.nlm.nih.gov/medlineplus/prostatecancer.html

  Sexual Health Issues
  http://www.nlm.nih.gov/medlineplus/sexualhealthissues.html

Within the health topic page dedicated to erectile dysfunction, the following was listed:

- General/Overview

  Endocrinology and Impotence (Erectile Dysfunction)
  Source: Endocrine Society
  http://www.endo-society.org/pubrelations/patientInfo/impotence.htm

  Impotence: Learning the Causes and What You Can Do
  Source: American Academy of Family Physicians
  http://familydoctor.org/healthfacts/109/index.html

- Diagnosis/Symptoms

  Testosterone Test
  Source: American Association for Clinical Chemistry
  http://www.labtestsonline.org/understanding/analytes/testosterone/test.html

- Treatment

  **FDA Assesses Irregularities Involving the Handling of Certain Unapproved
  Imported Viagra Products**
  Source: Food and Drug Administration
  http://www.fda.gov/bbs/topics/ANSWERS/2003/ANS01222.html

  Testosterone Replacement Therapy: Effective Treatments Are Available
  Source: Mayo Foundation for Medical Education and Research
  http://www.mayoclinic.com/invoke.cfm?id=MC00004

Viagra: Proper Use Can Restore Erections
Source: Mayo Foundation for Medical Education and Research
http://www.mayoclinic.com/invoke.cfm?id=MC00011

- Coping

JAMA Patient Page: Sexual Dysfunction -- Silence about Sexual Problems Can Hurt Relationships
Source: American Medical Association
http://www.medem.com/MedLB/article_detaillb.cfm?article_ID=ZZZSAC20NAC
&sub_cat=2

Where to Seek Professional Help: Sexuality and Cancer
Source: American Cancer Society
http://www.cancer.org/docroot/mit/content/mit_7_2x_where_to_seek_professio
nal_help_women.asp

- Specific Conditions/Aspects

Erectile Dysfunction in Diabetes: Keys to Prevention
Source: Mayo Foundation for Medical Education and Research
http://www.mayoclinic.com/invoke.cfm?id=DA00045

Male Sexual Problems
Source: American Association for Marriage and Family Therapy
http://www.aamft.org/families/consumer_updates/malesexualproblems.asp

Patient's Guide to Low Testosterone
Source: Endocrine Society, Hormone Foundation
http://www.medem.com/medlb/article_detaillb.cfm?article_ID=ZZZO7PDVDLC
&sub_cat=57

Peyronie's Disease
Source: National Kidney and Urologic Diseases Information Clearinghouse
http://kidney.niddk.nih.gov/kudiseases/pubs/peyronie/index.htm

What Is Peyronie's Disease?
Source: Mayo Foundation for Medical Education and Research
http://www.mayoclinic.com/invoke.cfm?id=DS00427

- From the National Institutes of Health

Erectile Dysfunction
Source: National Kidney and Urologic Diseases Information Clearinghouse
http://kidney.niddk.nih.gov/kudiseases/pubs/impotence/index.htm

- Latest News

FDA Approves Third Drug to Treat Erectile Dysfunction
Source: 11/21/2003, Food and Drug Administration
http://www.fda.gov/bbs/topics/ANSWERS/2003/ANS01265.html

New Erectile Awareness May Help Men's Hearts
Source: 11/11/2003, Reuters Health
http://www.nlm.nih.gov//www.nlm.nih.gov/medlineplus/news/fullstory_14610

.html

- Organizations

  American Foundation for Urologic Disease
  http://www.afud.org/

  National Institute of Diabetes and Digestive and Kidney Diseases
  http://www.niddk.nih.gov/

- Pictures/Diagrams

  Overview of the Male Anatomy
  Source: University of Utah, Health Sciences Center
  http://www.med.utah.edu/healthinfo/adult/men/maleanat.htm

- Research

  FDA Approves New Drug for Treatment of Erectile Dysfunction in Men
  Source: Food and Drug Administration
  http://www.fda.gov/bbs/topics/ANSWERS/2003/ANS01249.html

  FDA Approves Third Drug to Treat Erectile Dysfunction
  Source: Food and Drug Administration
  http://www.fda.gov/bbs/topics/ANSWERS/2003/ANS01265.html

  Nerve Grafting Restores Erectile Function After Prostatectomy: New Hope for Sex Life After Prostate Removal
  Source: American Cancer Society
  http://www.cancer.org/docroot/nws/content/nws_1_1x_nerve_grafting_restores
  _erectile_function_after_prostatectomy.asp

  Regular Cycling Can Improve Sexual Function in Men with Heart Failure
  Source: American Heart Association
  http://www.americanheart.org/presenter.jhtml?identifier=11999

  Risk of Erectile Dysfunction Similar for Different Prostate Cancer Treatments
  Source: American Cancer Society
  http://www.cancer.org/docroot/nws/content/nws_1_1x_risk_of_erectile_dysfunc
  tion_similar_for_different_prostate_cancer_treatments.asp

  Sexual Function in Men Older Than 50 Years of Age
  Source: American College of Physicians
  http://www.annals.org/cgi/content/full/139/3/I-22

- Statistics

  Kidney and Urologic Disease Statistics for the United States
  Source: National Kidney and Urologic Diseases Information Clearinghouse
  http://kidney.niddk.nih.gov/kudiseases/pubs/kustats/index.htm

You may also choose to use the search utility provided by MEDLINEplus at the following Web address: **http://www.nlm.nih.gov/medlineplus/**. Simply type a keyword into the search box and click "Search." This utility is similar to the NIH search utility, with the exception that it only includes materials that are linked within the MEDLINEplus system (mostly patient-oriented information). It also has the disadvantage of generating unstructured results. We recommend, therefore, that you use this method only if you have a very targeted search.

The Combined Health Information Database (CHID)

CHID Online is a reference tool that maintains a database directory of thousands of journal articles and patient education guidelines on erectile dysfunction. CHID offers summaries that describe the guidelines available, including contact information and pricing. CHID's general Web site is **http://chid.nih.gov/**. To search this database, go to **http://chid.nih.gov/detail/detail.html**. In particular, you can use the advanced search options to look up pamphlets, reports, brochures, and information kits. The following was recently posted in this archive:

- **Impotence?: A Guide to Understanding and Treating Erectile Dysfunction**

  Source: Minnetonka, MN: American Medical Systems. 2001. 29 p.

  Contact: Available from American Medical Systems. 10700 Bren Road West, Minnetonka, MN 55343. (800) 328-3881 or (612) 933-4666. Fax (612) 930-6592. Website: www.VisitAMS.com. PRICE: Single copy free. Order number 21600026.

  Summary: Erectile dysfunction (ED, or impotence) is the inability to maintain an erection that is firm enough or that lasts long enough to have successful sexual intercourse. It is a frustrating condition that may have either physical or psychological causes. This brochure offers a guide to understanding and treating ED. In more than half of all men with ED, the cause is physical; ED can be the result of diabetes, a hormone problem, blocked arteries, or other causes. And in many cases, physical causes can produce psychological side effects. Diagnosing the cause is the first step before determining an appropriate treatment. Psychological causes can include misinformation, performance anxiety, depression, or stress. Physical causes can include diabetes, vascular problems, pelvic surgery or trauma, neurological disorders, medications, alcoholism, or hormone problems. The brochure describes the physiology of the penis and how an erection occurs, including the stages of the flaccid state, the tumescent penis, and erection. The brochure describes what to expect at the urologist's examination, including the external physical (checking for the pulse to the penis), the rectal examination (to check for prostatitis), and checking for physical abnormalities such as Peyronie's disease (a curved and painful erection caused by scar tissue in the penis). Laboratory tests that may be called for include blood tests and urine analysis, penile blood flow studies, and sleep monitoring. The brochure briefly reviews treatment options, including counseling and sex therapy, oral medications, intraurethral suppositories, injection therapy, vacuum erection devices, venous and arterial surgery, and penile implants. Penile prostheses are described in some detail, including the advantages and disadvantages of the malleable prosthesis, the self contained inflatable prosthesis, the two piece inflatable prosthesis, and the three piece inflatable prosthesis. Diagrams are provided for each type of prosthesis. The brochure concludes with a self test: 23 questions that readers can ask themselves (and share with their urologists) to help ascertain the causes of ED. 26 figures.

- **What Every Man (and Woman) Should Know About Erectile Dysfunction**

  Source: New York, NY: Pfizer, Inc. 1999. (videocassette).

Contact: Available from Trigenesis Communications. 26 Main Street, Chatham, NJ 07928-2402. (800) 664-5484 or (877) 487-4436. Fax (973) 701-8896. PRICE: Single copy free.

Summary: For many men, the solution to erectile problems is a pill called Viagra (sildenafil). In this educational video, leading experts discuss the causes of erectile dysfunction (ED, also called impotence), dispel some common myths, and introduce how it is treated. The program interviews men who share their stories of how Viagra has helped them restore an important part of their lives. Viagra helps a man with erectile dysfunction get an erection only when he is sexually excited (taking the medication alone does not result in erection). The program reviews the most common side effects of Viagra, which include headache, facial flushing, and upset stomach. A small percentage of men (3 percent) reported mild and temporary visual effects. Viagra must not be taken by men who use drugs known as nitrates (most often used to control angina) in any form, at any time. The use of these drugs with Viagra can result in a sudden drop in blood pressure. In addition, viewers are advised to consult with their physicians about the cardiovascular stress of sexual activities. Accompanying the videotape program is a 24 page booklet that reviews the topics covered in the program and that summarizes the patient insert information that is packaged with the drug Viagra. Patients are encouraged to talk with their physicians and work cooperatively to address any issues of sexual dysfunction.

- **Key to Resolving Erectile Dysfunction**

Source: Baltimore, MD: American Foundation for Urologic Disease. 2000. 18 p.

Contact: Available from American Foundation for Urologic Disease (AFUD). 1128 North Charles Street, Baltimore, MD 21201. (800) 242-2383. Website: www.afud.org. PRICE: $13.00 for pack of 50; plus shipping and handling.

Summary: It is estimated that over 30 million men and their partners are affected by erectile dysfunction (ED), yet only a very small percentage seek help for this very treatable medical condition. This brochure is designed to help couples break down the barriers to communication both with each other and with their health care provider. Topics include myths about ED, how an erection occurs, the causes of ED, getting medical help for ED, what happens at the doctor's office, sex and cardiovascular function, treatment options for ED (treating reversible causes, sex education and counseling, and sildenafil, trade name Viagra), other treatments (vacuum erection devices, self injection therapy, transurethral therapy), surgical treatments (surgery to repair blood vessels and penile implants), and reclaiming one's sexuality. The brochure includes a sexual health inventory for men that asks readers to score their experiences on five simple questions related to sexual health. The score and the questionnaire may help men address the issue of ED with their health care provider. The brochure concludes with a list of resources for men with ED and their partners, including professional organizations, patient organizations, and government agencies. The brochure is illustrated with black and white photographs of couples and with medical illustrations of the penis, and some of the treatment options. 7 figures. 1 table.

- **Penile Self-Injection: Overcoming Erectile Dysfunction**

Source: San Bruno, CA: Krames Communications. 1995. 2 p.

Contact: Available from Krames Communications. Order Department, 1100 Grundy Lane, San Bruno, CA 94066-9821. (800) 333-3032. Fax (415) 244-4512. PRICE: $20.00 for 50. Order no. 1519.

Summary: This brochure describes penile self-injection and its role in creating an erection capable of sexual intercourse. The brochure presents a step-by-step guide to penile injection: preparing for injection; inserting the needle; injecting the medication; and gaining an erection. The brochure also includes brief information on warnings and complications. An additional section describes the anatomy of an erection and why injections can help. The brochure is illustrated with line drawings for each step of the self-injection procedure.

- **How to Treat Erectile Dysfunction: A Couple's Guide to Erectile Dysfunction**

  Source: Baltimore, MD: Sexual Function Health Council. American Foundation for Urologic Disease. 1998. [6 p.].

  Contact: Available from American Foundation for Urologic Disease. 1126 North Charles Street, Baltimore, MD 21201. (800) 242-2383 or (410) 468-1800. Fax (410) 468-1808. Website: www.afud.org. PRICE: Single copy free.

  Summary: This brochure provides basic information about the treatment options for erectile dysfunction (impotence). The brochure stresses that many sexual difficulties, including erectile dysfunction (ED), can be improved or resolved through open communication and a mutual commitment to learn about the condition and treatment options. ED is defined as the inability to achieve or to sustain an erection adequate for sexual intercourse. The brochure considers the causes of ED, including fatigue, temporary stress, or excessive alcohol consumption (for occasional erectile failures); physical causes, including blockage in the arteries, diabetes, neurological disorders, disease of the erectile tissue of the penis, pelvic surgery or trauma, side effects of medications, chronic disease, hormonal abnormalities, substance abuse (including heavy smoking) and Peyronie's disease; and psychological causes, including stress and anxiety, worry about poor sexual performance, marital discord, depression, and unresolved sexual orientation. The brochure stresses that, whether a man's erectile dysfunction is caused by physical or psychological factors or a combination of the two, it may become a source of mental, emotional, and physical stress. The brochure discusses the medical specialties that address ED, the impact of aging on treatment options for ED, how to decide if one's partner should be involved in treating ED, what to expect from the first visit to the physician, how men and their partners are affected by ED, and current treatment options. Treatments outlined include changing habits and medications, the use of oral medications, professional counseling, vacuum devices, hormone medications, injection therapy, intraurethral therapy, penile prostheses, and surgical treatment. The brochure concludes with a glossary of related terms; a pretest and answers are also included.

- **Managing Erectile Dysfunction with Vacuum Devices**

  Source: Washington, DC: Impotence Institute of America, Inc. 199x. 4 p.

  Contact: Available from Impotence Institute of America. 10400 Little Pawtuxent Parkway, Suite 485, Columbia, MD 21044. (410) 715-9605. PRICE: Contact organization directly.

  Summary: This fact sheet reviews the problem of erectile dysfunction in men with diabetes and summarizes the types of external management available for these men. The types of external devices discussed include vacuum devices, including ErecAid (Osbon Medical Systems), Response Unit (Mentor Urology), the VED Device (Mission Pharmacal), and the VTU System (Encore, Inc), and nonvacuum/entrapment devices, including Revive (Encore, Inc). The fact sheet concludes with general considerations for patient selection and education. The toll-free number of the Impotence Institute of America is included.

- **Patient Education: Erectile Dysfunction**

Source: Nurse Practitioner. 25(Supplement 6): 21. June 2000.

Contact: Available from Nurse Practitioner. Circulation Department, P.O. Box 5053, Brentwood, TN 37024-5053. (800) 490-6580. Fax (615) 377-0525.

Summary: This patient education handout discusses erectile dysfunction (ED), defined as the inability to achieve or maintain an erection satisfactory for sexual intercourse over a period of time. The handout covers the incidence of ED, the causes of ED, other factors that can affect ED, diagnostic methods, and treatment options. Some 80 percent of ED cases have an organic cause, which means it is caused by a physical condition such as diabetes, high blood pressure (hypertension), high cholesterol, or other physical problems; the other 20 percent are caused by psychological factors such as stress, depression, or anxiety. Many times, ED is caused by a combination of both types of factors. In addition, smoking tobacco or taking certain medications can decrease the likelihood of a man's experiencing adequate erections. Diagnosis includes a patient history (including sexual health and history) and a physical examination. ED can usually be easily treated in several different ways, depending on the underlying cause. The handout stresses that whatever the cause, ED is best resolved when the man and his partner are both involved in the treatment decision. Treatment options include lifestyle changes (such as quitting smoking), oral medications (sildenafil, trade name Viagra), penile vacuum devices, drug therapy (medications injected into the penis or inserted into the urethra), and penile implants. The handout concludes by reminding readers that one is never too old to have sex, and sex is an important part of one's overall health.

- **Diabetes and Erectile Dysfunction**

Source: Augusta, GA: Geddings D. Osbon, Sr. Foundation. 1995. 1 p.

Contact: Available from Geddings D. Osbon, Sr. Foundation. 121 Twelfth Street, P.O. Box 1593, Augusta, GA 30903. (800) 433-4215. PRICE: Single copy free.

Summary: This simple fact sheet lists facts about diabetes mellitus and erectile dysfunction. Topics include a definition of impotence; the epidemiology of erectile dysfunction; the evaluation of impotence; how autonomic and peripheral neuropathy can affect erection in men with diabetes; impotence related to arteriosclerosis; smoking as a risk factor for impotence; and treatment options. The fact sheet includes the toll-free telephone number of the Geddings Osbon Sr. Foundation, a resource organization on impotence.

- **Erectile Dysfunction**

Source: American Family Physician. 60(4): 1169. September 15, 1999.

Contact: Available from American Academy of Family Physicians. 11400 Tomahawk Creek Parkway, Leawood, KS 66211-2672. (800) 274-2237. Website: www.aafp.org.

Summary: With the introduction of effective drug treatment for erectile dysfunction (ED, previously called impotence), more men are seeking treatment. This patient education fact sheet accompanies an article that reviews the newer pharmacologic alternatives for ED. Written in question and answer format, the fact sheet discusses ED and its causes, the role of drug treatments, and other non-drug therapies for ED, including vacuum pump devices or surgery. Readers are reminded that ED does not have to be a part of aging, even though there are changes in erectile function that accompany aging. Medical problems that can cause ED include diabetes, high blood pressure (hypertension), and atherosclerosis (hardening of the arteries). Drinking too much, smoking too much, and abusing drugs can also cause ED.

The National Guideline Clearinghouse™

The National Guideline Clearinghouse™ offers hundreds of evidence-based clinical practice guidelines published in the United States and other countries. You can search this site located at **http://www.guideline.gov/** by using the keyword "erectile dysfunction" (or synonyms). The following was recently posted:

- **The primary care management of erectile dysfunction**

    Source: Department of Veterans Affairs - Federal Government Agency [U.S.]; 1999 June; 67 pages

    http://www.guideline.gov/summary/summary.aspx?doc_id=2577&nbr=1803&string=erectile+AND+dysfunction

Healthfinder™

Healthfinder™ is sponsored by the U.S. Department of Health and Human Services and offers links to hundreds of other sites that contain healthcare information. This Web site is located at **http://www.healthfinder.gov**. Again, keyword searches can be used to find guidelines. The following was recently found in this database:

- **Confronting Erectile Dysfunction as a Team**

    Summary: This fact sheet seeks to answer some of your questions about erectile dysfunction (ED), also known as impotence.

    Source: American Foundation for Urologic Disease

    http://www.healthfinder.gov/scripts/recordpass.asp?RecordType=0&RecordID=3949

The NIH Search Utility

The NIH search utility allows you to search for documents on over 100 selected Web sites that comprise the NIH-WEB-SPACE. Each of these servers is "crawled" and indexed on an ongoing basis. Your search will produce a list of various documents, all of which will relate in some way to erectile dysfunction. The drawbacks of this approach are that the information is not organized by theme and that the references are often a mix of information for professionals and patients. Nevertheless, a large number of the listed Web sites provide useful background information. We can only recommend this route, therefore, for relatively rare or specific disorders, or when using highly targeted searches. To use the NIH search utility, visit the following Web page: **http://search.nih.gov/index.html**

Additional Web Sources

A number of Web sites are available to the public that often link to government sites. These can also point you in the direction of essential information. The following is a representative sample:

- AOL: **http://search.aol.com/cat.adp?id=168&layer=&from=subcats**

- Family Village: **http://www.familyvillage.wisc.edu/specific.htm**

- Google: **http://directory.google.com/Top/Health/Conditions_and_Diseases/**

- Med Help International: **http://www.medhelp.org/HealthTopics/A.html**

- Open Directory Project: **http://dmoz.org/Health/Conditions_and_Diseases/**

- Yahoo.com: **http://dir.yahoo.com/Health/Diseases_and_Conditions/**

- WebMD®Health: **http://my.webmd.com/health_topics**

Finding Associations

There are several Internet directories that provide lists of medical associations with information on or resources relating to erectile dysfunction. By consulting all of associations listed in this chapter, you will have nearly exhausted all sources for patient associations concerned with erectile dysfunction.

The National Health Information Center (NHIC)

The National Health Information Center (NHIC) offers a free referral service to help people find organizations that provide information about erectile dysfunction. For more information, see the NHIC's Web site at **http://www.health.gov/NHIC/** or contact an information specialist by calling 1-800-336-4797.

Directory of Health Organizations

The Directory of Health Organizations, provided by the National Library of Medicine Specialized Information Services, is a comprehensive source of information on associations. The Directory of Health Organizations database can be accessed via the Internet at **http://www.sis.nlm.nih.gov/Dir/DirMain.html**. It is composed of two parts: DIRLINE and Health Hotlines.

The DIRLINE database comprises some 10,000 records of organizations, research centers, and government institutes and associations that primarily focus on health and biomedicine. To access DIRLINE directly, go to the following Web site: **http://dirline.nlm.nih.gov/**. Simply type in "erectile dysfunction" (or a synonym), and you will receive information on all relevant organizations listed in the database.

Health Hotlines directs you to toll-free numbers to over 300 organizations. You can access this database directly at **http://www.sis.nlm.nih.gov/hotlines/**. On this page, you are given the option to search by keyword or by browsing the subject list. When you have received your search results, click on the name of the organization for its description and contact information.

The Combined Health Information Database

Another comprehensive source of information on healthcare associations is the Combined Health Information Database. Using the "Detailed Search" option, you will need to limit your search to "Organizations" and "erectile dysfunction". Type the following hyperlink into your Web browser: **http://chid.nih.gov/detail/detail.html**. To find associations, use the drop boxes at the bottom of the search page where "You may refine your search by." For publication date, select "All Years." Then, select your preferred language and the format option "Organization Resource Sheet." Type "erectile dysfunction" (or synonyms) into the "For these words:" box. You should check back periodically with this database since it is updated every three months.

The National Organization for Rare Disorders, Inc.

The National Organization for Rare Disorders, Inc. has prepared a Web site that provides, at no charge, lists of associations organized by health topic. You can access this database at the following Web site: **http://www.rarediseases.org/search/orgsearch.html**. Type "erectile dysfunction" (or a synonym) into the search box, and click "Submit Query."

APPENDIX C. FINDING MEDICAL LIBRARIES

Overview

In this Appendix, we show you how to quickly find a medical library in your area.

Preparation

Your local public library and medical libraries have interlibrary loan programs with the National Library of Medicine (NLM), one of the largest medical collections in the world. According to the NLM, most of the literature in the general and historical collections of the National Library of Medicine is available on interlibrary loan to any library. If you would like to access NLM medical literature, then visit a library in your area that can request the publications for you.[24]

Finding a Local Medical Library

The quickest method to locate medical libraries is to use the Internet-based directory published by the National Network of Libraries of Medicine (NN/LM). This network includes 4626 members and affiliates that provide many services to librarians, health professionals, and the public. To find a library in your area, simply visit **http://nnlm.gov/members/adv.html** or call 1-800-338-7657.

Medical Libraries in the U.S. and Canada

In addition to the NN/LM, the National Library of Medicine (NLM) lists a number of libraries with reference facilities that are open to the public. The following is the NLM's list and includes hyperlinks to each library's Web site. These Web pages can provide information on hours of operation and other restrictions. The list below is a small sample of

---

[24] Adapted from the NLM: **http://www.nlm.nih.gov/psd/cas/interlibrary.html**.

libraries recommended by the National Library of Medicine (sorted alphabetically by name of the U.S. state or Canadian province where the library is located)[25]:

- **Alabama:** Health InfoNet of Jefferson County (Jefferson County Library Cooperative, Lister Hill Library of the Health Sciences), **http://www.uab.edu/infonet/**

- **Alabama:** Richard M. Scrushy Library (American Sports Medicine Institute)

- **Arizona:** Samaritan Regional Medical Center: The Learning Center (Samaritan Health System, Phoenix, Arizona), **http://www.samaritan.edu/library/bannerlibs.htm**

- **California:** Kris Kelly Health Information Center (St. Joseph Health System, Humboldt), **http://www.humboldt1.com/~kkhic/index.html**

- **California:** Community Health Library of Los Gatos, **http://www.healthlib.org/orgresources.html**

- **California:** Consumer Health Program and Services (CHIPS) (County of Los Angeles Public Library, Los Angeles County Harbor-UCLA Medical Center Library) - Carson, CA, **http://www.colapublib.org/services/chips.html**

- **California:** Gateway Health Library (Sutter Gould Medical Foundation)

- **California:** Health Library (Stanford University Medical Center), **http://www-med.stanford.edu/healthlibrary/**

- **California:** Patient Education Resource Center - Health Information and Resources (University of California, San Francisco), **http://sfghdean.ucsf.edu/barnett/PERC/default.asp**

- **California:** Redwood Health Library (Petaluma Health Care District), **http://www.phcd.org/rdwdlib.html**

- **California:** Los Gatos PlaneTree Health Library, **http://planetreesanjose.org/**

- **California:** Sutter Resource Library (Sutter Hospitals Foundation, Sacramento), **http://suttermedicalcenter.org/library/**

- **California:** Health Sciences Libraries (University of California, Davis), **http://www.lib.ucdavis.edu/healthsci/**

- **California:** ValleyCare Health Library & Ryan Comer Cancer Resource Center (ValleyCare Health System, Pleasanton), **http://gaelnet.stmarys-ca.edu/other.libs/gbal/east/vchl.html**

- **California:** Washington Community Health Resource Library (Fremont), **http://www.healthlibrary.org/**

- **Colorado:** William V. Gervasini Memorial Library (Exempla Healthcare), **http://www.saintjosephdenver.org/yourhealth/libraries/**

- **Connecticut:** Hartford Hospital Health Science Libraries (Hartford Hospital), **http://www.harthosp.org/library/**

- **Connecticut:** Healthnet: Connecticut Consumer Health Information Center (University of Connecticut Health Center, Lyman Maynard Stowe Library), **http://library.uchc.edu/departm/hnet/**

[25] Abstracted from **http://www.nlm.nih.gov/medlineplus/libraries.html**.

- **Connecticut:** Waterbury Hospital Health Center Library (Waterbury Hospital, Waterbury), **http://www.waterburyhospital.com/library/consumer.shtml**

- **Delaware:** Consumer Health Library (Christiana Care Health System, Eugene du Pont Preventive Medicine & Rehabilitation Institute, Wilmington), **http://www.christianacare.org/health_guide/health_guide_pmri_health_info.cfm**

- **Delaware:** Lewis B. Flinn Library (Delaware Academy of Medicine, Wilmington), **http://www.delamed.org/chls.html**

- **Georgia:** Family Resource Library (Medical College of Georgia, Augusta), **http://cmc.mcg.edu/kids_families/fam_resources/fam_res_lib/frl.htm**

- **Georgia:** Health Resource Center (Medical Center of Central Georgia, Macon), **http://www.mccg.org/hrc/hrchome.asp**

- **Hawaii:** Hawaii Medical Library: Consumer Health Information Service (Hawaii Medical Library, Honolulu), **http://hml.org/CHIS/**

- **Idaho:** DeArmond Consumer Health Library (Kootenai Medical Center, Coeur d'Alene), **http://www.nicon.org/DeArmond/index.htm**

- **Illinois:** Health Learning Center of Northwestern Memorial Hospital (Chicago), **http://www.nmh.org/health_info/hlc.html**

- **Illinois:** Medical Library (OSF Saint Francis Medical Center, Peoria), **http://www.osfsaintfrancis.org/general/library/**

- **Kentucky:** Medical Library - Services for Patients, Families, Students & the Public (Central Baptist Hospital, Lexington), **http://www.centralbap.com/education/community/library.cfm**

- **Kentucky:** University of Kentucky - Health Information Library (Chandler Medical Center, Lexington), **http://www.mc.uky.edu/PatientEd/**

- **Louisiana:** Alton Ochsner Medical Foundation Library (Alton Ochsner Medical Foundation, New Orleans), **http://www.ochsner.org/library/**

- **Louisiana:** Louisiana State University Health Sciences Center Medical Library-Shreveport, **http://lib-sh.lsuhsc.edu/**

- **Maine:** Franklin Memorial Hospital Medical Library (Franklin Memorial Hospital, Farmington), **http://www.fchn.org/fmh/lib.htm**

- **Maine:** Gerrish-True Health Sciences Library (Central Maine Medical Center, Lewiston), **http://www.cmmc.org/library/library.html**

- **Maine:** Hadley Parrot Health Science Library (Eastern Maine Healthcare, Bangor), **http://www.emh.org/hll/hpl/guide.htm**

- **Maine:** Maine Medical Center Library (Maine Medical Center, Portland), **http://www.mmc.org/library/**

- **Maine:** Parkview Hospital (Brunswick), **http://www.parkviewhospital.org/**

- **Maine:** Southern Maine Medical Center Health Sciences Library (Southern Maine Medical Center, Biddeford), **http://www.smmc.org/services/service.php3?choice=10**

- **Maine:** Stephens Memorial Hospital's Health Information Library (Western Maine Health, Norway), **http://www.wmhcc.org/Library/**

- **Manitoba, Canada:** Consumer & Patient Health Information Service (University of Manitoba Libraries), **http://www.umanitoba.ca/libraries/units/health/reference/chis.html**

- **Manitoba, Canada:** J.W. Crane Memorial Library (Deer Lodge Centre, Winnipeg), **http://www.deerlodge.mb.ca/crane_library/about.asp**

- **Maryland:** Health Information Center at the Wheaton Regional Library (Montgomery County, Dept. of Public Libraries, Wheaton Regional Library), **http://www.mont.lib.md.us/healthinfo/hic.asp**

- **Massachusetts:** Baystate Medical Center Library (Baystate Health System), **http://www.baystatehealth.com/1024/**

- **Massachusetts:** Boston University Medical Center Alumni Medical Library (Boston University Medical Center), **http://med-libwww.bu.edu/library/lib.html**

- **Massachusetts:** Lowell General Hospital Health Sciences Library (Lowell General Hospital, Lowell), **http://www.lowellgeneral.org/library/HomePageLinks/WWW.htm**

- **Massachusetts:** Paul E. Woodard Health Sciences Library (New England Baptist Hospital, Boston), **http://www.nebh.org/health_lib.asp**

- **Massachusetts:** St. Luke's Hospital Health Sciences Library (St. Luke's Hospital, Southcoast Health System, New Bedford), **http://www.southcoast.org/library/**

- **Massachusetts:** Treadwell Library Consumer Health Reference Center (Massachusetts General Hospital), **http://www.mgh.harvard.edu/library/chrcindex.html**

- **Massachusetts:** UMass HealthNet (University of Massachusetts Medical School, Worchester), **http://healthnet.umassmed.edu/**

- **Michigan:** Botsford General Hospital Library - Consumer Health (Botsford General Hospital, Library & Internet Services), **http://www.botsfordlibrary.org/consumer.htm**

- **Michigan:** Helen DeRoy Medical Library (Providence Hospital and Medical Centers), **http://www.providence-hospital.org/library/**

- **Michigan:** Marquette General Hospital - Consumer Health Library (Marquette General Hospital, Health Information Center), **http://www.mgh.org/center.html**

- **Michigan:** Patient Education Resouce Center - University of Michigan Cancer Center (University of Michigan Comprehensive Cancer Center, Ann Arbor), **http://www.cancer.med.umich.edu/learn/leares.htm**

- **Michigan:** Sladen Library & Center for Health Information Resources - Consumer Health Information (Detroit), **http://www.henryford.com/body.cfm?id=39330**

- **Montana:** Center for Health Information (St. Patrick Hospital and Health Sciences Center, Missoula)

- **National:** Consumer Health Library Directory (Medical Library Association, Consumer and Patient Health Information Section), **http://caphis.mlanet.org/directory/index.html**

- **National:** National Network of Libraries of Medicine (National Library of Medicine) - provides library services for health professionals in the United States who do not have access to a medical library, **http://nnlm.gov/**

- **National:** NN/LM List of Libraries Serving the Public (National Network of Libraries of Medicine), **http://nnlm.gov/members/**

- **Nevada:** Health Science Library, West Charleston Library (Las Vegas-Clark County Library District, Las Vegas), **http://www.lvccld.org/special_collections/medical/index.htm**

- **New Hampshire:** Dartmouth Biomedical Libraries (Dartmouth College Library, Hanover), **http://www.dartmouth.edu/~biomed/resources.htmld/conshealth.htmld/**

- **New Jersey:** Consumer Health Library (Rahway Hospital, Rahway), **http://www.rahwayhospital.com/library.htm**

- **New Jersey:** Dr. Walter Phillips Health Sciences Library (Englewood Hospital and Medical Center, Englewood), **http://www.englewoodhospital.com/links/index.htm**

- **New Jersey:** Meland Foundation (Englewood Hospital and Medical Center, Englewood), **http://www.geocities.com/ResearchTriangle/9360/**

- **New York:** Choices in Health Information (New York Public Library) - NLM Consumer Pilot Project participant, **http://www.nypl.org/branch/health/links.html**

- **New York:** Health Information Center (Upstate Medical University, State University of New York, Syracuse), **http://www.upstate.edu/library/hic/**

- **New York:** Health Sciences Library (Long Island Jewish Medical Center, New Hyde Park), **http://www.lij.edu/library/library.html**

- **New York:** ViaHealth Medical Library (Rochester General Hospital), **http://www.nyam.org/library/**

- **Ohio:** Consumer Health Library (Akron General Medical Center, Medical & Consumer Health Library), **http://www.akrongeneral.org/hwlibrary.htm**

- **Oklahoma:** The Health Information Center at Saint Francis Hospital (Saint Francis Health System, Tulsa), **http://www.sfh-tulsa.com/services/healthinfo.asp**

- **Oregon:** Planetree Health Resource Center (Mid-Columbia Medical Center, The Dalles), **http://www.mcmc.net/phrc/**

- **Pennsylvania:** Community Health Information Library (Milton S. Hershey Medical Center, Hershey), **http://www.hmc.psu.edu/commhealth/**

- **Pennsylvania:** Community Health Resource Library (Geisinger Medical Center, Danville), **http://www.geisinger.edu/education/commlib.shtml**

- **Pennsylvania:** HealthInfo Library (Moses Taylor Hospital, Scranton), **http://www.mth.org/healthwellness.html**

- **Pennsylvania:** Hopwood Library (University of Pittsburgh, Health Sciences Library System, Pittsburgh), **http://www.hsls.pitt.edu/guides/chi/hopwood/index_html**

- **Pennsylvania:** Koop Community Health Information Center (College of Physicians of Philadelphia), **http://www.collphyphil.org/kooppg1.shtml**

- **Pennsylvania:** Learning Resources Center - Medical Library (Susquehanna Health System, Williamsport), **http://www.shscares.org/services/lrc/index.asp**

- **Pennsylvania:** Medical Library (UPMC Health System, Pittsburgh), **http://www.upmc.edu/passavant/library.htm**

- **Quebec, Canada:** Medical Library (Montreal General Hospital), **http://www.mghlib.mcgill.ca/**

- **South Dakota:** Rapid City Regional Hospital Medical Library (Rapid City Regional Hospital), **http://www.rcrh.org/Services/Library/Default.asp**

- **Texas:** Houston HealthWays (Houston Academy of Medicine-Texas Medical Center Library), **http://hhw.library.tmc.edu/**

- **Washington:** Community Health Library (Kittitas Valley Community Hospital), **http://www.kvch.com/**

- **Washington:** Southwest Washington Medical Center Library (Southwest Washington Medical Center, Vancouver), **http://www.swmedicalcenter.com/body.cfm?id=72**

ONLINE GLOSSARIES

The Internet provides access to a number of free-to-use medical dictionaries. The National Library of Medicine has compiled the following list of online dictionaries:

- ADAM Medical Encyclopedia (A.D.A.M., Inc.), comprehensive medical reference: **http://www.nlm.nih.gov/medlineplus/encyclopedia.html**

- MedicineNet.com Medical Dictionary (MedicineNet, Inc.): **http://www.medterms.com/Script/Main/hp.asp**

- Merriam-Webster Medical Dictionary (Inteli-Health, Inc.): **http://www.intelihealth.com/IH/**

- Multilingual Glossary of Technical and Popular Medical Terms in Eight European Languages (European Commission) - Danish, Dutch, English, French, German, Italian, Portuguese, and Spanish: **http://allserv.rug.ac.be/~rvdstich/eugloss/welcome.html**

- On-line Medical Dictionary (CancerWEB): **http://cancerweb.ncl.ac.uk/omd/**

- Rare Diseases Terms (Office of Rare Diseases): **http://ord.aspensys.com/asp/diseases/diseases.asp**

- Technology Glossary (National Library of Medicine) - Health Care Technology: **http://www.nlm.nih.gov/nichsr/ta101/ta10108.htm**

Beyond these, MEDLINEplus contains a very patient-friendly encyclopedia covering every aspect of medicine (licensed from A.D.A.M., Inc.). The ADAM Medical Encyclopedia can be accessed at **http://www.nlm.nih.gov/medlineplus/encyclopedia.html**. ADAM is also available on commercial Web sites such as drkoop.com (**http://www.drkoop.com/**) and Web MD (**http://my.webmd.com/adam/asset/adam_disease_articles/a_to_z/a**).

Online Dictionary Directories

The following are additional online directories compiled by the National Library of Medicine, including a number of specialized medical dictionaries:

- Medical Dictionaries: Medical & Biological (World Health Organization): **http://www.who.int/hlt/virtuallibrary/English/diction.htm#Medical**

- MEL-Michigan Electronic Library List of Online Health and Medical Dictionaries (Michigan Electronic Library): **http://mel.lib.mi.us/health/health-dictionaries.html**

- Patient Education: Glossaries (DMOZ Open Directory Project): **http://dmoz.org/Health/Education/Patient_Education/Glossaries/**

- Web of Online Dictionaries (Bucknell University): **http://www.yourdictionary.com/diction5.html#medicine**

ERECTILE DYSFUNCTION DICTIONARY

The definitions below are derived from official public sources, including the National Institutes of Health [NIH] and the European Union [EU].

Abdomen: That portion of the body that lies between the thorax and the pelvis. [NIH]

Abdominal: Having to do with the abdomen, which is the part of the body between the chest and the hips that contains the pancreas, stomach, intestines, liver, gallbladder, and other organs. [NIH]

Abdominal Pain: Sensation of discomfort, distress, or agony in the abdominal region. [NIH]

Ablation: The removal of an organ by surgery. [NIH]

Acceptor: A substance which, while normally not oxidized by oxygen or reduced by hydrogen, can be oxidized or reduced in presence of a substance which is itself undergoing oxidation or reduction. [NIH]

Acetohexamide: A sulfonylurea hypoglycemic agent that is metabolized in the liver to 1-hydrohexamide. [NIH]

Acetylcholine: A neurotransmitter. Acetylcholine in vertebrates is the major transmitter at neuromuscular junctions, autonomic ganglia, parasympathetic effector junctions, a subset of sympathetic effector junctions, and at many sites in the central nervous system. It is generally not used as an administered drug because it is broken down very rapidly by cholinesterases, but it is useful in some ophthalmological applications. [NIH]

Acetyltransferases: Enzymes catalyzing the transfer of an acetyl group, usually from acetyl coenzyme A, to another compound. EC 2.3.1. [NIH]

Acidosis: A pathologic condition resulting from accumulation of acid or depletion of the alkaline reserve (bicarbonate content) in the blood and body tissues, and characterized by an increase in hydrogen ion concentration. [EU]

Actin: Essential component of the cell skeleton. [NIH]

Adaptation: 1. The adjustment of an organism to its environment, or the process by which it enhances such fitness. 2. The normal ability of the eye to adjust itself to variations in the intensity of light; the adjustment to such variations. 3. The decline in the frequency of firing of a neuron, particularly of a receptor, under conditions of constant stimulation. 4. In dentistry, (a) the proper fitting of a denture, (b) the degree of proximity and interlocking of restorative material to a tooth preparation, (c) the exact adjustment of bands to teeth. 5. In microbiology, the adjustment of bacterial physiology to a new environment. [EU]

Adenine: A purine base and a fundamental unit of adenine nucleotides. [NIH]

Adenocarcinoma: A malignant epithelial tumor with a glandular organization. [NIH]

Adenoma: A benign epithelial tumor with a glandular organization. [NIH]

Adenosine: A nucleoside that is composed of adenine and d-ribose. Adenosine or adenosine derivatives play many important biological roles in addition to being components of DNA and RNA. Adenosine itself is a neurotransmitter. [NIH]

Adenylate Cyclase: An enzyme of the lyase class that catalyzes the formation of cyclic AMP and pyrophosphate from ATP. EC 4.6.1.1. [NIH]

Adipose Tissue: Connective tissue composed of fat cells lodged in the meshes of areolar tissue. [NIH]

Adjustment: The dynamic process wherein the thoughts, feelings, behavior, and biophysiological mechanisms of the individual continually change to adjust to the environment. [NIH]

Adjuvant: A substance which aids another, such as an auxiliary remedy; in immunology, nonspecific stimulator (e.g., BCG vaccine) of the immune response. [EU]

Adrenal Cortex: The outer layer of the adrenal gland. It secretes mineralocorticoids, androgens, and glucocorticoids. [NIH]

Adrenal Medulla: The inner part of the adrenal gland; it synthesizes, stores and releases catecholamines. [NIH]

Adrenaline: A hormone. Also called epinephrine. [NIH]

Adrenergic: Activated by, characteristic of, or secreting epinephrine or substances with similar activity; the term is applied to those nerve fibres that liberate norepinephrine at a synapse when a nerve impulse passes, i.e., the sympathetic fibres. [EU]

Adrenergic Agents: Drugs that act on adrenergic receptors or affect the life cycle of adrenergic transmitters. Included here are adrenergic agonists and antagonists and agents that affect the synthesis, storage, uptake, metabolism, or release of adrenergic transmitters. [NIH]

Adrenoreceptor: Receptors specifically sensitive to and operated by adrenaline and/or noradrenaline and related sympathomimetic drugs. Adrenoreceptor is an alternative name. [NIH]

Adverse Effect: An unwanted side effect of treatment. [NIH]

Aerosol: A solution of a drug which can be atomized into a fine mist for inhalation therapy. [EU]

Aetiology: Study of the causes of disease. [EU]

Affinity: 1. Inherent likeness or relationship. 2. A special attraction for a specific element, organ, or structure. 3. Chemical affinity; the force that binds atoms in molecules; the tendency of substances to combine by chemical reaction. 4. The strength of noncovalent chemical binding between two substances as measured by the dissociation constant of the complex. 5. In immunology, a thermodynamic expression of the strength of interaction between a single antigen-binding site and a single antigenic determinant (and thus of the stereochemical compatibility between them), most accurately applied to interactions among simple, uniform antigenic determinants such as haptens. Expressed as the association constant (K litres mole -1), which, owing to the heterogeneity of affinities in a population of antibody molecules of a given specificity, actually represents an average value (mean intrinsic association constant). 6. The reciprocal of the dissociation constant. [EU]

Agar: A complex sulfated polymer of galactose units, extracted from Gelidium cartilagineum, Gracilaria confervoides, and related red algae. It is used as a gel in the preparation of solid culture media for microorganisms, as a bulk laxative, in making emulsions, and as a supporting medium for immunodiffusion and immunoelectrophoresis. [NIH]

Age Factors: Age as a constituent element or influence contributing to the production of a result. It may be applicable to the cause or the effect of a circumstance. It is used with human or animal concepts but should be differentiated from aging, a physiological process, and time factors which refers only to the passage of time. [NIH]

Age of Onset: The age or period of life at which a disease or the initial symptoms or manifestations of a disease appear in an individual. [NIH]

Age-Adjusted: Summary measures of rates of morbidity or mortality in a population using statistical procedures to remove the effect of age differences in populations that are being compared. Age is probably the most important and the most common variable in determining the risk of morbidity and mortality. [NIH]

Ageing: A physiological or morphological change in the life of an organism or its parts, generally irreversible and typically associated with a decline in growth and reproductive vigor. [NIH]

Agonist: In anatomy, a prime mover. In pharmacology, a drug that has affinity for and stimulates physiologic activity at cell receptors normally stimulated by naturally occurring substances. [EU]

Airway: A device for securing unobstructed passage of air into and out of the lungs during general anesthesia. [NIH]

Albumin: 1. Any protein that is soluble in water and moderately concentrated salt solutions and is coagulable by heat. 2. Serum albumin; the major plasma protein (approximately 60 per cent of the total), which is responsible for much of the plasma colloidal osmotic pressure and serves as a transport protein carrying large organic anions, such as fatty acids, bilirubin, and many drugs, and also carrying certain hormones, such as cortisol and thyroxine, when their specific binding globulins are saturated. Albumin is synthesized in the liver. Low serum levels occur in protein malnutrition, active inflammation and serious hepatic and renal disease. [EU]

Aldehyde Dehydrogenase: An enzyme that oxidizes an aldehyde in the presence of NAD+ and water to an acid and NADH. EC 1.2.1.3. Before 1978, it was classified as EC 1.1.1.70. [NIH]

Aldehydes: Organic compounds containing a carbonyl group in the form -CHO. [NIH]

Aldosterone: (11 beta)-11,21-Dihydroxy-3,20-dioxopregn-4-en-18-al. A hormone secreted by the adrenal cortex that functions in the regulation of electrolyte and water balance by increasing the renal retention of sodium and the excretion of potassium. [NIH]

Alertness: A state of readiness to detect and respond to certain specified small changes occurring at random intervals in the environment. [NIH]

Algorithms: A procedure consisting of a sequence of algebraic formulas and/or logical steps to calculate or determine a given task. [NIH]

Alimentary: Pertaining to food or nutritive material, or to the organs of digestion. [EU]

Alkaline: Having the reactions of an alkali. [EU]

Alkaloid: A member of a large group of chemicals that are made by plants and have nitrogen in them. Some alkaloids have been shown to work against cancer. [NIH]

Allergen: An antigenic substance capable of producing immediate-type hypersensitivity (allergy). [EU]

Allosteric Site: A site on an enzyme which upon binding of a modulator, causes the protein to undergo a conformational change that may alter the catalytic or binding properties of the enzyme. [NIH]

Allylamine: Possesses an unusual and selective cytotoxicity for vascular smooth muscle cells in dogs and rats. Useful for experiments dealing with arterial injury, myocardial fibrosis or cardiac decompensation. [NIH]

Alpha Particles: Positively charged particles composed of two protons and two neutrons, i.e., helium nuclei, emitted during disintegration of very heavy isotopes; a beam of alpha particles or an alpha ray has very strong ionizing power, but weak penetrability. [NIH]

Alpha-1: A protein with the property of inactivating proteolytic enzymes such as leucocyte collagenase and elastase. [NIH]

Alprenolol: 1-((1-Methylethyl)amino)-3-(2-(2-propenyl)phenoxy)-2-propanol. Adrenergic beta-blocker used as an antihypertensive, anti-anginal, and anti-arrhythmic agent. [NIH]

Alprostadil: A potent vasodilator agent that increases peripheral blood flow. It inhibits platelet aggregation and has many other biological effects such as bronchodilation, mediation of inflammation, etc. [NIH]

Alternative medicine: Practices not generally recognized by the medical community as standard or conventional medical approaches and used instead of standard treatments. Alternative medicine includes the taking of dietary supplements, megadose vitamins, and herbal preparations; the drinking of special teas; and practices such as massage therapy, magnet therapy, spiritual healing, and meditation. [NIH]

Alternative Splicing: A process whereby multiple protein isoforms are generated from a single gene. Alternative splicing involves the splicing together of nonconsecutive exons during the processing of some, but not all, transcripts of the gene. Thus a particular exon may be connected to any one of several alternative exons to form messenger RNA. The alternative forms produce proteins in which one part is common while the other part is different. [NIH]

Ameliorated: A changeable condition which prevents the consequence of a failure or accident from becoming as bad as it otherwise would. [NIH]

Ameliorating: A changeable condition which prevents the consequence of a failure or accident from becoming as bad as it otherwise would. [NIH]

Amenorrhea: Absence of menstruation. [NIH]

Amine: An organic compound containing nitrogen; any member of a group of chemical compounds formed from ammonia by replacement of one or more of the hydrogen atoms by organic (hydrocarbon) radicals. The amines are distinguished as primary, secondary, and tertiary, according to whether one, two, or three hydrogen atoms are replaced. The amines include allylamine, amylamine, ethylamine, methylamine, phenylamine, propylamine, and many other compounds. [EU]

Amino Acid Sequence: The order of amino acids as they occur in a polypeptide chain. This is referred to as the primary structure of proteins. It is of fundamental importance in determining protein conformation. [NIH]

Amino Acids: Organic compounds that generally contain an amino (-NH2) and a carboxyl (-COOH) group. Twenty alpha-amino acids are the subunits which are polymerized to form proteins. [NIH]

Amino Acids: Organic compounds that generally contain an amino (-NH2) and a carboxyl (-COOH) group. Twenty alpha-amino acids are the subunits which are polymerized to form proteins. [NIH]

Ammonia: A colorless alkaline gas. It is formed in the body during decomposition of organic materials during a large number of metabolically important reactions. [NIH]

Amphetamine: A powerful central nervous system stimulant and sympathomimetic. Amphetamine has multiple mechanisms of action including blocking uptake of adrenergics and dopamine, stimulation of release of monamines, and inhibiting monoamine oxidase. Amphetamine is also a drug of abuse and a psychotomimetic. The l- and the d,l-forms are included here. The l-form has less central nervous system activity but stronger cardiovascular effects. The d-form is dextroamphetamine. [NIH]

Ampulla: A sac-like enlargement of a canal or duct. [NIH]

Amputation: Surgery to remove part or all of a limb or appendage. [NIH]

Amyloid: A general term for a variety of different proteins that accumulate as extracellular fibrils of 7-10 nm and have common structural features, including a beta-pleated sheet conformation and the ability to bind such dyes as Congo red and thioflavine (Kandel, Schwartz, and Jessel, Principles of Neural Science, 3rd ed). [NIH]

Anaesthesia: Loss of feeling or sensation. Although the term is used for loss of tactile sensibility, or of any of the other senses, it is applied especially to loss of the sensation of pain, as it is induced to permit performance of surgery or other painful procedures. [EU]

Anal: Having to do with the anus, which is the posterior opening of the large bowel. [NIH]

Analgesic: An agent that alleviates pain without causing loss of consciousness. [EU]

Analog: In chemistry, a substance that is similar, but not identical, to another. [NIH]

Analytes: A component of a test sample the presence of which has to be demonstrated. The term "analyte" includes where appropriate formed from the analyte during the analyses. [NIH]

Anaphylatoxins: The family of peptides C3a, C4a, C5a, and C5a des-arginine produced in the serum during complement activation. They produce smooth muscle contraction, mast cell histamine release, affect platelet aggregation, and act as mediators of the local inflammatory process. The order of anaphylatoxin activity from strongest to weakest is C5a, C3a, C4a, and C5a des-arginine. The latter is the so-called "classical" anaphylatoxin but shows no spasmogenic activity though it contains some chemotactic ability. [NIH]

Anaplasia: Loss of structural differentiation and useful function of neoplastic cells. [NIH]

Anatomical: Pertaining to anatomy, or to the structure of the organism. [EU]

Androgen suppression: Treatment to suppress or block the production of male hormones. Androgen suppression is achieved by surgical removal of the testicles, by taking female sex hormones, or by taking other drugs. Also called androgen ablation. [NIH]

Androgenic: Producing masculine characteristics. [EU]

Androgens: A class of sex hormones associated with the development and maintenance of the secondary male sex characteristics, sperm induction, and sexual differentiation. In addition to increasing virility and libido, they also increase nitrogen and water retention and stimulate skeletal growth. [NIH]

Anemia: A reduction in the number of circulating erythrocytes or in the quantity of hemoglobin. [NIH]

Anesthesia: A state characterized by loss of feeling or sensation. This depression of nerve function is usually the result of pharmacologic action and is induced to allow performance of surgery or other painful procedures. [NIH]

Aneurysm: A sac formed by the dilatation of the wall of an artery, a vein, or the heart. [NIH]

Angina: Chest pain that originates in the heart. [NIH]

Angina Pectoris: The symptom of paroxysmal pain consequent to myocardial ischemia usually of distinctive character, location and radiation, and provoked by a transient stressful situation during which the oxygen requirements of the myocardium exceed the capacity of the coronary circulation to supply it. [NIH]

Angiogenesis: Blood vessel formation. Tumor angiogenesis is the growth of blood vessels from surrounding tissue to a solid tumor. This is caused by the release of chemicals by the tumor. [NIH]

Angiopathy: Disease of the blood vessels (arteries, veins, and capillaries) that occurs when someone has diabetes for a long time. There are two types of angiopathy: macroangiopathy and microangiopathy. In macroangiopathy, fat and blood clots build up in the large blood vessels, stick to the vessel walls, and block the flow of blood. In microangiopathy, the walls of the smaller blood vessels become so thick and weak that they bleed, leak protein, and slow the flow of blood through the body. Then the cells, for example, the ones in the center of the eye, do not get enough blood and may be damaged. [NIH]

Angioplasty: Endovascular reconstruction of an artery, which may include the removal of atheromatous plaque and/or the endothelial lining as well as simple dilatation. These are procedures performed by catheterization. When reconstruction of an artery is performed surgically, it is called endarterectomy. [NIH]

Animal model: An animal with a disease either the same as or like a disease in humans. Animal models are used to study the development and progression of diseases and to test new treatments before they are given to humans. Animals with transplanted human cancers or other tissues are called xenograft models. [NIH]

Anionic: Pertaining to or containing an anion. [EU]

Anorexia: Lack or loss of appetite for food. Appetite is psychologic, dependent on memory and associations. Anorexia can be brought about by unattractive food, surroundings, or company. [NIH]

Antagonism: Interference with, or inhibition of, the growth of a living organism by another living organism, due either to creation of unfavorable conditions (e. g. exhaustion of food supplies) or to production of a specific antibiotic substance (e. g. penicillin). [NIH]

Antiandrogen therapy: Treatment with drugs used to block production or interfere with the action of male sex hormones. [NIH]

Antiandrogens: Drugs used to block the production or interfere with the action of male sex hormones. [NIH]

Antibiotic: A drug used to treat infections caused by bacteria and other microorganisms. [NIH]

Antibodies: Immunoglobulin molecules having a specific amino acid sequence by virtue of which they interact only with the antigen that induced their synthesis in cells of the lymphoid series (especially plasma cells), or with an antigen closely related to it. [NIH]

Antibody: A type of protein made by certain white blood cells in response to a foreign substance (antigen). Each antibody can bind to only a specific antigen. The purpose of this binding is to help destroy the antigen. Antibodies can work in several ways, depending on the nature of the antigen. Some antibodies destroy antigens directly. Others make it easier for white blood cells to destroy the antigen. [NIH]

Anticoagulant: A drug that helps prevent blood clots from forming. Also called a blood thinner. [NIH]

Antidepressant: A drug used to treat depression. [NIH]

Antidiabetic: An agent that prevents or alleviates diabetes. [EU]

Antiemetic: An agent that prevents or alleviates nausea and vomiting. Also antinauseant. [EU]

Antifungal: Destructive to fungi, or suppressing their reproduction or growth; effective against fungal infections. [EU]

Antigen: Any substance which is capable, under appropriate conditions, of inducing a specific immune response and of reacting with the products of that response, that is, with specific antibody or specifically sensitized T-lymphocytes, or both. Antigens may be soluble substances, such as toxins and foreign proteins, or particulate, such as bacteria and tissue cells; however, only the portion of the protein or polysaccharide molecule known as the antigenic determinant (q.v.) combines with antibody or a specific receptor on a lymphocyte. Abbreviated Ag. [EU]

Antigen-Antibody Complex: The complex formed by the binding of antigen and antibody molecules. The deposition of large antigen-antibody complexes leading to tissue damage causes immune complex diseases. [NIH]

Antihypertensive: An agent that reduces high blood pressure. [EU]

Anti-infective: An agent that so acts. [EU]

Anti-inflammatory: Having to do with reducing inflammation. [NIH]

Antioxidant: A substance that prevents damage caused by free radicals. Free radicals are highly reactive chemicals that often contain oxygen. They are produced when molecules are split to give products that have unpaired electrons. This process is called oxidation. [NIH]

Antipyretic: An agent that relieves or reduces fever. Called also antifebrile, antithermic and febrifuge. [EU]

Antispasmodic: An agent that relieves spasm. [EU]

Anuria: Inability to form or excrete urine. [NIH]

Anus: The opening of the rectum to the outside of the body. [NIH]

Anxiety: Persistent feeling of dread, apprehension, and impending disaster. [NIH]

Anxiety Disorders: Disorders in which anxiety (persistent feelings of apprehension, tension, or uneasiness) is the predominant disturbance. [NIH]

Aorta: The main trunk of the systemic arteries. [NIH]

Apnea: A transient absence of spontaneous respiration. [NIH]

Apolipoproteins: The protein components of lipoproteins which remain after the lipids to which the proteins are bound have been removed. They play an important role in lipid transport and metabolism. [NIH]

Apomorphine: A derivative of morphine that is a dopamine D2 agonist. It is a powerful emetic and has been used for that effect in acute poisoning. It has also been used in the diagnosis and treatment of parkinsonism, but its adverse effects limit its use. [NIH]

Apoptosis: One of the two mechanisms by which cell death occurs (the other being the pathological process of necrosis). Apoptosis is the mechanism responsible for the physiological deletion of cells and appears to be intrinsically programmed. It is characterized by distinctive morphologic changes in the nucleus and cytoplasm, chromatin cleavage at regularly spaced sites, and the endonucleolytic cleavage of genomic DNA (DNA fragmentation) at internucleosomal sites. This mode of cell death serves as a balance to mitosis in regulating the size of animal tissues and in mediating pathologic processes associated with tumor growth. [NIH]

Aqueous: Having to do with water. [NIH]

Arachidonic Acid: An unsaturated, essential fatty acid. It is found in animal and human fat as well as in the liver, brain, and glandular organs, and is a constituent of animal phosphatides. It is formed by the synthesis from dietary linoleic acid and is a precursor in the biosynthesis of prostaglandins, thromboxanes, and leukotrienes. [NIH]

Arginase: A ureahydrolase that catalyzes the hydrolysis of arginine or canavanine to yield L-ORNITHINE and urea. Deficiency of this enzyme causes hyperargininemia. EC 3.5.3.1. [NIH]

Arginine: An essential amino acid that is physiologically active in the L-form. [NIH]

Aromatic: Having a spicy odour. [EU]

Arrhythmia: Any variation from the normal rhythm or rate of the heart beat. [NIH]

Arterial: Pertaining to an artery or to the arteries. [EU]

Arteries: The vessels carrying blood away from the heart. [NIH]

Arterioles: The smallest divisions of the arteries located between the muscular arteries and the capillaries. [NIH]

Arteriolosclerosis: Sclerosis and thickening of the walls of the smaller arteries (arterioles). Hyaline arteriolosclerosis, in which there is homogeneous pink hyaline thickening of the arteriolar walls, is associated with benign nephrosclerosis. Hyperplastic arteriolosclerosis, in which there is a concentric thickening with progressive narrowing of the lumina may be associated with malignant hypertension, nephrosclerosis, and scleroderma. [EU]

Arteriosclerosis: Thickening and loss of elasticity of arterial walls. Atherosclerosis is the most common form of arteriosclerosis and involves lipid deposition and thickening of the intimal cell layers within arteries. Additional forms of arteriosclerosis involve calcification of the media of muscular arteries (Monkeberg medial calcific sclerosis) and thickening of the walls of small arteries or arterioles due to cell proliferation or hyaline deposition (arteriolosclerosis). [NIH]

Arteriovenous: Both arterial and venous; pertaining to or affecting an artery and a vein. [EU]

Articular: Of or pertaining to a joint. [EU]

Aspergillosis: Infections with fungi of the genus Aspergillus. [NIH]

Assay: Determination of the amount of a particular constituent of a mixture, or of the biological or pharmacological potency of a drug. [EU]

Astrocytes: The largest and most numerous neuroglial cells in the brain and spinal cord. Astrocytes (from "star" cells) are irregularly shaped with many long processes, including those with "end feet" which form the glial (limiting) membrane and directly and indirectly contribute to the blood brain barrier. They regulate the extracellular ionic and chemical environment, and "reactive astrocytes" (along with microglia) respond to injury. Astrocytes have high-affinity transmitter uptake systems, voltage-dependent and transmitter-gated ion channels, and can release transmitter, but their role in signaling (as in many other functions) is not well understood. [NIH]

Autoimmune disease: A condition in which the body recognizes its own tissues as foreign and directs an immune response against them. [NIH]

Autonomic: Self-controlling; functionally independent. [EU]

Autonomic Nervous System: The enteric, parasympathetic, and sympathetic nervous systems taken together. Generally speaking, the autonomic nervous system regulates the internal environment during both peaceful activity and physical or emotional stress. Autonomic activity is controlled and integrated by the central nervous system, especially the hypothalamus and the solitary nucleus, which receive information relayed from visceral afferents; these and related central and sensory structures are sometimes (but not here) considered to be part of the autonomic nervous system itself. [NIH]

Autonomic Neuropathy: A disease of the nerves affecting mostly the internal organs such as the bladder muscles, the cardiovascular system, the digestive tract, and the genital organs. These nerves are not under a person's conscious control and function automatically. Also called visceral neuropathy. [NIH]

Babesiosis: A group of tick-borne diseases of mammals including zoonoses in humans. They are caused by protozoans of the genus babesia, which parasitize erythrocytes, producing hemolysis. In the U.S., the organism's natural host is mice and transmission is by the deer tick ixodes scapularis. [NIH]

Bacteria: Unicellular prokaryotic microorganisms which generally possess rigid cell walls, multiply by cell division, and exhibit three principal forms: round or coccal, rodlike or bacillary, and spiral or spirochetal. [NIH]

Bacteriophage: A virus whose host is a bacterial cell; A virus that exclusively infects bacteria. It generally has a protein coat surrounding the genome (DNA or RNA). One of the coliphages most extensively studied is the lambda phage, which is also one of the most important. [NIH]

Bacteriostatic: 1. Inhibiting the growth or multiplication of bacteria. 2. An agent that inhibits the growth or multiplication of bacteria. [EU]

Bacterium: Microscopic organism which may have a spherical, rod-like, or spiral unicellular or non-cellular body. Bacteria usually reproduce through asexual processes. [NIH]

Bacteriuria: The presence of bacteria in the urine with or without consequent urinary tract infection. Since bacteriuria is a clinical entity, the term does not preclude the use of urine/microbiology for technical discussions on the isolation and segregation of bacteria in the urine. [NIH]

Balanitis: Inflammation of the glans penis. [NIH]

Base: In chemistry, the nonacid part of a salt; a substance that combines with acids to form salts; a substance that dissociates to give hydroxide ions in aqueous solutions; a substance whose molecule or ion can combine with a proton (hydrogen ion); a substance capable of donating a pair of electrons (to an acid) for the formation of a coordinate covalent bond. [EU]

Basophils: Granular leukocytes characterized by a relatively pale-staining, lobate nucleus and cytoplasm containing coarse dark-staining granules of variable size and stainable by basic dyes. [NIH]

Benign: Not cancerous; does not invade nearby tissue or spread to other parts of the body. [NIH]

Benign prostatic hyperplasia: A benign (noncancerous) condition in which an overgrowth of prostate tissue pushes against the urethra and the bladder, blocking the flow of urine. Also called benign prostatic hypertrophy or BPH. [NIH]

Benzoic Acid: A fungistatic compound that is widely used as a food preservative. It is conjugated to glycine in the liver and excreted as hippuric acid. [NIH]

Beta Rays: A stream of positive or negative electrons ejected with high energy from a disintegrating atomic nucleus; most biomedically used isotopes emit negative particles (electrons or negatrons, rather than positrons). Cathode rays are low-energy negative electrons produced in cathode ray tubes, also called television tubes or oscilloscopes. [NIH]

Beta-pleated: Particular three-dimensional pattern of amyloidoses. [NIH]

Bifida: A defect in development of the vertebral column in which there is a central deficiency of the vertebral lamina. [NIH]

Bile: An emulsifying agent produced in the liver and secreted into the duodenum. Its composition includes bile acids and salts, cholesterol, and electrolytes. It aids digestion of fats in the duodenum. [NIH]

Bile Acids: Acids made by the liver that work with bile to break down fats. [NIH]

Binding Sites: The reactive parts of a macromolecule that directly participate in its specific combination with another molecule. [NIH]

Bioavailability: The degree to which a drug or other substance becomes available to the target tissue after administration. [EU]

Biochemical: Relating to biochemistry; characterized by, produced by, or involving chemical reactions in living organisms. [EU]

Biological Transport: The movement of materials (including biochemical substances and drugs) across cell membranes and epithelial layers, usually by passive diffusion. [NIH]

Biopsy: Removal and pathologic examination of specimens in the form of small pieces of tissue from the living body. [NIH]

Biosynthesis: The building up of a chemical compound in the physiologic processes of a living organism. [EU]

Biotechnology: Body of knowledge related to the use of organisms, cells or cell-derived constituents for the purpose of developing products which are technically, scientifically and clinically useful. Alteration of biologic function at the molecular level (i.e., genetic engineering) is a central focus; laboratory methods used include transfection and cloning technologies, sequence and structure analysis algorithms, computer databases, and gene and protein structure function analysis and prediction. [NIH]

Bladder: The organ that stores urine. [NIH]

Blastocyst: The mammalian embryo in the post-morula stage in which a fluid-filled cavity, enclosed primarily by trophoblast, contains an inner cell mass which becomes the embryonic disc. [NIH]

Blastomycosis: A fungal infection that may appear in two forms: 1) a primary lesion characterized by the formation of a small cutaneous nodule and small nodules along the lymphatics that may heal within several months; and 2) chronic granulomatous lesions characterized by thick crusts, warty growths, and unusual vascularity and infection in the middle or upper lobes of the lung. [NIH]

Bloating: Fullness or swelling in the abdomen that often occurs after meals. [NIH]

Blood Coagulation: The process of the interaction of blood coagulation factors that results in an insoluble fibrin clot. [NIH]

Blood Glucose: Glucose in blood. [NIH]

Blood Platelets: Non-nucleated disk-shaped cells formed in the megakaryocyte and found in the blood of all mammals. They are mainly involved in blood coagulation. [NIH]

Blood pressure: The pressure of blood against the walls of a blood vessel or heart chamber. Unless there is reference to another location, such as the pulmonary artery or one of the heart chambers, it refers to the pressure in the systemic arteries, as measured, for example, in the forearm. [NIH]

Blood vessel: A tube in the body through which blood circulates. Blood vessels include a network of arteries, arterioles, capillaries, venules, and veins. [NIH]

Blot: To transfer DNA, RNA, or proteins to an immobilizing matrix such as nitrocellulose. [NIH]

Body Fluids: Liquid components of living organisms. [NIH]

Body Mass Index: One of the anthropometric measures of body mass; it has the highest correlation with skinfold thickness or body density. [NIH]

Bone Marrow: The soft tissue filling the cavities of bones. Bone marrow exists in two types, yellow and red. Yellow marrow is found in the large cavities of large bones and consists mostly of fat cells and a few primitive blood cells. Red marrow is a hematopoietic tissue and is the site of production of erythrocytes and granular leukocytes. Bone marrow is made up of a framework of connective tissue containing branching fibers with the frame being filled with marrow cells. [NIH]

Bone Resorption: Bone loss due to osteoclastic activity. [NIH]

Bowel: The long tube-shaped organ in the abdomen that completes the process of digestion. There is both a small and a large bowel. Also called the intestine. [NIH]

Bowel Movement: Body wastes passed through the rectum and anus. [NIH]

Brachytherapy: A collective term for interstitial, intracavity, and surface radiotherapy. It uses small sealed or partly-sealed sources that may be placed on or near the body surface or within a natural body cavity or implanted directly into the tissues. [NIH]

Bradykinin: A nonapeptide messenger that is enzymatically produced from kallidin in the blood where it is a potent but short-lived agent of arteriolar dilation and increased capillary permeability. Bradykinin is also released from mast cells during asthma attacks, from gut walls as a gastrointestinal vasodilator, from damaged tissues as a pain signal, and may be a neurotransmitter. [NIH]

Brain Ischemia: Localized reduction of blood flow to brain tissue due to arterial obtruction or systemic hypoperfusion. This frequently occurs in conjuction with brain hypoxia. Prolonged ischemia is associated with brain infarction. [NIH]

Brain Stem: The part of the brain that connects the cerebral hemispheres with the spinal cord. It consists of the mesencephalon, pons, and medulla oblongata. [NIH]

Branch: Most commonly used for branches of nerves, but applied also to other structures. [NIH]

Breakdown: A physical, metal, or nervous collapse. [NIH]

Breeding: The science or art of changing the constitution of a population of plants or animals through sexual reproduction. [NIH]

Bromocriptine: A semisynthetic ergot alkaloid that is a dopamine D2 agonist. It suppresses prolactin secretion and is used to treat amenorrhea, galactorrhea, and female infertility, and has been proposed for Parkinson disease. [NIH]

Bronchi: The larger air passages of the lungs arising from the terminal bifurcation of the trachea. [NIH]

Bronchial: Pertaining to one or more bronchi. [EU]

Buccal: Pertaining to or directed toward the cheek. In dental anatomy, used to refer to the buccal surface of a tooth. [EU]

Bupivacaine: A widely used local anesthetic agent. [NIH]

Caffeine: A methylxanthine naturally occurring in some beverages and also used as a pharmacological agent. Caffeine's most notable pharmacological effect is as a central nervous system stimulant, increasing alertness and producing agitation. It also relaxes smooth muscle, stimulates cardiac muscle, stimulates diuresis, and appears to be useful in the treatment of some types of headache. Several cellular actions of caffeine have been observed, but it is not entirely clear how each contributes to its pharmacological profile. Among the most important are inhibition of cyclic nucleotide phosphodiesterases, antagonism of adenosine receptors, and modulation of intracellular calcium handling. [NIH]

Calcification: Deposits of calcium in the tissues of the breast. Calcification in the breast can be seen on a mammogram, but cannot be detected by touch. There are two types of breast calcification, macrocalcification and microcalcification. Macrocalcifications are large deposits and are usually not related to cancer. Microcalcifications are specks of calcium that may be found in an area of rapidly dividing cells. Many microcalcifications clustered together may be a sign of cancer. [NIH]

Calcitonin Gene-Related Peptide: Calcitonin gene-related peptide. A 37-amino acid peptide derived from the calcitonin gene. It occurs as a result of alternative processing of mRNA from the calcitonin gene. The neuropeptide is widely distributed in neural tissue of the brain, gut, perivascular nerves, and other tissue. The peptide produces multiple biological effects and has both circulatory and neurotransmitter modes of action. In particular, it is a potent endogenous vasodilator. [NIH]

Calcium: A basic element found in nearly all organized tissues. It is a member of the alkaline earth family of metals with the atomic symbol Ca, atomic number 20, and atomic weight 40. Calcium is the most abundant mineral in the body and combines with phosphorus to form calcium phosphate in the bones and teeth. It is essential for the normal functioning of nerves and muscles and plays a role in blood coagulation (as factor IV) and in many enzymatic processes. [NIH]

Calcium channel blocker: A drug used to relax the blood vessel and heart muscle, causing pressure inside blood vessels to drop. It also can regulate heart rhythm. [NIH]

Calcium Channel Blockers: A class of drugs that act by selective inhibition of calcium influx through cell membranes or on the release and binding of calcium in intracellular pools. Since they are inducers of vascular and other smooth muscle relaxation, they are used in the drug therapy of hypertension and cerebrovascular spasms, as myocardial protective agents, and in the relaxation of uterine spasms. [NIH]

Calcium Channels: Voltage-dependent cell membrane glycoproteins selectively permeable to calcium ions. They are categorized as L-, T-, N-, P-, Q-, and R-types based on the activation and inactivation kinetics, ion specificity, and sensitivity to drugs and toxins. The L- and T-types are present throughout the cardiovascular and central nervous systems and the N-, P-, Q-, & R-types are located in neuronal tissue. [NIH]

Calculi: An abnormal concretion occurring mostly in the urinary and biliary tracts, usually composed of mineral salts. Also called stones. [NIH]

Callus: A callosity or hard, thick skin; the bone-like reparative substance that is formed round the edges and fragments of broken bone. [NIH]

Calmodulin: A heat-stable, low-molecular-weight activator protein found mainly in the brain and heart. The binding of calcium ions to this protein allows this protein to bind to cyclic nucleotide phosphodiesterases and to adenyl cyclase with subsequent activation. Thereby this protein modulates cyclic AMP and cyclic GMP levels. [NIH]

Capillary: Any one of the minute vessels that connect the arterioles and venules, forming a network in nearly all parts of the body. Their walls act as semipermeable membranes for the interchange of various substances, including fluids, between the blood and tissue fluid; called also vas capillare. [EU]

Capsules: Hard or soft soluble containers used for the oral administration of medicine. [NIH]

Carbohydrate: An aldehyde or ketone derivative of a polyhydric alcohol, particularly of the pentahydric and hexahydric alcohols. They are so named because the hydrogen and oxygen are usually in the proportion to form water, $(CH2O)n$. The most important carbohydrates are the starches, sugars, celluloses, and gums. They are classified into mono-, di-, tri-, poly- and heterosaccharides. [EU]

Carbon Dioxide: A colorless, odorless gas that can be formed by the body and is necessary for the respiration cycle of plants and animals. [NIH]

Carboxy: Cannabinoid. [NIH]

Carcinogenic: Producing carcinoma. [EU]

Carcinogens: Substances that increase the risk of neoplasms in humans or animals. Both genotoxic chemicals, which affect DNA directly, and nongenotoxic chemicals, which induce neoplasms by other mechanism, are included. [NIH]

Carcinoma: Cancer that begins in the skin or in tissues that line or cover internal organs. [NIH]

Cardiac: Having to do with the heart. [NIH]

Cardiac Output: The volume of blood passing through the heart per unit of time. It is usually expressed as liters (volume) per minute so as not to be confused with stroke volume (volume per beat). [NIH]

Cardiopathy: Any disorder or disease of the heart. In addition to heart disease of inflammatory origin, there are arteriosclerotic cardiopathy, due to arteriosclerosis; fatty cardiopathy, due to growth of fatty tissue; hypertensive cardiopathy, due to high blood pressure; nephropathic cardiopathy, due to kidney disease, thyrotoxic cardiopathy, due to thyroid intoxication; toxic cardiopathy, due to the effect of some toxin; and valvular cardiopathy, due to faulty valve action. [EU]

Cardiotonic: 1. Having a tonic effect on the heart. 2. An agent that has a tonic effect on the heart. [EU]

Cardiotonic Agents: Agents that have a tonic effect on the heart or increase cardiac output. They may be glycosidic steroids related to Digitalis products, sympathomimetics, or other drugs and are used after myocardial infarcts, cardiac surgery, in shock, or in congestive heart failure. [NIH]

Cardiovascular: Having to do with the heart and blood vessels. [NIH]

Cardiovascular disease: Any abnormal condition characterized by dysfunction of the heart and blood vessels. CVD includes atherosclerosis (especially coronary heart disease, which can lead to heart attacks), cerebrovascular disease (e.g., stroke), and hypertension (high blood pressure). [NIH]

Cardiovascular System: The heart and the blood vessels by which blood is pumped and circulated through the body. [NIH]

Carotene: The general name for a group of pigments found in green, yellow, and leafy vegetables, and yellow fruits. The pigments are fat-soluble, unsaturated aliphatic hydrocarbons functioning as provitamins and are converted to vitamin A through enzymatic processes in the intestinal wall. [NIH]

Catalytic Domain: The region of an enzyme that interacts with its substrate to cause the enzymatic reaction. [NIH]

Cataract: An opacity, partial or complete, of one or both eyes, on or in the lens or capsule, especially an opacity impairing vision or causing blindness. The many kinds of cataract are classified by their morphology (size, shape, location) or etiology (cause and time of occurrence). [EU]

Catecholamine: A group of chemical substances manufactured by the adrenal medulla and secreted during physiological stress. [NIH]

Catheterization: Use or insertion of a tubular device into a duct, blood vessel, hollow organ, or body cavity for injecting or withdrawing fluids for diagnostic or therapeutic purposes. It differs from intubation in that the tube here is used to restore or maintain patency in obstructions. [NIH]

Catheters: A small, flexible tube that may be inserted into various parts of the body to inject or remove liquids. [NIH]

Cathode: An electrode, usually an incandescent filament of tungsten, which emits electrons in an X-ray tube. [NIH]

Caudal: Denoting a position more toward the cauda, or tail, than some specified point of reference; same as inferior, in human anatomy. [EU]

Cell: The individual unit that makes up all of the tissues of the body. All living things are made up of one or more cells. [NIH]

Cell Adhesion: Adherence of cells to surfaces or to other cells. [NIH]

Cell Communication: Any of several ways in which living cells of an organism communicate with one another, whether by direct contact between cells or by means of chemical signals carried by neurotransmitter substances, hormones, and cyclic AMP. [NIH]

Cell Cycle: The complex series of phenomena, occurring between the end of one cell division and the end of the next, by which cellular material is divided between daughter cells. [NIH]

Cell Death: The termination of the cell's ability to carry out vital functions such as metabolism, growth, reproduction, responsiveness, and adaptability. [NIH]

Cell Differentiation: Progressive restriction of the developmental potential and increasing specialization of function which takes place during the development of the embryo and leads to the formation of specialized cells, tissues, and organs. [NIH]

Cell Division: The fission of a cell. [NIH]

Cell membrane: Cell membrane = plasma membrane. The structure enveloping a cell, enclosing the cytoplasm, and forming a selective permeability barrier; it consists of lipids, proteins, and some carbohydrates, the lipids thought to form a bilayer in which integral proteins are embedded to varying degrees. [EU]

Cell motility: The ability of a cell to move. [NIH]

Cell proliferation: An increase in the number of cells as a result of cell growth and cell division. [NIH]

Central Nervous System: The main information-processing organs of the nervous system, consisting of the brain, spinal cord, and meninges. [NIH]

Central Nervous System Infections: Pathogenic infections of the brain, spinal cord, and meninges. DNA virus infections; RNA virus infections; bacterial infections; mycoplasma infections; Spirochaetales infections; fungal infections; protozoan infections; helminthiasis; and prion diseases may involve the central nervous system as a primary or secondary process. [NIH]

Centrifugation: A method of separating organelles or large molecules that relies upon differential sedimentation through a preformed density gradient under the influence of a gravitational field generated in a centrifuge. [NIH]

Cerebellum: Part of the metencephalon that lies in the posterior cranial fossa behind the brain stem. It is concerned with the coordination of movement. [NIH]

Cerebral: Of or pertaining of the cerebrum or the brain. [EU]

Cerebral hemispheres: The two halves of the cerebrum, the part of the brain that controls muscle functions of the body and also controls speech, emotions, reading, writing, and learning. The right hemisphere controls muscle movement on the left side of the body, and the left hemisphere controls muscle movement on the right side of the body. [NIH]

Cerebral Infarction: The formation of an area of necrosis in the cerebrum caused by an insufficiency of arterial or venous blood flow. Infarcts of the cerebrum are generally classified by hemisphere (i.e., left vs. right), lobe (e.g., frontal lobe infarction), arterial distribution (e.g., infarction, anterior cerebral artery), and etiology (e.g., embolic infarction). [NIH]

Cerebrospinal: Pertaining to the brain and spinal cord. [EU]

Cerebrospinal fluid: CSF. The fluid flowing around the brain and spinal cord. Cerebrospinal fluid is produced in the ventricles in the brain. [NIH]

Cerebrovascular: Pertaining to the blood vessels of the cerebrum, or brain. [EU]

Cerebrovascular Disorders: A broad category of disorders characterized by impairment of blood flow in the arteries and veins which supply the brain. These include cerebral infarction; brain ischemia; hypoxia, brain; intracranial embolism and thrombosis; intracranial arteriovenous malformations; and vasculitis, central nervous system. In common usage, the term cerebrovascular disorders is not limited to conditions that affect the cerebrum, but refers to vascular disorders of the entire brain including the diencephalon; brain stem; and cerebellum. [NIH]

Cerebrum: The largest part of the brain. It is divided into two hemispheres, or halves, called the cerebral hemispheres. The cerebrum controls muscle functions of the body and also controls speech, emotions, reading, writing, and learning. [NIH]

Character: In current usage, approximately equivalent to personality. The sum of the relatively fixed personality traits and habitual modes of response of an individual. [NIH]

Chemotactic Factors: Chemical substances that attract or repel cells or organisms. The concept denotes especially those factors released as a result of tissue injury, invasion, or immunologic activity, that attract leukocytes, macrophages, or other cells to the site of infection or insult. [NIH]

Chemotherapy: Treatment with anticancer drugs. [NIH]

Chlorine: A greenish-yellow, diatomic gas that is a member of the halogen family of elements. It has the atomic symbol Cl, atomic number 17, and atomic weight 70.906. It is a powerful irritant that can cause fatal pulmonary edema. Chlorine is used in manufacturing, as a reagent in synthetic chemistry, for water purification, and in the production of chlorinated lime, which is used in fabric bleaching. [NIH]

Cholesterol: The principal sterol of all higher animals, distributed in body tissues, especially the brain and spinal cord, and in animal fats and oils. [NIH]

Cholesterol Esters: Fatty acid esters of cholesterol which constitute about two-thirds of the cholesterol in the plasma. The accumulation of cholesterol esters in the arterial intima is a characteristic feature of atherosclerosis. [NIH]

Chromaffin System: The cells of the body which stain with chromium salts. They occur along the sympathetic nerves, in the adrenal gland, and in various other organs. [NIH]

Chromatin: The material of chromosomes. It is a complex of DNA, histones, and nonhistone proteins (chromosomal proteins, non-histone) found within the nucleus of a cell. [NIH]

Chromium: A trace element that plays a role in glucose metabolism. It has the atomic symbol Cr, atomic number 24, and atomic weight 52. According to the Fourth Annual Report on Carcinogens (NTP85-002,1985), chromium and some of its compounds have been listed as known carcinogens. [NIH]

Chromosome: Part of a cell that contains genetic information. Except for sperm and eggs, all human cells contain 46 chromosomes. [NIH]

Chronic: A disease or condition that persists or progresses over a long period of time. [NIH]

Chronic Disease: Disease or ailment of long duration. [NIH]

Chronic prostatitis: Inflammation of the prostate gland, developing slowly and lasting a long time. [NIH]

Chronic renal: Slow and progressive loss of kidney function over several years, often resulting in end-stage renal disease. People with end-stage renal disease need dialysis or transplantation to replace the work of the kidneys. [NIH]

Chylomicrons: A class of lipoproteins that carry dietary cholesterol and triglycerides from the small intestines to the tissues. [NIH]

Cimetidine: A histamine congener, it competitively inhibits histamine binding to H2 receptors. Cimetidine has a range of pharmacological actions. It inhibits gastric acid secretion, as well as pepsin and gastrin output. It also blocks the activity of cytochrome P-450. [NIH]

Cinchona: A genus of rubiaceous South American trees that yields the toxic cinchona alkaloids from their bark; quinine, quinidine, chinconine, cinchonidine and others are used to treat malaria and cardiac arrhythmias. [NIH]

Circulatory system: The system that contains the heart and the blood vessels and moves blood throughout the body. This system helps tissues get enough oxygen and nutrients, and it helps them get rid of waste products. The lymph system, which connects with the blood system, is often considered part of the circulatory system. [NIH]

Circumcision: Excision of the prepuce or part of it. [NIH]

CIS: Cancer Information Service. The CIS is the National Cancer Institute's link to the public, interpreting and explaining research findings in a clear and understandable manner, and providing personalized responses to specific questions about cancer. Access the CIS by calling 1-800-4-CANCER, or by using the Web site at http://cis.nci.nih.gov. [NIH]

Clamp: A u-shaped steel rod used with a pin or wire for skeletal traction in the treatment of certain fractures. [NIH]

Claudication: Limping or lameness. [EU]

Clinical study: A research study in which patients receive treatment in a clinic or other medical facility. Reports of clinical studies can contain results for single patients (case reports) or many patients (case series or clinical trials). [NIH]

Clinical trial: A research study that tests how well new medical treatments or other interventions work in people. Each study is designed to test new methods of screening, prevention, diagnosis, or treatment of a disease. [NIH]

Cloning: The production of a number of genetically identical individuals; in genetic engineering, a process for the efficient replication of a great number of identical DNA molecules. [NIH]

Coagulation: 1. The process of clot formation. 2. In colloid chemistry, the solidification of a sol into a gelatinous mass; an alteration of a disperse phase or of a dissolved solid which causes the separation of the system into a liquid phase and an insoluble mass called the clot or curd. Coagulation is usually irreversible. 3. In surgery, the disruption of tissue by physical means to form an amorphous residuum, as in electrocoagulation and photocoagulation. [EU]

Cobalt: A trace element that is a component of vitamin B12. It has the atomic symbol Co, atomic number 27, and atomic weight 58.93. It is used in nuclear weapons, alloys, and pigments. Deficiency in animals leads to anemia; its excess in humans can lead to erythrocytosis. [NIH]

Cochlear: Of or pertaining to the cochlea. [EU]

Cochlear Diseases: Diseases of the cochlea, the part of the inner ear that is concerned with hearing. [NIH]

Coenzyme: An organic nonprotein molecule, frequently a phosphorylated derivative of a water-soluble vitamin, that binds with the protein molecule (apoenzyme) to form the active enzyme (holoenzyme). [EU]

Cofactor: A substance, microorganism or environmental factor that activates or enhances the action of another entity such as a disease-causing agent. [NIH]

Coitus: Sexual intercourse. [NIH]

Colitis: Inflammation of the colon. [NIH]

Collagen: A polypeptide substance comprising about one third of the total protein in mammalian organisms. It is the main constituent of skin, connective tissue, and the organic substance of bones and teeth. Different forms of collagen are produced in the body but all consist of three alpha-polypeptide chains arranged in a triple helix. Collagen is differentiated from other fibrous proteins, such as elastin, by the content of proline, hydroxyproline, and hydroxylysine; by the absence of tryptophan; and particularly by the high content of polar groups which are responsible for its swelling properties. [NIH]

Collapse: 1. A state of extreme prostration and depression, with failure of circulation. 2. Abnormal falling in of the walls of any part of organ. [EU]

Combination Therapy: Association of 3 drugs to treat AIDS (AZT + DDC or DDI + protease inhibitor). [NIH]

Combinatorial: A cut-and-paste process that churns out thousands of potentially valuable compounds at once. [NIH]

Complement: A term originally used to refer to the heat-labile factor in serum that causes immune cytolysis, the lysis of antibody-coated cells, and now referring to the entire functionally related system comprising at least 20 distinct serum proteins that is the effector not only of immune cytolysis but also of other biologic functions. Complement activation occurs by two different sequences, the classic and alternative pathways. The proteins of the classic pathway are termed 'components of complement' and are designated by the symbols C1 through C9. C1 is a calcium-dependent complex of three distinct proteins C1q, C1r and C1s. The proteins of the alternative pathway (collectively referred to as the properdin system) and complement regulatory proteins are known by semisystematic or trivial names. Fragments resulting from proteolytic cleavage of complement proteins are designated with lower-case letter suffixes, e.g., C3a. Inactivated fragments may be designated with the suffix 'i', e.g. C3bi. Activated components or complexes with biological activity are designated by a bar over the symbol e.g. C1 or C4b,2a. The classic pathway is activated by the binding of C1 to classic pathway activators, primarily antigen-antibody complexes containing IgM, IgG1, IgG3; C1q binds to a single IgM molecule or two adjacent IgG molecules. The alternative pathway can be activated by IgA immune complexes and also by nonimmunologic materials including bacterial endotoxins, microbial polysaccharides, and cell walls. Activation of the classic pathway triggers an enzymatic cascade involving C1, C4, C2 and C3; activation of the alternative pathway triggers a cascade involving C3 and factors B, D and P. Both result in the cleavage of C5 and the formation of the membrane attack complex. Complement activation also results in the formation of many biologically active complement fragments that act as anaphylatoxins, opsonins, or chemotactic factors. [EU]

Complementary and alternative medicine: CAM. Forms of treatment that are used in addition to (complementary) or instead of (alternative) standard treatments. These practices are not considered standard medical approaches. CAM includes dietary supplements, megadose vitamins, herbal preparations, special teas, massage therapy, magnet therapy, spiritual healing, and meditation. [NIH]

Complementary medicine: Practices not generally recognized by the medical community as standard or conventional medical approaches and used to enhance or complement the standard treatments. Complementary medicine includes the taking of dietary supplements, megadose vitamins, and herbal preparations; the drinking of special teas; and practices such as massage therapy, magnet therapy, spiritual healing, and meditation. [NIH]

Complementation: The production of a wild-type phenotype when two different mutations are combined in a diploid or a heterokaryon and tested in trans-configuration. [NIH]

Comprehensive Health Care: Providing for the full range of personal health services for diagnosis, treatment, follow-up and rehabilitation of patients. [NIH]

Computational Biology: A field of biology concerned with the development of techniques for the collection and manipulation of biological data, and the use of such data to make biological discoveries or predictions. This field encompasses all computational methods and theories applicable to molecular biology and areas of computer-based techniques for solving biological problems including manipulation of models and datasets. [NIH]

Computed tomography: CT scan. A series of detailed pictures of areas inside the body, taken from different angles; the pictures are created by a computer linked to an x-ray machine. Also called computerized tomography and computerized axial tomography (CAT) scan. [NIH]

Computerized axial tomography: A series of detailed pictures of areas inside the body, taken from different angles; the pictures are created by a computer linked to an x-ray machine. Also called CAT scan, computed tomography (CT scan), or computerized tomography. [NIH]

Computerized tomography: A series of detailed pictures of areas inside the body, taken from different angles; the pictures are created by a computer linked to an x-ray machine. Also called computerized axial tomography (CAT) scan and computed tomography (CT scan). [NIH]

Concomitant: Accompanying; accessory; joined with another. [EU]

Cone: One of the special retinal receptor elements which are presumed to be primarily concerned with perception of light and color stimuli when the eye is adapted to light. [NIH]

Confounding: Extraneous variables resulting in outcome effects that obscure or exaggerate the "true" effect of an intervention. [NIH]

Confusion: A mental state characterized by bewilderment, emotional disturbance, lack of clear thinking, and perceptual disorientation. [NIH]

Congenita: Displacement, subluxation, or malposition of the crystalline lens. [NIH]

Congestion: Excessive or abnormal accumulation of blood in a part. [EU]

Congestive heart failure: Weakness of the heart muscle that leads to a buildup of fluid in body tissues. [NIH]

Conjugated: Acting or operating as if joined; simultaneous. [EU]

Conjugation: 1. The act of joining together or the state of being conjugated. 2. A sexual process seen in bacteria, ciliate protozoa, and certain fungi in which nuclear material is exchanged during the temporary fusion of two cells (conjugants). In bacterial genetics a form of sexual reproduction in which a donor bacterium (male) contributes some, or all, of its DNA (in the form of a replicated set) to a recipient (female) which then incorporates differing genetic information into its own chromosome by recombination and passes the recombined set on to its progeny by replication. In ciliate protozoa, two conjugants of separate mating types exchange micronuclear material and then separate, each now being a fertilized cell. In certain fungi, the process involves fusion of two gametes, resulting in union of their nuclei and formation of a zygote. 3. In chemistry, the joining together of two compounds to produce another compound, such as the combination of a toxic product with some substance in the body to form a detoxified product, which is then eliminated. [EU]

Connective Tissue: Tissue that supports and binds other tissues. It consists of connective tissue cells embedded in a large amount of extracellular matrix. [NIH]

Connective Tissue: Tissue that supports and binds other tissues. It consists of connective tissue cells embedded in a large amount of extracellular matrix. [NIH]

Connective Tissue Cells: A group of cells that includes fibroblasts, cartilage cells, adipocytes, smooth muscle cells, and bone cells. [NIH]

Connexins: A group of homologous proteins which form the intermembrane channels of gap junctions. The connexins are the products of an identified gene family which has both highly conserved and highly divergent regions. The variety contributes to the wide range of functional properties of gap junctions. [NIH]

Consciousness: Sense of awareness of self and of the environment. [NIH]

Constipation: Infrequent or difficult evacuation of feces. [NIH]

Constriction: The act of constricting. [NIH]

Constriction, Pathologic: The condition of an anatomical structure's being constricted beyond normal dimensions. [NIH]

Consumption: Pulmonary tuberculosis. [NIH]

Continence: The ability to hold in a bowel movement or urine. [NIH]

Contractility: Capacity for becoming short in response to a suitable stimulus. [EU]

Contracture: A condition of fixed high resistance to passive stretch of a muscle, resulting from fibrosis of the tissues supporting the muscles or the joints, or from disorders of the muscle fibres. [EU]

Contraindications: Any factor or sign that it is unwise to pursue a certain kind of action or treatment, e. g. giving a general anesthetic to a person with pneumonia. [NIH]

Control group: In a clinical trial, the group that does not receive the new treatment being studied. This group is compared to the group that receives the new treatment, to see if the new treatment works. [NIH]

Controlled clinical trial: A clinical study that includes a comparison (control) group. The comparison group receives a placebo, another treatment, or no treatment at all. [NIH]

Controlled study: An experiment or clinical trial that includes a comparison (control) group. [NIH]

Coordination: Muscular or motor regulation or the harmonious cooperation of muscles or groups of muscles, in a complex action or series of actions. [NIH]

Cornea: The transparent part of the eye that covers the iris and the pupil and allows light to enter the inside. [NIH]

Coronary: Encircling in the manner of a crown; a term applied to vessels; nerves, ligaments, etc. The term usually denotes the arteries that supply the heart muscle and, by extension, a pathologic involvement of them. [EU]

Coronary Circulation: The circulation of blood through the coronary vessels of the heart. [NIH]

Coronary heart disease: A type of heart disease caused by narrowing of the coronary arteries that feed the heart, which needs a constant supply of oxygen and nutrients carried by the blood in the coronary arteries. When the coronary arteries become narrowed or clogged by fat and cholesterol deposits and cannot supply enough blood to the heart, CHD results. [NIH]

Coronary Thrombosis: Presence of a thrombus in a coronary artery, often causing a myocardial infarction. [NIH]

Corpus: The body of the uterus. [NIH]

Corpus Luteum: The yellow glandular mass formed in the ovary by an ovarian follicle that has ruptured and discharged its ovum [NIH]

Cortex: The outer layer of an organ or other body structure, as distinguished from the internal substance. [EU]

Corticosteroids: Hormones that have antitumor activity in lymphomas and lymphoid leukemias; in addition, corticosteroids (steroids) may be used for hormone replacement and for the management of some of the complications of cancer and its treatment. [NIH]

Cortisol: A steroid hormone secreted by the adrenal cortex as part of the body's response to stress. [NIH]

Cost Savings: Reductions in all or any portion of the costs of providing goods or services. Savings may be incurred by the provider or the consumer. [NIH]

Cranial: Pertaining to the cranium, or to the anterior (in animals) or superior (in humans) end of the body. [EU]

Craniocerebral Trauma: Traumatic injuries involving the cranium and intracranial structures (i.e., brain; cranial nerves; meninges; and other structures). Injuries may be classified by whether or not the skull is penetrated (i.e., penetrating vs. nonpenetrating) or whether there is an associated hemorrhage. [NIH]

Croton Oil: Viscous, nauseating oil obtained from the shrub Croton tiglium (Euphorbaceae). It is a vesicant and skin irritant used as pharmacologic standard for skin inflammation and allergy and causes skin cancer. It was formerly used as an emetic and cathartic with frequent mortality. [NIH]

Cryptorchidism: A condition in which one or both testicles fail to move from the abdomen, where they develop before birth, into the scrotum. Cryptorchidism may increase the risk for development of testicular cancer. Also called undescended testicles. [NIH]

Curative: Tending to overcome disease and promote recovery. [EU]

Cutaneous: Having to do with the skin. [NIH]

Cyclic: Pertaining to or occurring in a cycle or cycles; the term is applied to chemical compounds that contain a ring of atoms in the nucleus. [EU]

Cyclosporine: A drug used to help reduce the risk of rejection of organ and bone marrow transplants by the body. It is also used in clinical trials to make cancer cells more sensitive to anticancer drugs. [NIH]

Cystine: A covalently linked dimeric nonessential amino acid formed by the oxidation of cysteine. Two molecules of cysteine are joined together by a disulfide bridge to form cystine. [NIH]

Cystitis: Inflammation of the urinary bladder. [EU]

Cytochrome: Any electron transfer hemoprotein having a mode of action in which the transfer of a single electron is effected by a reversible valence change of the central iron atom of the heme prosthetic group between the +2 and +3 oxidation states; classified as cytochromes a in which the heme contains a formyl side chain, cytochromes b, which contain protoheme or a closely similar heme that is not covalently bound to the protein, cytochromes c in which protoheme or other heme is covalently bound to the protein, and cytochromes d in which the iron-tetrapyrrole has fewer conjugated double bonds than the hemes have. Well-known cytochromes have been numbered consecutively within groups and are designated by subscripts (beginning with no subscript), e.g. cytochromes c, c1, C2, . New cytochromes are named according to the wavelength in nanometres of the absorption maximum of the a-band of the iron (II) form in pyridine, e.g., c-555. [EU]

Cytokine: Small but highly potent protein that modulates the activity of many cell types, including T and B cells. [NIH]

Cytokinesis: Division of the rest of cell. [NIH]

Cytoplasm: The protoplasm of a cell exclusive of that of the nucleus; it consists of a continuous aqueous solution (cytosol) and the organelles and inclusions suspended in it (phaneroplasm), and is the site of most of the chemical activities of the cell. [EU]

Cytoskeleton: The network of filaments, tubules, and interconnecting filamentous bridges which give shape, structure, and organization to the cytoplasm. [NIH]

Cytotoxic: Cell-killing. [NIH]

Cytotoxicity: Quality of being capable of producing a specific toxic action upon cells of special organs. [NIH]

Data Collection: Systematic gathering of data for a particular purpose from various sources, including questionnaires, interviews, observation, existing records, and electronic devices. The process is usually preliminary to statistical analysis of the data. [NIH]

Databases, Bibliographic: Extensive collections, reputedly complete, of references and citations to books, articles, publications, etc., generally on a single subject or specialized subject area. Databases can operate through automated files, libraries, or computer disks. The concept should be differentiated from factual databases which is used for collections of data and facts apart from bibliographic references to them. [NIH]

Deamination: The removal of an amino group (NH2) from a chemical compound. [NIH]

Decidua: The epithelial lining of the endometrium that is formed before the fertilized ovum reaches the uterus. The fertilized ovum embeds in the decidua. If the ovum is not fertilized, the decidua is shed during menstruation. [NIH]

Decision Making: The process of making a selective intellectual judgment when presented with several complex alternatives consisting of several variables, and usually defining a course of action or an idea. [NIH]

Decubitus: An act of lying down; also the position assumed in lying down. [EU]

Decubitus Ulcer: An ulceration caused by prolonged pressure in patients permitted to lie too still for a long period of time. The bony prominences of the body are the most frequently affected sites. The ulcer is caused by ischemia of the underlying structures of the skin, fat, and muscles as a result of the sustained and constant pressure. [NIH]

Degenerative: Undergoing degeneration : tending to degenerate; having the character of or involving degeneration; causing or tending to cause degeneration. [EU]

Dehydroepiandrosterone: DHEA. A substance that is being studied as a cancer prevention drug. It belongs to the family of drugs called steroids. [NIH]

Deletion: A genetic rearrangement through loss of segments of DNA (chromosomes), bringing sequences, which are normally separated, into close proximity. [NIH]

Dementia: An acquired organic mental disorder with loss of intellectual abilities of sufficient severity to interfere with social or occupational functioning. The dysfunction is multifaceted and involves memory, behavior, personality, judgment, attention, spatial relations, language, abstract thought, and other executive functions. The intellectual decline is usually progressive, and initially spares the level of consciousness. [NIH]

Dendrites: Extensions of the nerve cell body. They are short and branched and receive stimuli from other neurons. [NIH]

Dendritic: 1. Branched like a tree. 2. Pertaining to or possessing dendrites. [EU]

Density: The logarithm to the base 10 of the opacity of an exposed and processed film. [NIH]

Depersonalization: Alteration in the perception of the self so that the usual sense of one's own reality is lost, manifested in a sense of unreality or self-estrangement, in changes of body image, or in a feeling that one does not control his own actions and speech; seen in depersonalization disorder, schizophrenic disorders, and schizotypal personality disorder. Some do not draw a distinction between depersonalization and derealization, using depersonalization to include both. [EU]

Depolarization: The process or act of neutralizing polarity. In neurophysiology, the reversal of the resting potential in excitable cell membranes when stimulated, i.e., the tendency of the cell membrane potential to become positive with respect to the potential outside the cell. [EU]

Derealization: Is characterized by the loss of the sense of reality concerning one's surroundings. [NIH]

Dermal: Pertaining to or coming from the skin. [NIH]

Designer Drugs: Drugs designed and synthesized, often for illegal street use, by modification of existing drug structures (e.g., amphetamines). Of special interest are MPTP (a reverse ester of meperidine), MDA (3,4-methylenedioxyamphetamine), and MDMA (3,4-methylenedioxymethamphetamine). Many drugs act on the aminergic system, the physiologically active biogenic amines. [NIH]

Detergents: Purifying or cleansing agents, usually salts of long-chain aliphatic bases or acids, that exert cleansing (oil-dissolving) and antimicrobial effects through a surface action that depends on possessing both hydrophilic and hydrophobic properties. [NIH]

Deuterium: Deuterium. The stable isotope of hydrogen. It has one neutron and one proton in the nucleus. [NIH]

DHEA: Dehydroepiandrosterone. A substance that is being studied as a cancer prevention drug. It belongs to the family of drugs called steroids. [NIH]

Diabetes Mellitus: A heterogeneous group of disorders that share glucose intolerance in common. [NIH]

Diabetes, Gestational: Either symptomatic diabetes or impaired glucose tolerance induced by pregnancy but resolved at the end of pregnancy. It does not include previously diagnosed diabetics who become pregnant (pregnancy in diabetics). [NIH]

Diabetic Ketoacidosis: Complication of diabetes resulting from severe insulin deficiency coupled with an absolute or relative increase in glucagon concentration. The metabolic acidosis is caused by the breakdown of adipose stores and resulting increased levels of free fatty acids. Glucagon accelerates the oxidation of the free fatty acids producing excess ketone bodies (ketosis). [NIH]

Diabetic Retinopathy: Retinopathy associated with diabetes mellitus, which may be of the background type, progressively characterized by microaneurysms, interretinal punctuate macular edema, or of the proliferative type, characterized by neovascularization of the retina and optic disk, which may project into the vitreous, proliferation of fibrous tissue, vitreous hemorrhage, and retinal detachment. [NIH]

Diagnostic procedure: A method used to identify a disease. [NIH]

Dialyzer: A part of the hemodialysis machine. (See hemodialysis under dialysis.) The dialyzer has two sections separated by a membrane. One section holds dialysate. The other holds the patient's blood. [NIH]

Diarrhea: Passage of excessively liquid or excessively frequent stools. [NIH]

Diastolic: Of or pertaining to the diastole. [EU]

Diencephalon: The paired caudal parts of the prosencephalon from which the thalamus, hypothalamus, epithalamus, and subthalamus are derived. [NIH]

Diffusion: The tendency of a gas or solute to pass from a point of higher pressure or concentration to a point of lower pressure or concentration and to distribute itself throughout the available space; a major mechanism of biological transport. [NIH]

Digestion: The process of breakdown of food for metabolism and use by the body. [NIH]

Digestive system: The organs that take in food and turn it into products that the body can use to stay healthy. Waste products the body cannot use leave the body through bowel movements. The digestive system includes the salivary glands, mouth, esophagus, stomach, liver, pancreas, gallbladder, small and large intestines, and rectum. [NIH]

Digestive tract: The organs through which food passes when food is eaten. These organs are the mouth, esophagus, stomach, small and large intestines, and rectum. [NIH]

Dihydrotestosterone: Anabolic agent. [NIH]

Dilatation: The act of dilating. [NIH]

Dilatation, Pathologic: The condition of an anatomical structure's being dilated beyond normal dimensions. [NIH]

Dilation: A process by which the pupil is temporarily enlarged with special eye drops (mydriatic); allows the eye care specialist to better view the inside of the eye. [NIH]

Dilator: A device used to stretch or enlarge an opening. [NIH]

Dimethyl: A volatile metabolite of the amino acid methionine. [NIH]

Diploid: Having two sets of chromosomes. [NIH]

Direct: 1. Straight; in a straight line. 2. Performed immediately and without the intervention of subsidiary means. [EU]

Discrimination: The act of qualitative and/or quantitative differentiation between two or more stimuli. [NIH]

Dissociation: 1. The act of separating or state of being separated. 2. The separation of a molecule into two or more fragments (atoms, molecules, ions, or free radicals) produced by the absorption of light or thermal energy or by solvation. 3. In psychology, a defense mechanism in which a group of mental processes are segregated from the rest of a person's mental activity in order to avoid emotional distress, as in the dissociative disorders (q.v.), or in which an idea or object is segregated from its emotional significance; in the first sense it is roughly equivalent to splitting, in the second, to isolation. 4. A defect of mental integration in which one or more groups of mental processes become separated off from normal consciousness and, thus separated, function as a unitary whole. [EU]

Distal: Remote; farther from any point of reference; opposed to proximal. In dentistry, used to designate a position on the dental arch farther from the median line of the jaw. [EU]

Diuresis: Increased excretion of urine. [EU]

Diuretic: A drug that increases the production of urine. [NIH]

Dizziness: An imprecise term which may refer to a sense of spatial disorientation, motion of the environment, or lightheadedness. [NIH]

Dopamine: An endogenous catecholamine and prominent neurotransmitter in several systems of the brain. In the synthesis of catecholamines from tyrosine, it is the immediate precursor to norepinephrine and epinephrine. Dopamine is a major transmitter in the extrapyramidal system of the brain, and important in regulating movement. A family of dopaminergic receptor subtypes mediate its action. Dopamine is used pharmacologically for its direct (beta adrenergic agonist) and indirect (adrenergic releasing) sympathomimetic effects including its actions as an inotropic agent and as a renal vasodilator. [NIH]

Dorsal: 1. Pertaining to the back or to any dorsum. 2. Denoting a position more toward the back surface than some other object of reference; same as posterior in human anatomy; superior in the anatomy of quadrupeds. [EU]

Dorsum: A plate of bone which forms the posterior boundary of the sella turcica. [NIH]

Dosage Forms: Completed forms of the pharmaceutical preparation in which prescribed doses of medication are included. They are designed to resist action by gastric fluids, prevent vomiting and nausea, reduce or alleviate the undesirable taste and smells associated with oral administration, achieve a high concentration of drug at target site, or produce a delayed or long-acting drug effect. They include capsules, liniments, ointments, pharmaceutical solutions, powders, tablets, etc. [NIH]

Drive: A state of internal activity of an organism that is a necessary condition before a given stimulus will elicit a class of responses; e.g., a certain level of hunger (drive) must be present before food will elicit an eating response. [NIH]

Drug Interactions: The action of a drug that may affect the activity, metabolism, or toxicity of another drug. [NIH]

Drug Tolerance: Progressive diminution of the susceptibility of a human or animal to the effects of a drug, resulting from its continued administration. It should be differentiated from drug resistance wherein an organism, disease, or tissue fails to respond to the intended effectiveness of a chemical or drug. It should also be differentiated from maximum tolerated dose and no-observed-adverse-effect level. [NIH]

Duct: A tube through which body fluids pass. [NIH]

Duke: A lamp which produces ultraviolet radiations for certain ophthalmologic therapy. [NIH]

Duodenum: The first part of the small intestine. [NIH]

Dyes: Chemical substances that are used to stain and color other materials. The coloring may or may not be permanent. Dyes can also be used as therapeutic agents and test reagents in medicine and scientific research. [NIH]

Dyslipidemia: Disorders in the lipoprotein metabolism; classified as hypercholesterolemia, hypertriglyceridemia, combined hyperlipidemia, and low levels of high-density lipoprotein (HDL) cholesterol. All of the dyslipidemias can be primary or secondary. Both elevated levels of low-density lipoprotein (LDL) cholesterol and low levels of HDL cholesterol predispose to premature atherosclerosis. [NIH]

Dysmenorrhea: Painful menstruation. [NIH]

Dyspepsia: Impaired digestion, especially after eating. [NIH]

Dysphagia: Difficulty in swallowing. [EU]

Dyspnea: Difficult or labored breathing. [NIH]

Dysprosium: Dysprosium. An element of the rare earth family that has the atomic symbol Dy, atomic number 66, and atomic weight 162.50. Dysprosium is a silvery metal used primarily in the form of various salts. [NIH]

Eating Disorders: A group of disorders characterized by physiological and psychological disturbances in appetite or food intake. [NIH]

Edema: Excessive amount of watery fluid accumulated in the intercellular spaces, most commonly present in subcutaneous tissue. [NIH]

Effector: It is often an enzyme that converts an inactive precursor molecule into an active second messenger. [NIH]

Effector cell: A cell that performs a specific function in response to a stimulus; usually used to describe cells in the immune system. [NIH]

Efficacy: The extent to which a specific intervention, procedure, regimen, or service produces a beneficial result under ideal conditions. Ideally, the determination of efficacy is based on the results of a randomized control trial. [NIH]

Ejaculation: The release of semen through the penis during orgasm. [NIH]

Elasticity: Resistance and recovery from distortion of shape. [NIH]

Elastin: The protein that gives flexibility to tissues. [NIH]

Elective: Subject to the choice or decision of the patient or physician; applied to procedures that are advantageous to the patient but not urgent. [EU]

Electrolyte: A substance that dissociates into ions when fused or in solution, and thus becomes capable of conducting electricity; an ionic solute. [EU]

Electrons: Stable elementary particles having the smallest known negative charge, present in all elements; also called negatrons. Positively charged electrons are called positrons. The numbers, energies and arrangement of electrons around atomic nuclei determine the chemical identities of elements. Beams of electrons are called cathode rays or beta rays, the latter being a high-energy biproduct of nuclear decay. [NIH]

Electrophysiological: Pertaining to electrophysiology, that is a branch of physiology that is concerned with the electric phenomena associated with living bodies and involved in their functional activity. [EU]

Elementary Particles: Individual components of atoms, usually subatomic; subnuclear particles are usually detected only when the atomic nucleus decays and then only transiently, as most of them are unstable, often yielding pure energy without substance, i.e., radiation. [NIH]

Embryo: The prenatal stage of mammalian development characterized by rapid morphological changes and the differentiation of basic structures. [NIH]

Embryogenesis: The process of embryo or embryoid formation, whether by sexual (zygotic) or asexual means. In asexual embryogenesis embryoids arise directly from the explant or on intermediary callus tissue. In some cases they arise from individual cells (somatic cell embryoge). [NIH]

Emetic: An agent that causes vomiting. [EU]

Encapsulated: Confined to a specific, localized area and surrounded by a thin layer of tissue. [NIH]

Endarterectomy: Surgical excision, performed under general anesthesia, of the atheromatous tunica intima of an artery. When reconstruction of an artery is performed as an endovascular procedure through a catheter, it is called atherectomy. [NIH]

Endocrine Glands: Ductless glands that secrete substances which are released directly into the circulation and which influence metabolism and other body functions. [NIH]

Endocrine System: The system of glands that release their secretions (hormones) directly into the circulatory system. In addition to the endocrine glands, included are the chromaffin system and the neurosecretory systems. [NIH]

Endocrinologist: A doctor that specializes in diagnosing and treating hormone disorders. [NIH]

Endocrinology: A subspecialty of internal medicine concerned with the metabolism, physiology, and disorders of the endocrine system. [NIH]

Endoscope: A thin, lighted tube used to look at tissues inside the body. [NIH]

Endoscopic: A technique where a lateral-view endoscope is passed orally to the duodenum for visualization of the ampulla of Vater. [NIH]

Endothelial cell: The main type of cell found in the inside lining of blood vessels, lymph vessels, and the heart. [NIH]

Endothelium: A layer of epithelium that lines the heart, blood vessels (endothelium, vascular), lymph vessels (endothelium, lymphatic), and the serous cavities of the body. [NIH]

Endothelium, Lymphatic: Unbroken cellular lining (intima) of the lymph vessels (e.g., the high endothelial lymphatic venules). It is more permeable than vascular endothelium, lacking selective absorption and functioning mainly to remove plasma proteins that have filtered through the capillaries into the tissue spaces. [NIH]

Endothelium, Vascular: Single pavement layer of cells which line the luminal surface of the entire vascular system and regulate the transport of macromolecules and blood components from interstitium to lumen; this function has been most intensively studied in the blood capillaries. [NIH]

Endothelium-derived: Small molecule that diffuses to the adjacent muscle layer and relaxes it. [NIH]

Endotoxic: Of, relating to, or acting as an endotoxin (= a heat-stable toxin, associated with the outer membranes of certain gram-negative bacteria. Endotoxins are not secreted and are released only when the cells are disrupted). [EU]

Endotoxin: Toxin from cell walls of bacteria. [NIH]

End-stage renal: Total chronic kidney failure. When the kidneys fail, the body retains fluid and harmful wastes build up. A person with ESRD needs treatment to replace the work of the failed kidneys. [NIH]

Enhancer: Transcriptional element in the virus genome. [NIH]

Enterotoxins: Substances that are toxic to the intestinal tract causing vomiting, diarrhea, etc.; most common enterotoxins are produced by bacteria. [NIH]

Enuresis: Involuntary discharge of urine after the age at which urinary control should have been achieved; often used alone with specific reference to involuntary discharge of urine occurring during sleep at night (bed-wetting, nocturnal enuresis). [EU]

Environmental Health: The science of controlling or modifying those conditions, influences, or forces surrounding man which relate to promoting, establishing, and maintaining health. [NIH]

Enzymatic: Phase where enzyme cuts the precursor protein. [NIH]

Enzyme: A protein that speeds up chemical reactions in the body. [NIH]

Enzyme Inhibitors: Compounds or agents that combine with an enzyme in such a manner as to prevent the normal substrate-enzyme combination and the catalytic reaction. [NIH]

Eosinophils: Granular leukocytes with a nucleus that usually has two lobes connected by a slender thread of chromatin, and cytoplasm containing coarse, round granules that are uniform in size and stainable by eosin. [NIH]

Epidemiological: Relating to, or involving epidemiology. [EU]

Epigastric: Having to do with the upper middle area of the abdomen. [NIH]

Epinephrine: The active sympathomimetic hormone from the adrenal medulla in most species. It stimulates both the alpha- and beta- adrenergic systems, causes systemic vasoconstriction and gastrointestinal relaxation, stimulates the heart, and dilates bronchi and cerebral vessels. It is used in asthma and cardiac failure and to delay absorption of local anesthetics. [NIH]

Epithelial: Refers to the cells that line the internal and external surfaces of the body. [NIH]

Epithelium: One or more layers of epithelial cells, supported by the basal lamina, which covers the inner or outer surfaces of the body. [NIH]

Erectile: The inability to get or maintain an erection for satisfactory sexual intercourse. Also called impotence. [NIH]

Erection: The condition of being made rigid and elevated; as erectile tissue when filled with blood. [EU]

Ergot: Cataract due to ergot poisoning caused by eating of rye cereals contaminated by a fungus. [NIH]

Erythrocytes: Red blood cells. Mature erythrocytes are non-nucleated, biconcave disks containing hemoglobin whose function is to transport oxygen. [NIH]

Erythromycin: A bacteriostatic antibiotic substance produced by Streptomyces erythreus. Erythromycin A is considered its major active component. In sensitive organisms, it inhibits protein synthesis by binding to 50S ribosomal subunits. This binding process inhibits peptidyl transferase activity and interferes with translocation of amino acids during translation and assembly of proteins. [NIH]

Erythropoietin: Glycoprotein hormone, secreted chiefly by the kidney in the adult and the liver in the fetus, that acts on erythroid stem cells of the bone marrow to stimulate proliferation and differentiation. [NIH]

Escalation: Progressive use of more harmful drugs. [NIH]

Esophageal: Having to do with the esophagus, the muscular tube through which food passes from the throat to the stomach. [NIH]

Esophageal Spasms: Muscle cramps in the esophagus that cause pain in the chest. [NIH]

Esophagus: The muscular tube through which food passes from the throat to the stomach. [NIH]

Estrogen: One of the two female sex hormones. [NIH]

Eukaryotic Cells: Cells of the higher organisms, containing a true nucleus bounded by a nuclear membrane. [NIH]

Evacuation: An emptying, as of the bowels. [EU]

Evoke: The electric response recorded from the cerebral cortex after stimulation of a peripheral sense organ. [NIH]

Excipient: Any more or less inert substance added to a prescription in order to confer a suitable consistency or form to the drug; a vehicle. [EU]

Excitation: An act of irritation or stimulation or of responding to a stimulus; the addition of energy, as the excitation of a molecule by absorption of photons. [EU]

Excrete: To get rid of waste from the body. [NIH]

Exocrine: Secreting outwardly, via a duct. [EU]

Exogenous: Developed or originating outside the organism, as exogenous disease. [EU]

Exon: The part of the DNA that encodes the information for the actual amino acid sequence of the protein. In many eucaryotic genes, the coding sequences consist of a series of exons alternating with intron sequences. [NIH]

External-beam radiation: Radiation therapy that uses a machine to aim high-energy rays at the cancer. Also called external radiation. [NIH]

Extracellular: Outside a cell or cells. [EU]

Extracellular Matrix: A meshwork-like substance found within the extracellular space and in association with the basement membrane of the cell surface. It promotes cellular proliferation and provides a supporting structure to which cells or cell lysates in culture dishes adhere. [NIH]

Extracorporeal: Situated or occurring outside the body. [EU]

Extrapyramidal: Outside of the pyramidal tracts. [EU]

Extremity: A limb; an arm or leg (membrum); sometimes applied specifically to a hand or foot. [EU]

Facial: Of or pertaining to the face. [EU]

Fallopian Tubes: Two long muscular tubes that transport ova from the ovaries to the uterus. They extend from the horn of the uterus to the ovaries and consist of an ampulla, an infundibulum, an isthmus, two ostia, and a pars uterina. The walls of the tubes are composed of three layers: mucosal, muscular, and serosal. [NIH]

Family Planning: Programs or services designed to assist the family in controlling reproduction by either improving or diminishing fertility. [NIH]

Family Relations: Behavioral, psychological, and social relations among various members of the nuclear family and the extended family. [NIH]

Fast Neutrons: Neutrons, the energy of which exceeds some arbitrary level, usually around one million electron volts. [NIH]

Fat: Total lipids including phospholipids. [NIH]

Fatigue: The state of weariness following a period of exertion, mental or physical, characterized by a decreased capacity for work and reduced efficiency to respond to stimuli. [NIH]

Fatty acids: A major component of fats that are used by the body for energy and tissue development. [NIH]

Fecal Incontinence: Failure of voluntary control of the anal sphincters, with involuntary passage of feces and flatus. [NIH]

Feces: The excrement discharged from the intestines, consisting of bacteria, cells exfoliated from the intestines, secretions, chiefly of the liver, and a small amount of food residue. [EU]

Femoral: Pertaining to the femur, or to the thigh. [EU]

Femoral Artery: The main artery of the thigh, a continuation of the external iliac artery. [NIH]

Femoral Vein: The vein accompanying the femoral artery in the same sheath; it is a continuation of the popliteal vein and becomes the external iliac vein. [NIH]

Femur: The longest and largest bone of the skeleton, it is situated between the hip and the knee. [NIH]

Fetus: The developing offspring from 7 to 8 weeks after conception until birth. [NIH]

Fibrin: A protein derived from fibrinogen in the presence of thrombin, which forms part of the blood clot. [NIH]

Fibroblast Growth Factor: Peptide isolated from the pituitary gland and from the brain. It is a potent mitogen which stimulates growth of a variety of mesodermal cells including chondrocytes, granulosa, and endothelial cells. The peptide may be active in wound healing and animal limb regeneration. [NIH]

Fibroblasts: Connective tissue cells which secrete an extracellular matrix rich in collagen and other macromolecules. [NIH]

Fibrosis: Any pathological condition where fibrous connective tissue invades any organ, usually as a consequence of inflammation or other injury. [NIH]

Finasteride: An orally active testosterone 5-alpha-reductase inhibitor. It is used as a surgical alternative for treatment of benign prostatic hyperplasia. [NIH]

Fistula: Abnormal communication most commonly seen between two internal organs, or between an internal organ and the surface of the body. [NIH]

Fixation: 1. The act or operation of holding, suturing, or fastening in a fixed position. 2. The condition of being held in a fixed position. 3. In psychiatry, a term with two related but distinct meanings : (1) arrest of development at a particular stage, which like regression (return to an earlier stage), if temporary is a normal reaction to setbacks and difficulties but if protracted or frequent is a cause of developmental failures and emotional problems, and (2) a close and suffocating attachment to another person, especially a childhood figure, such as one's mother or father. Both meanings are derived from psychoanalytic theory and refer to 'fixation' of libidinal energy either in a specific erogenous zone, hence fixation at the oral, anal, or phallic stage, or in a specific object, hence mother or father fixation. 4. The use of a fixative (q.v.) to preserve histological or cytological specimens. 5. In chemistry, the process whereby a substance is removed from the gaseous or solution phase and localized, as in carbon dioxide fixation or nitrogen fixation. 6. In ophthalmology, direction of the gaze so that the visual image of the object falls on the fovea centralis. 7. In film processing, the chemical removal of all undeveloped salts of the film emulsion, leaving only the developed silver to form a permanent image. [EU]

Flaccid: Weak, lax and soft. [EU]

Flatus: Gas passed through the rectum. [NIH]

Flushing: A transient reddening of the face that may be due to fever, certain drugs, exertion, stress, or a disease process. [NIH]

Folate: A B-complex vitamin that is being studied as a cancer prevention agent. Also called folic acid. [NIH]

Fold: A plication or doubling of various parts of the body. [NIH]

Folic Acid: N-(4-(((2-Amino-1,4-dihydro-4-oxo-6-pteridinyl)methyl)amino)benzoyl)-L-glutamic acid. A member of the vitamin B family that stimulates the hematopoietic system. It is present in the liver and kidney and is found in mushrooms, spinach, yeast, green leaves, and grasses. Folic acid is used in the treatment and prevention of folate deficiencies and megaloblastic anemia. [NIH]

Foot Ulcer: Lesion on the surface of the skin of the foot, usually accompanied by inflammation. The lesion may become infected or necrotic and is frequently associated with diabetes or leprosy. [NIH]

Forearm: The part between the elbow and the wrist. [NIH]

Fossa: A cavity, depression, or pit. [NIH]

Frostbite: Damage to tissues as the result of low environmental temperatures. [NIH]

Fructose: A type of sugar found in many fruits and vegetables and in honey. Fructose is used to sweeten some diet foods. It is considered a nutritive sweetener because it has calories. [NIH]

Functional Disorders: Disorders such as irritable bowel syndrome. These conditions result from poor nerve and muscle function. Symptoms such as gas, pain, constipation, and diarrhea come back again and again, but there are no signs of disease or damage. Emotional stress can trigger symptoms. Also called motility disorders. [NIH]

Fungi: A kingdom of eukaryotic, heterotrophic organisms that live as saprobes or parasites, including mushrooms, yeasts, smuts, molds, etc. They reproduce either sexually or asexually, and have life cycles that range from simple to complex. Filamentous fungi refer to those that grow as multicelluar colonies (mushrooms and molds). [NIH]

Fungistatic : Inhibiting the growth of fungi. [EU]

Gadolinium: An element of the rare earth family of metals. It has the atomic symbol Gd, atomic number 64, and atomic weight 157.25. Its oxide is used in the control rods of some nuclear reactors. [NIH]

Gallbladder: The pear-shaped organ that sits below the liver. Bile is concentrated and stored in the gallbladder. [NIH]

Gamma Rays: Very powerful and penetrating, high-energy electromagnetic radiation of shorter wavelength than that of x-rays. They are emitted by a decaying nucleus, usually between 0.01 and 10 MeV. They are also called nuclear x-rays. [NIH]

Ganglia: Clusters of multipolar neurons surrounded by a capsule of loosely organized connective tissue located outside the central nervous system. [NIH]

Ganglion: 1. A knot, or knotlike mass. 2. A general term for a group of nerve cell bodies located outside the central nervous system; occasionally applied to certain nuclear groups within the brain or spinal cord, e.g. basal ganglia. 3. A benign cystic tumour occurring on a aponeurosis or tendon, as in the wrist or dorsum of the foot; it consists of a thin fibrous capsule enclosing a clear mucinous fluid. [EU]

Gangrene: Death and putrefaction of tissue usually due to a loss of blood supply. [NIH]

Gap Junctions: Connections between cells which allow passage of small molecules and electric current. Gap junctions were first described anatomically as regions of close apposition between cells with a narrow (1-2 nm) gap between cell membranes. The variety in the properties of gap junctions is reflected in the number of connexins, the family of proteins which form the junctions. [NIH]

Gas: Air that comes from normal breakdown of food. The gases are passed out of the body through the rectum (flatus) or the mouth (burp). [NIH]

Gas exchange: Primary function of the lungs; transfer of oxygen from inhaled air into the blood and of carbon dioxide from the blood into the lungs. [NIH]

Gastric: Having to do with the stomach. [NIH]

Gastric Acid: Hydrochloric acid present in gastric juice. [NIH]

Gastric Emptying: The evacuation of food from the stomach into the duodenum. [NIH]

Gastrin: A hormone released after eating. Gastrin causes the stomach to produce more acid. [NIH]

Gastrointestinal: Refers to the stomach and intestines. [NIH]

Gastrointestinal tract: The stomach and intestines. [NIH]

Gastroparesis: Nerve or muscle damage in the stomach. Causes slow digestion and emptying, vomiting, nausea, or bloating. Also called delayed gastric emptying. [NIH]

Gelatin: A product formed from skin, white connective tissue, or bone collagen. It is used as a protein food adjuvant, plasma substitute, hemostatic, suspending agent in pharmaceutical preparations, and in the manufacturing of capsules and suppositories. [NIH]

Gene: The functional and physical unit of heredity passed from parent to offspring. Genes are pieces of DNA, and most genes contain the information for making a specific protein. [NIH]

Gene Expression: The phenotypic manifestation of a gene or genes by the processes of gene action. [NIH]

Genetic Code: The specifications for how information, stored in nucleic acid sequence (base sequence), is translated into protein sequence (amino acid sequence). The start, stop, and order of amino acids of a protein is specified by consecutive triplets of nucleotides called codons (codon). [NIH]

Genetic Counseling: Advising families of the risks involved pertaining to birth defects, in order that they may make an informed decision on current or future pregnancies. [NIH]

Genetics: The biological science that deals with the phenomena and mechanisms of heredity. [NIH]

Genital: Pertaining to the genitalia. [EU]

Genitourinary: Pertaining to the genital and urinary organs; urogenital; urinosexual. [EU]

Genotype: The genetic constitution of the individual; the characterization of the genes. [NIH]

Geriatric: Pertaining to the treatment of the aged. [EU]

Gestation: The period of development of the young in viviparous animals, from the time of fertilization of the ovum until birth. [EU]

Gestational: Psychosis attributable to or occurring during pregnancy. [NIH]

Ginseng: An araliaceous genus of plants that contains a number of pharmacologically active agents used as stimulants, sedatives, and tonics, especially in traditional medicine. [NIH]

Gland: An organ that produces and releases one or more substances for use in the body. Some glands produce fluids that affect tissues or organs. Others produce hormones or participate in blood production. [NIH]

Gliclazide: An oral sulfonylurea hypoglycemic agent which stimulates insulin secretion. [NIH]

Glipizide: An oral hypoglycemic agent which is rapidly absorbed and completely metabolized. [NIH]

Glomerular: Pertaining to or of the nature of a glomerulus, especially a renal glomerulus. [EU]

Glomeruli: Plural of glomerulus. [NIH]

Glomerulonephritis: Glomerular disease characterized by an inflammatory reaction, with leukocyte infiltration and cellular proliferation of the glomeruli, or that appears to be the result of immune glomerular injury. [NIH]

Glomerulosclerosis: Scarring of the glomeruli. It may result from diabetes mellitus (diabetic glomerulosclerosis) or from deposits in parts of the glomerulus (focal segmental glomerulosclerosis). The most common signs of glomerulosclerosis are proteinuria and kidney failure. [NIH]

Glomerulus: A tiny set of looping blood vessels in the nephron where blood is filtered in the kidney. [NIH]

Glucocorticoid: A compound that belongs to the family of compounds called corticosteroids (steroids). Glucocorticoids affect metabolism and have anti-inflammatory and immunosuppressive effects. They may be naturally produced (hormones) or synthetic (drugs). [NIH]

Glucose: D-Glucose. A primary source of energy for living organisms. It is naturally occurring and is found in fruits and other parts of plants in its free state. It is used therapeutically in fluid and nutrient replacement. [NIH]

Glucose Intolerance: A pathological state in which the fasting plasma glucose level is less than 140 mg per deciliter and the 30-, 60-, or 90-minute plasma glucose concentration following a glucose tolerance test exceeds 200 mg per deciliter. This condition is seen frequently in diabetes mellitus but also occurs with other diseases. [NIH]

Glucose tolerance: The power of the normal liver to absorb and store large quantities of glucose and the effectiveness of intestinal absorption of glucose. The glucose tolerance test is a metabolic test of carbohydrate tolerance that measures active insulin, a hepatic function based on the ability of the liver to absorb glucose. The test consists of ingesting 100 grams of glucose into a fasting stomach; blood sugar should return to normal in 2 to 21 hours after ingestion. [NIH]

Glucose Tolerance Test: Determination of whole blood or plasma sugar in a fasting state before and at prescribed intervals (usually 1/2 hr, 1 hr, 3 hr, 4 hr) after taking a specified amount (usually 100 gm orally) of glucose. [NIH]

Glucuronic Acid: Derivatives of uronic acid found throughout the plant and animal kingdoms. They detoxify drugs and toxins by conjugating with them to form glucuronides in the liver which are more water-soluble metabolites that can be easily eliminated from the body. [NIH]

Glutamic Acid: A non-essential amino acid naturally occurring in the L-form. Glutamic acid (glutamate) is the most common excitatory neurotransmitter in the central nervous system. [NIH]

Glyburide: An antidiabetic sulfonylurea derivative with actions similar to those of chlorpropamide. [NIH]

Glycine: A non-essential amino acid. It is found primarily in gelatin and silk fibroin and used therapeutically as a nutrient. It is also a fast inhibitory neurotransmitter. [NIH]

Glycosidic: Formed by elimination of water between the anomeric hydroxyl of one sugar and a hydroxyl of another sugar molecule. [NIH]

Gonad: A sex organ, such as an ovary or a testicle, which produces the gametes in most multicellular animals. [NIH]

Gonadal: Pertaining to a gonad. [EU]

Governing Board: The group in which legal authority is vested for the control of health-related institutions and organizations. [NIH]

Government Agencies: Administrative units of government responsible for policy making and management of governmental activities in the U.S. and abroad. [NIH]

Graft: Healthy skin, bone, or other tissue taken from one part of the body and used to replace diseased or injured tissue removed from another part of the body. [NIH]

Grafting: The operation of transfer of tissue from one site to another. [NIH]

Gram-negative: Losing the stain or decolorized by alcohol in Gram's method of staining, a primary characteristic of bacteria having a cell wall composed of a thin layer of peptidoglycan covered by an outer membrane of lipoprotein and lipopolysaccharide. [EU]

Gram-Negative Bacteria: Bacteria which lose crystal violet stain but are stained pink when treated by Gram's method. [NIH]

Granulocytes: Leukocytes with abundant granules in the cytoplasm. They are divided into three groups: neutrophils, eosinophils, and basophils. [NIH]

Grasses: A large family, Gramineae, of narrow-leaved herbaceous monocots. Many grasses produce highly allergenic pollens and are hosts to cattle parasites and toxic fungi. [NIH]

Groin: The external junctural region between the lower part of the abdomen and the thigh. [NIH]

Growth: The progressive development of a living being or part of an organism from its earliest stage to maturity. [NIH]

Guanylate Cyclase: An enzyme that catalyzes the conversion of GTP to 3',5'-cyclic GMP and pyrophosphate. It also acts on ITP and dGTP. (From Enzyme Nomenclature, 1992) EC 4.6.1.2. [NIH]

Haematological: Relating to haematology, that is that branch of medical science which treats of the morphology of the blood and blood-forming tissues. [EU]

Haematology: The science of the blood, its nature, functions, and diseases. [NIH]

Half-Life: The time it takes for a substance (drug, radioactive nuclide, or other) to lose half of its pharmacologic, physiologic, or radiologic activity. [NIH]

Haptens: Small antigenic determinants capable of eliciting an immune response only when coupled to a carrier. Haptens bind to antibodies but by themselves cannot elicit an antibody response. [NIH]

Headache: Pain in the cranial region that may occur as an isolated and benign symptom or as a manifestation of a wide variety of conditions including subarachnoid hemorrhage; craniocerebral trauma; central nervous system infections; intracranial hypertension; and other disorders. In general, recurrent headaches that are not associated with a primary disease process are referred to as headache disorders (e.g., migraine). [NIH]

Headache Disorders: Common conditions characterized by persistent or recurrent headaches. Headache syndrome classification systems may be based on etiology (e.g., vascular headache, post-traumatic headaches, etc.), temporal pattern (e.g., cluster headache, paroxysmal hemicrania, etc.), and precipitating factors (e.g., cough headache). [NIH]

Heart attack: A seizure of weak or abnormal functioning of the heart. [NIH]

Heart failure: Loss of pumping ability by the heart, often accompanied by fatigue, breathlessness, and excess fluid accumulation in body tissues. [NIH]

Heartburn: Substernal pain or burning sensation, usually associated with regurgitation of gastric juice into the esophagus. [NIH]

Hematuria: Presence of blood in the urine. [NIH]

Heme: The color-furnishing portion of hemoglobin. It is found free in tissues and as the prosthetic group in many hemeproteins. [NIH]

Hemodialysis: The use of a machine to clean wastes from the blood after the kidneys have failed. The blood travels through tubes to a dialyzer, which removes wastes and extra fluid. The cleaned blood then flows through another set of tubes back into the body. [NIH]

Hemodynamics: The movements of the blood and the forces involved in systemic or regional blood circulation. [NIH]

Hemoglobin: One of the fractions of glycosylated hemoglobin A1c. Glycosylated hemoglobin is formed when linkages of glucose and related monosaccharides bind to hemoglobin A and its concentration represents the average blood glucose level over the previous several weeks. HbA1c levels are used as a measure of long-term control of plasma glucose (normal, 4 to 6 percent). In controlled diabetes mellitus, the concentration of glycosylated hemoglobin A is within the normal range, but in uncontrolled cases the level may be 3 to 4 times the normal conentration. Generally, complications are substantially lower among patients with Hb levels of 7 percent or less than in patients with HbA1c levels of 9 percent or more. [NIH]

Hemorrhage: Bleeding or escape of blood from a vessel. [NIH]

Hemostasis: The process which spontaneously arrests the flow of blood from vessels carrying blood under pressure. It is accomplished by contraction of the vessels, adhesion and aggregation of formed blood elements, and the process of blood or plasma coagulation. [NIH]

Heparin: Heparinic acid. A highly acidic mucopolysaccharide formed of equal parts of sulfated D-glucosamine and D-glucuronic acid with sulfaminic bridges. The molecular weight ranges from six to twenty thousand. Heparin occurs in and is obtained from liver, lung, mast cells, etc., of vertebrates. Its function is unknown, but it is used to prevent blood clotting in vivo and vitro, in the form of many different salts. [NIH]

Hepatic: Refers to the liver. [NIH]

Heredity: 1. The genetic transmission of a particular quality or trait from parent to offspring. 2. The genetic constitution of an individual. [EU]

Heterodimer: Zippered pair of nonidentical proteins. [NIH]

Heterogeneity: The property of one or more samples or populations which implies that they are not identical in respect of some or all of their parameters, e. g. heterogeneity of variance. [NIH]

Hirsutism: Excess hair in females and children with an adult male pattern of distribution. The concept does not include hypertrichosis, which is localized or generalized excess hair. [NIH]

Histamine: 1H-Imidazole-4-ethanamine. A depressor amine derived by enzymatic decarboxylation of histidine. It is a powerful stimulant of gastric secretion, a constrictor of bronchial smooth muscle, a vasodilator, and also a centrally acting neurotransmitter. [NIH]

Homeostasis: The processes whereby the internal environment of an organism tends to remain balanced and stable. [NIH]

Homologous: Corresponding in structure, position, origin, etc., as (a) the feathers of a bird and the scales of a fish, (b) antigen and its specific antibody, (c) allelic chromosomes. [EU]

Hormonal: Pertaining to or of the nature of a hormone. [EU]

Hormonal therapy: Treatment of cancer by removing, blocking, or adding hormones. Also called hormone therapy or endocrine therapy. [NIH]

Hormone: A substance in the body that regulates certain organs. Hormones such as gastrin help in breaking down food. Some hormones come from cells in the stomach and small intestine. [NIH]

Hormone Replacement Therapy: Therapeutic use of hormones to alleviate the effects of hormone deficiency. [NIH]

Hormone therapy: Treatment of cancer by removing, blocking, or adding hormones. Also called endocrine therapy. [NIH]

Host: Any animal that receives a transplanted graft. [NIH]

Humoral: Of, relating to, proceeding from, or involving a bodily humour - now often used of endocrine factors as opposed to neural or somatic. [EU]

Humour: 1. A normal functioning fluid or semifluid of the body (as the blood, lymph or bile) especially of vertebrates. 2. A secretion that is itself an excitant of activity (as certain hormones). [EU]

Hydrocephalus: Excessive accumulation of cerebrospinal fluid within the cranium which may be associated with dilation of cerebral ventricles, intracranial hypertension; headache; lethargy; urinary incontinence; and ataxia (and in infants macrocephaly). This condition may be caused by obstruction of cerebrospinal fluid pathways due to neurologic abnormalities, intracranial hemorrhages; central nervous system infections; brain neoplasms; craniocerebral trauma; and other conditions. Impaired resorption of cerebrospinal fluid from the arachnoid villi results in a communicating form of hydrocephalus. Hydrocephalus ex-vacuo refers to ventricular dilation that occurs as a result of brain substance loss from cerebral infarction and other conditions. [NIH]

Hydrogel: A network of cross-linked hydrophilic macromolecules used in biomedical applications. [NIH]

Hydrogen: The first chemical element in the periodic table. It has the atomic symbol H, atomic number 1, and atomic weight 1. It exists, under normal conditions, as a colorless, odorless, tasteless, diatomic gas. Hydrogen ions are protons. Besides the common H1 isotope, hydrogen exists as the stable isotope deuterium and the unstable, radioactive isotope tritium. [NIH]

Hydrolysis: The process of cleaving a chemical compound by the addition of a molecule of water. [NIH]

Hydronephrosis: Abnormal enlargement of a kidney, which may be caused by blockage of the ureter (such as by a kidney stone) or chronic kidney disease that prevents urine from draining into the bladder. [NIH]

Hydrophilic: Readily absorbing moisture; hygroscopic; having strongly polar groups that readily interact with water. [EU]

Hydrophobic: Not readily absorbing water, or being adversely affected by water, as a hydrophobic colloid. [EU]

Hydroxylysine: A hydroxylated derivative of the amino acid lysine that is present in certain collagens. [NIH]

Hydroxyproline: A hydroxylated form of the imino acid proline. A deficiency in ascorbic acid can result in impaired hydroxyproline formation. [NIH]

Hygienic: Pertaining to hygiene, or conducive to health. [EU]

Hyperandrogenism: A state characterized or caused by an excessive secretion of androgens by the adrenal cortex, ovaries, or testes. The clinical significance in males is negligible, so the term is used most commonly with reference to the female. The common manifestations in women are hirsutism and virilism. It is often caused by ovarian disease (particularly the polycystic ovary syndrome) and by adrenal diseases (particularly adrenal gland hyperfunction). [NIH]

Hypercalcemia: Abnormally high level of calcium in the blood. [NIH]

Hypercholesterolemia: Abnormally high levels of cholesterol in the blood. [NIH]

Hyperglycemia: Abnormally high blood sugar. [NIH]

Hyperlipidaemia: A general term for elevated concentrations of any or all of the lipids in the plasma, including hyperlipoproteinaemia, hypercholesterolaemia, etc. [EU]

Hyperlipidemia: An excess of lipids in the blood. [NIH]

Hyperlipoproteinemia: Metabolic disease characterized by elevated plasma cholesterol and/or triglyceride levels. The inherited form is attributed to a single gene mechanism. [NIH]

Hyperphagia: Ingestion of a greater than optimal quantity of food. [NIH]

Hyperplasia: An increase in the number of cells in a tissue or organ, not due to tumor formation. It differs from hypertrophy, which is an increase in bulk without an increase in the number of cells. [NIH]

Hypersensitivity: Altered reactivity to an antigen, which can result in pathologic reactions upon subsequent exposure to that particular antigen. [NIH]

Hypertension: Persistently high arterial blood pressure. Currently accepted threshold levels are 140 mm Hg systolic and 90 mm Hg diastolic pressure. [NIH]

Hypertension, Pulmonary: Increased pressure within the pulmonary circulation, usually secondary to cardiac or pulmonary disease. [NIH]

Hypertension, Renovascular: Hypertension due to compression or obstruction of the renal artery or its branches. [NIH]

Hypertriglyceridemia: Condition of elevated triglyceride concentration in the blood; an inherited form occurs in familial hyperlipoproteinemia IIb and hyperlipoproteinemia type IV. It has been linked to higher risk of heart disease and arteriosclerosis. [NIH]

Hypertrophy: General increase in bulk of a part or organ, not due to tumor formation, nor to an increase in the number of cells. [NIH]

Hypoglycemia: Abnormally low blood sugar [NIH]

Hypoglycemic: An orally active drug that produces a fall in blood glucose concentration. [NIH]

Hypoglycemic Agents: Agents which lower the blood glucose level. [NIH]

Hypogonadism: Condition resulting from or characterized by abnormally decreased functional activity of the gonads, with retardation of growth and sexual development. [NIH]

Hypophyseal: Hypophysial. [EU]

Hypotension: Abnormally low blood pressure. [NIH]

Hypothalamic: Of or involving the hypothalamus. [EU]

Hypothalamus: Ventral part of the diencephalon extending from the region of the optic chiasm to the caudal border of the mammillary bodies and forming the inferior and lateral walls of the third ventricle. [NIH]

Hypothyroidism: Deficiency of thyroid activity. In adults, it is most common in women and is characterized by decrease in basal metabolic rate, tiredness and lethargy, sensitivity to cold, and menstrual disturbances. If untreated, it progresses to full-blown myxoedema. In infants, severe hypothyroidism leads to cretinism. In juveniles, the manifestations are intermediate, with less severe mental and developmental retardation and only mild symptoms of the adult form. When due to pituitary deficiency of thyrotropin secretion it is called secondary hypothyroidism. [EU]

Hypoxanthine: A purine and a reaction intermediate in the metabolism of adenosine and in the formation of nucleic acids by the salvage pathway. [NIH]

Hypoxia: Reduction of oxygen supply to tissue below physiological levels despite adequate perfusion of the tissue by blood. [EU]

Id: The part of the personality structure which harbors the unconscious instinctive desires and strivings of the individual. [NIH]

Iliac Artery: Either of two large arteries originating from the abdominal aorta; they supply blood to the pelvis, abdominal wall and legs. [NIH]

Iliac Vein: A vein on either side of the body which is formed by the union of the external and internal iliac veins and passes upward to join with its fellow of the opposite side to form the inferior vena cava. [NIH]

Immune response: The activity of the immune system against foreign substances (antigens). [NIH]

Immune system: The organs, cells, and molecules responsible for the recognition and disposal of foreign ("non-self") material which enters the body. [NIH]

Immunization: Deliberate stimulation of the host's immune response. Active immunization involves administration of antigens or immunologic adjuvants. Passive immunization involves administration of immune sera or lymphocytes or their extracts (e.g., transfer factor, immune RNA) or transplantation of immunocompetent cell producing tissue (thymus or bone marrow). [NIH]

Immunoglobulin: A protein that acts as an antibody. [NIH]

Immunohistochemistry: Histochemical localization of immunoreactive substances using labeled antibodies as reagents. [NIH]

Immunologic: The ability of the antibody-forming system to recall a previous experience with an antigen and to respond to a second exposure with the prompt production of large amounts of antibody. [NIH]

Immunology: The study of the body's immune system. [NIH]

Immunophilins: Members of a family of highly conserved proteins which are all cis-trans peptidyl-prolyl isomerases (peptidylprolyl isomerase). They bind the immunosuppressant drugs cyclosporine; tacrolimus and sirolimus. They possess rotomase activity, which is inhibited by the immunosuppressant drugs that bind to them. EC 5.2.1.- [NIH]

Immunosuppressant: An agent capable of suppressing immune responses. [EU]

Immunosuppressive: Describes the ability to lower immune system responses. [NIH]

Impairment: In the context of health experience, an impairment is any loss or abnormality of psychological, physiological, or anatomical structure or function. [NIH]

Implant radiation: A procedure in which radioactive material sealed in needles, seeds, wires, or catheters is placed directly into or near the tumor. Also called [NIH]

Implantation: The insertion or grafting into the body of biological, living, inert, or radioactive material. [EU]

Impotence: The inability to perform sexual intercourse. [NIH]

Impotency: Lack of power in the male to copulate, i. e. inability to achieve penile erection; the cause may be exposure to organic solvents or other toxic substances. [NIH]

Impotent: Unable to have an erection adequate for sexual intercourse. [NIH]

In situ: In the natural or normal place; confined to the site of origin without invasion of neighbouring tissues. [EU]

In Situ Hybridization: A technique that localizes specific nucleic acid sequences within intact chromosomes, eukaryotic cells, or bacterial cells through the use of specific nucleic acid-labeled probes. [NIH]

In vitro: In the laboratory (outside the body). The opposite of in vivo (in the body). [NIH]

In vivo: In the body. The opposite of in vitro (outside the body or in the laboratory). [NIH]

Incision: A cut made in the body during surgery. [NIH]

Incompetence: Physical or mental inadequacy or insufficiency. [EU]

Incontinence: Inability to control the flow of urine from the bladder (urinary incontinence) or the escape of stool from the rectum (fecal incontinence). [NIH]

Indicative: That indicates; that points out more or less exactly; that reveals fairly clearly. [EU]

Indigestion: Poor digestion. Symptoms include heartburn, nausea, bloating, and gas. Also called dyspepsia. [NIH]

Induction: The act or process of inducing or causing to occur, especially the production of a specific morphogenetic effect in the developing embryo through the influence of evocators or organizers, or the production of anaesthesia or unconsciousness by use of appropriate agents. [EU]

Infarction: A pathological process consisting of a sudden insufficient blood supply to an area, which results in necrosis of that area. It is usually caused by a thrombus, an embolus, or a vascular torsion. [NIH]

Infection: 1. Invasion and multiplication of microorganisms in body tissues, which may be clinically unapparent or result in local cellular injury due to competitive metabolism, toxins, intracellular replication, or antigen-antibody response. The infection may remain localized, subclinical, and temporary if the body's defensive mechanisms are effective. A local infection may persist and spread by extension to become an acute, subacute, or chronic clinical infection or disease state. A local infection may also become systemic when the microorganisms gain access to the lymphatic or vascular system. 2. An infectious disease. [EU]

Infertility: The diminished or absent ability to conceive or produce an offspring while sterility is the complete inability to conceive or produce an offspring. [NIH]

Infiltration: The diffusion or accumulation in a tissue or cells of substances not normal to it or in amounts of the normal. Also, the material so accumulated. [EU]

Inflammation: A pathological process characterized by injury or destruction of tissues caused by a variety of cytologic and chemical reactions. It is usually manifested by typical signs of pain, heat, redness, swelling, and loss of function. [NIH]

Inflammatory bowel disease: A general term that refers to the inflammation of the colon and rectum. Inflammatory bowel disease includes ulcerative colitis and Crohn's disease. [NIH]

Infusion: A method of putting fluids, including drugs, into the bloodstream. Also called intravenous infusion. [NIH]

Ingestion: Taking into the body by mouth [NIH]

Inhalation: The drawing of air or other substances into the lungs. [EU]

Initiation: Mutation induced by a chemical reactive substance causing cell changes; being a step in a carcinogenic process. [NIH]

Innervation: 1. The distribution or supply of nerves to a part. 2. The supply of nervous energy or of nerve stimulus sent to a part. [EU]

Inotropic: Affecting the force or energy of muscular contractions. [EU]

Insecticides: Pesticides designed to control insects that are harmful to man. The insects may be directly harmful, as those acting as disease vectors, or indirectly harmful, as destroyers of crops, food products, or textile fabrics. [NIH]

Insight: The capacity to understand one's own motives, to be aware of one's own psychodynamics, to appreciate the meaning of symbolic behavior. [NIH]

Insomnia: Difficulty in going to sleep or getting enough sleep. [NIH]

Instillation: . [EU]

Insulator: Material covering the metal conductor of the lead. It is usually polyurethane or silicone. [NIH]

Insulin: A protein hormone secreted by beta cells of the pancreas. Insulin plays a major role in the regulation of glucose metabolism, generally promoting the cellular utilization of glucose. It is also an important regulator of protein and lipid metabolism. Insulin is used as a drug to control insulin-dependent diabetes mellitus. [NIH]

Insulin-dependent diabetes mellitus: A disease characterized by high levels of blood glucose resulting from defects in insulin secretion, insulin action, or both. Autoimmune, genetic, and environmental factors are involved in the development of type I diabetes. [NIH]

Intermittent: Occurring at separated intervals; having periods of cessation of activity. [EU]

Internal Medicine: A medical specialty concerned with the diagnosis and treatment of diseases of the internal organ systems of adults. [NIH]

Internal radiation: A procedure in which radioactive material sealed in needles, seeds, wires, or catheters is placed directly into or near the tumor. Also called brachytherapy, implant radiation, or interstitial radiation therapy. [NIH]

Interstitial: Pertaining to or situated between parts or in the interspaces of a tissue. [EU]

Intestinal: Having to do with the intestines. [NIH]

Intestine: A long, tube-shaped organ in the abdomen that completes the process of digestion. There is both a large intestine and a small intestine. Also called the bowel. [NIH]

Intoxication: Poisoning, the state of being poisoned. [EU]

Intracellular: Inside a cell. [NIH]

Intracranial Embolism: The sudden obstruction of a blood vessel by an embolus. [NIH]

Intracranial Embolism and Thrombosis: Embolism or thrombosis involving blood vessels which supply intracranial structures. Emboli may originate from extracranial or intracranial sources. Thrombosis may occur in arterial or venous structures. [NIH]

Intracranial Hypertension: Increased pressure within the cranial vault. This may result from several conditions, including hydrocephalus; brain edema; intracranial masses; severe systemic hypertension; pseudotumor cerebri; and other disorders. [NIH]

Intramuscular: IM. Within or into muscle. [NIH]

Intraperitoneal: IP. Within the peritoneal cavity (the area that contains the abdominal organs). [NIH]

Intrathecal: Describes the fluid-filled space between the thin layers of tissue that cover the brain and spinal cord. Drugs can be injected into the fluid or a sample of the fluid can be removed for testing. [NIH]

Intravenous: IV. Into a vein. [NIH]

Intrinsic: Situated entirely within or pertaining exclusively to a part. [EU]

Intubation: Introduction of a tube into a hollow organ to restore or maintain patency if obstructed. It is differentiated from catheterization in that the insertion of a catheter is usually performed for the introducing or withdrawing of fluids from the body. [NIH]

Invasive: 1. Having the quality of invasiveness. 2. Involving puncture or incision of the skin or insertion of an instrument or foreign material into the body; said of diagnostic techniques. [EU]

Involuntary: Reaction occurring without intention or volition. [NIH]

Ion Channels: Gated, ion-selective glycoproteins that traverse membranes. The stimulus for channel gating can be a membrane potential, drug, transmitter, cytoplasmic messenger, or a mechanical deformation. Ion channels which are integral parts of ionotropic neurotransmitter receptors are not included. [NIH]

Ionizing: Radiation comprising charged particles, e. g. electrons, protons, alpha-particles, etc., having sufficient kinetic energy to produce ionization by collision. [NIH]

Ions: An atom or group of atoms that have a positive or negative electric charge due to a gain (negative charge) or loss (positive charge) of one or more electrons. Atoms with a positive charge are known as cations; those with a negative charge are anions. [NIH]

Irritable Bowel Syndrome: A disorder that comes and goes. Nerves that control the muscles in the GI tract are too active. The GI tract becomes sensitive to food, stool, gas, and stress. Causes abdominal pain, bloating, and constipation or diarrhea. Also called spastic colon or mucous colitis. [NIH]

Ischemia: Deficiency of blood in a part, due to functional constriction or actual obstruction of a blood vessel. [EU]

Isomerases: A class of enzymes that catalyze geometric or structural changes within a molecule to form a single product. The reactions do not involve a net change in the concentrations of compounds other than the substrate and the product.(from Dorland, 28th ed) EC 5. [NIH]

Isosorbide: 1,4:3,6-Dianhydro D-glucitol. Chemically inert osmotic diuretic used mainly to treat hydrocephalus; also used in glaucoma. [NIH]

Itraconazole: An antifungal agent that has been used in the treatment of histoplasmosis, blastomycosis, cryptococcal meningitis, and aspergillosis. [NIH]

Joint: The point of contact between elements of an animal skeleton with the parts that surround and support it. [NIH]

Kb: A measure of the length of DNA fragments, 1 Kb = 1000 base pairs. The largest DNA fragments are up to 50 kilobases long. [NIH]

Ketanserin: A selective serotonin receptor antagonist with weak adrenergic receptor blocking properties. The drug is effective in lowering blood pressure in essential hypertension. It also inhibits platelet aggregation. It is well tolerated and is particularly effective in older patients. [NIH]

Ketoconazole: Broad spectrum antifungal agent used for long periods at high doses, especially in immunosuppressed patients. [NIH]

Ketone Bodies: Chemicals that the body makes when there is not enough insulin in the blood and it must break down fat for its energy. Ketone bodies can poison and even kill body cells. When the body does not have the help of insulin, the ketones build up in the blood and then "spill" over into the urine so that the body can get rid of them. The body can also rid itself of one type of ketone, called acetone, through the lungs. This gives the breath a fruity odor. Ketones that build up in the body for a long time lead to serious illness and coma. [NIH]

Ketosis: A condition of having ketone bodies build up in body tissues and fluids. The signs of ketosis are nausea, vomiting, and stomach pain. Ketosis can lead to ketoacidosis. [NIH]

Kidney Disease: Any one of several chronic conditions that are caused by damage to the cells of the kidney. People who have had diabetes for a long time may have kidney damage. Also called nephropathy. [NIH]

Kidney Failure: The inability of a kidney to excrete metabolites at normal plasma levels under conditions of normal loading, or the inability to retain electrolytes under conditions of normal intake. In the acute form (kidney failure, acute), it is marked by uremia and usually by oliguria or anuria, with hyperkalemia and pulmonary edema. The chronic form (kidney failure, chronic) is irreversible and requires hemodialysis. [NIH]

Kidney Failure, Acute: A clinical syndrome characterized by a sudden decrease in glomerular filtration rate, often to values of less than 1 to 2 ml per minute. It is usually associated with oliguria (urine volumes of less than 400 ml per day) and is always associated with biochemical consequences of the reduction in glomerular filtration rate such as a rise in blood urea nitrogen (BUN) and serum creatinine concentrations. [NIH]

Kidney Failure, Chronic: An irreversible and usually progressive reduction in renal function in which both kidneys have been damaged by a variety of diseases to the extent that they are unable to adequately remove the metabolic products from the blood and regulate the body's electrolyte composition and acid-base balance. Chronic kidney failure requires hemodialysis or surgery, usually kidney transplantation. [NIH]

Kidney stone: A stone that develops from crystals that form in urine and build up on the inner surfaces of the kidney, in the renal pelvis, or in the ureters. [NIH]

Knee Prosthesis: Replacement for a knee joint. [NIH]

Labile: 1. Gliding; moving from point to point over the surface; unstable; fluctuating. 2.

Chemically unstable. [EU]

Lactation: The period of the secretion of milk. [EU]

Large Intestine: The part of the intestine that goes from the cecum to the rectum. The large intestine absorbs water from stool and changes it from a liquid to a solid form. The large intestine is 5 feet long and includes the appendix, cecum, colon, and rectum. Also called colon. [NIH]

Latent: Phoria which occurs at one distance or another and which usually has no troublesome effect. [NIH]

Lens: The transparent, double convex (outward curve on both sides) structure suspended between the aqueous and vitreous; helps to focus light on the retina. [NIH]

Leprosy: A chronic granulomatous infection caused by Mycobacterium leprae. The granulomatous lesions are manifested in the skin, the mucous membranes, and the peripheral nerves. Two polar or principal types are lepromatous and tuberculoid. [NIH]

Lesion: An area of abnormal tissue change. [NIH]

Lethargy: Abnormal drowsiness or stupor; a condition of indifference. [EU]

Leukocytes: White blood cells. These include granular leukocytes (basophils, eosinophils, and neutrophils) as well as non-granular leukocytes (lymphocytes and monocytes). [NIH]

Libido: The psychic drive or energy associated with sexual instinct in the broad sense (pleasure and love-object seeking). It may also connote the psychic energy associated with instincts in general that motivate behavior. [NIH]

Library Services: Services offered to the library user. They include reference and circulation. [NIH]

Lidocaine: A local anesthetic and cardiac depressant used as an antiarrhythmia agent. Its actions are more intense and its effects more prolonged than those of procaine but its duration of action is shorter than that of bupivacaine or prilocaine. [NIH]

Life cycle: The successive stages through which an organism passes from fertilized ovum or spore to the fertilized ovum or spore of the next generation. [NIH]

Life Expectancy: A figure representing the number of years, based on known statistics, to which any person of a given age may reasonably expect to live. [NIH]

Ligament: A band of fibrous tissue that connects bones or cartilages, serving to support and strengthen joints. [EU]

Ligands: A RNA simulation method developed by the MIT. [NIH]

Ligation: Application of a ligature to tie a vessel or strangulate a part. [NIH]

Linkages: The tendency of two or more genes in the same chromosome to remain together from one generation to the next more frequently than expected according to the law of independent assortment. [NIH]

Lipid: Fat. [NIH]

Lipid Peroxidation: Peroxidase catalyzed oxidation of lipids using hydrogen peroxide as an electron acceptor. [NIH]

Lipophilic: Having an affinity for fat; pertaining to or characterized by lipophilia. [EU]

Lipoprotein: Any of the lipid-protein complexes in which lipids are transported in the blood; lipoprotein particles consist of a spherical hydrophobic core of triglycerides or cholesterol esters surrounded by an amphipathic monolayer of phospholipids, cholesterol, and apolipoproteins; the four principal classes are high-density, low-density, and very-low-density lipoproteins and chylomicrons. [EU]

Lithotripsy: The destruction of a calculus of the kidney, ureter, bladder, or gallbladder by physical forces, including crushing with a lithotriptor through a catheter. Focused percutaneous ultrasound and focused hydraulic shock waves may be used without surgery. Lithotripsy does not include the dissolving of stones by acids or litholysis. Lithotripsy by laser is laser lithotripsy. [NIH]

Liver: A large, glandular organ located in the upper abdomen. The liver cleanses the blood and aids in digestion by secreting bile. [NIH]

Localization: The process of determining or marking the location or site of a lesion or disease. May also refer to the process of keeping a lesion or disease in a specific location or site. [NIH]

Localized: Cancer which has not metastasized yet. [NIH]

Longitudinal study: Also referred to as a "cohort study" or "prospective study"; the analytic method of epidemiologic study in which subsets of a defined population can be identified who are, have been, or in the future may be exposed or not exposed, or exposed in different degrees, to a factor or factors hypothesized to influence the probability of occurrence of a given disease or other outcome. The main feature of this type of study is to observe large numbers of subjects over an extended time, with comparisons of incidence rates in groups that differ in exposure levels. [NIH]

Loop: A wire usually of platinum bent at one end into a small loop (usually 4 mm inside diameter) and used in transferring microorganisms. [NIH]

Low-density lipoprotein: Lipoprotein that contains most of the cholesterol in the blood. LDL carries cholesterol to the tissues of the body, including the arteries. A high level of LDL increases the risk of heart disease. LDL typically contains 60 to 70 percent of the total serum cholesterol and both are directly correlated with CHD risk. [NIH]

Lumbar: Pertaining to the loins, the part of the back between the thorax and the pelvis. [EU]

Lumen: The cavity or channel within a tube or tubular organ. [EU]

Lupus: A form of cutaneous tuberculosis. It is seen predominantly in women and typically involves the nasal, buccal, and conjunctival mucosa. [NIH]

Lupus Nephritis: Glomerulonephritis associated with systemic lupus erythematosus. It is classified into four histologic types: mesangial, focal, diffuse, and membranous. [NIH]

Lutein Cells: The cells of the corpus luteum which are derived from the granulosa cells and the theca cells of the Graafian follicle. [NIH]

Lycopene: A red pigment found in tomatoes and some fruits. [NIH]

Lymph: The almost colorless fluid that travels through the lymphatic system and carries cells that help fight infection and disease. [NIH]

Lymphatic: The tissues and organs, including the bone marrow, spleen, thymus, and lymph nodes, that produce and store cells that fight infection and disease. [NIH]

Lymphatic system: The tissues and organs that produce, store, and carry white blood cells that fight infection and other diseases. This system includes the bone marrow, spleen, thymus, lymph nodes and a network of thin tubes that carry lymph and white blood cells. These tubes branch, like blood vessels, into all the tissues of the body. [NIH]

Lymphocyte: A white blood cell. Lymphocytes have a number of roles in the immune system, including the production of antibodies and other substances that fight infection and diseases. [NIH]

Lymphoid: Referring to lymphocytes, a type of white blood cell. Also refers to tissue in which lymphocytes develop. [NIH]

Lysine: An essential amino acid. It is often added to animal feed. [NIH]

Macula: A stain, spot, or thickening. Often used alone to refer to the macula retinae. [EU]

Macula Lutea: An oval area in the retina, 3 to 5 mm in diameter, usually located temporal to the superior pole of the eye and slightly below the level of the optic disk. [NIH]

Macular Degeneration: Degenerative changes in the macula lutea of the retina. [NIH]

Malignancy: A cancerous tumor that can invade and destroy nearby tissue and spread to other parts of the body. [NIH]

Malignant: Cancerous; a growth with a tendency to invade and destroy nearby tissue and spread to other parts of the body. [NIH]

Mammary: Pertaining to the mamma, or breast. [EU]

Manifest: Being the part or aspect of a phenomenon that is directly observable : concretely expressed in behaviour. [EU]

Masturbation: Sexual stimulation or gratification of the self. [NIH]

Medial: Lying near the midsaggital plane of the body; opposed to lateral. [NIH]

Mediate: Indirect; accomplished by the aid of an intervening medium. [EU]

Mediator: An object or substance by which something is mediated, such as (1) a structure of the nervous system that transmits impulses eliciting a specific response; (2) a chemical substance (transmitter substance) that induces activity in an excitable tissue, such as nerve or muscle; or (3) a substance released from cells as the result of the interaction of antigen with antibody or by the action of antigen with a sensitized lymphocyte. [EU]

Medical Illustration: The field which deals with illustrative clarification of biomedical concepts, as in the use of diagrams and drawings. The illustration may be produced by hand, photography, computer, or other electronic or mechanical methods. [NIH]

Medical Records: Recording of pertinent information concerning patient's illness or illnesses. [NIH]

Medicament: A medicinal substance or agent. [EU]

MEDLINE: An online database of MEDLARS, the computerized bibliographic Medical Literature Analysis and Retrieval System of the National Library of Medicine. [NIH]

Megaloblastic: A large abnormal red blood cell appearing in the blood in pernicious anaemia. [EU]

Meiosis: A special method of cell division, occurring in maturation of the germ cells, by means of which each daughter nucleus receives half the number of chromosomes characteristic of the somatic cells of the species. [NIH]

Melanin: The substance that gives the skin its color. [NIH]

Melanocytes: Epidermal dendritic pigment cells which control long-term morphological color changes by alteration in their number or in the amount of pigment they produce and store in the pigment containing organelles called melanosomes. Melanophores are larger cells which do not exist in mammals. [NIH]

Melanosomes: Melanin-containing organelles found in melanocytes and melanophores. [NIH]

Membrane: A very thin layer of tissue that covers a surface. [NIH]

Memory: Complex mental function having four distinct phases: (1) memorizing or learning, (2) retention, (3) recall, and (4) recognition. Clinically, it is usually subdivided into immediate, recent, and remote memory. [NIH]

Meninges: The three membranes that cover and protect the brain and spinal cord. [NIH]

Meningitis: Inflammation of the meninges. When it affects the dura mater, the disease is termed pachymeningitis; when the arachnoid and pia mater are involved, it is called leptomeningitis, or meningitis proper. [EU]

Menopause: Permanent cessation of menstruation. [NIH]

Menstrual Cycle: The period of the regularly recurring physiologic changes in the endometrium occurring during the reproductive period in human females and some primates and culminating in partial sloughing of the endometrium (menstruation). [NIH]

Menstruation: The normal physiologic discharge through the vagina of blood and mucosal tissues from the nonpregnant uterus. [NIH]

Mental Disorders: Psychiatric illness or diseases manifested by breakdowns in the adaptational process expressed primarily as abnormalities of thought, feeling, and behavior producing either distress or impairment of function. [NIH]

Mental Health: The state wherein the person is well adjusted. [NIH]

Mental Processes: Conceptual functions or thinking in all its forms. [NIH]

Meperidine: 1-Methyl-4-phenyl-4-piperidinecarboxylic acid ethyl ester. A narcotic analgesic that can be used for the relief of most types of moderate to severe pain, including postoperative pain and the pain of labor. Prolonged use may lead to dependence of the morphine type; withdrawal symptoms appear more rapidly than with morphine and are of shorter duration. [NIH]

Mesenchymal: Refers to cells that develop into connective tissue, blood vessels, and lymphatic tissue. [NIH]

Meta-Analysis: A quantitative method of combining the results of independent studies (usually drawn from the published literature) and synthesizing summaries and conclusions which may be used to evaluate therapeutic effectiveness, plan new studies, etc., with application chiefly in the areas of research and medicine. [NIH]

Metabolic disorder: A condition in which normal metabolic processes are disrupted, usually because of a missing enzyme. [NIH]

Metabolite: Any substance produced by metabolism or by a metabolic process. [EU]

Metastasis: The spread of cancer from one part of the body to another. Tumors formed from cells that have spread are called "secondary tumors" and contain cells that are like those in the original (primary) tumor. The plural is metastases. [NIH]

Methionine: A sulfur containing essential amino acid that is important in many body functions. It is a chelating agent for heavy metals. [NIH]

Metoprolol: Adrenergic beta-1-blocking agent with no stimulatory action. It is less bound to plasma albumin than alprenolol and may be useful in angina pectoris, hypertension, or cardiac arrhythmias. [NIH]

MI: Myocardial infarction. Gross necrosis of the myocardium as a result of interruption of the blood supply to the area; it is almost always caused by atherosclerosis of the coronary arteries, upon which coronary thrombosis is usually superimposed. [NIH]

Mianserin: A tetracyclic compound with antidepressant effects. It may cause drowsiness and hematological problems. Its mechanism of therapeutic action is not well understood, although it apparently blocks alpha-adrenergic, histamine H1, and some types of serotonin receptors. [NIH]

Mibefradil: A benzimidazoyl-substituted tetraline that binds selectively to and inhibits calcium channels, T-type. [NIH]

Microbe: An organism which cannot be observed with the naked eye; e. g. unicellular animals, lower algae, lower fungi, bacteria. [NIH]

Microcirculation: The vascular network lying between the arterioles and venules; includes capillaries, metarterioles and arteriovenous anastomoses. Also, the flow of blood through this network. [NIH]

Microsomal: Of or pertaining to microsomes : vesicular fragments of endoplasmic reticulum formed after disruption and centrifugation of cells. [EU]

Migration: The systematic movement of genes between populations of the same species, geographic race, or variety. [NIH]

Mineralocorticoids: A group of corticosteroids primarily associated with the regulation of water and electrolyte balance. This is accomplished through the effect on ion transport in renal tubules, resulting in retention of sodium and loss of potassium. Mineralocorticoid secretion is itself regulated by plasma volume, serum potassium, and angiotensin II. [NIH]

Mitochondrial Swelling: Increase in volume of mitochondria due to an influx of fluid; it occurs in hypotonic solutions due to osmotic pressure and in isotonic solutions as a result of altered permeability of the membranes of respiring mitochondria. [NIH]

Mitosis: A method of indirect cell division by means of which the two daughter nuclei normally receive identical complements of the number of chromosomes of the somatic cells of the species. [NIH]

Modeling: A treatment procedure whereby the therapist presents the target behavior which the learner is to imitate and make part of his repertoire. [NIH]

Modification: A change in an organism, or in a process in an organism, that is acquired from its own activity or environment. [NIH]

Modulator: A specific inductor that brings out characteristics peculiar to a definite region. [EU]

Molecular: Of, pertaining to, or composed of molecules : a very small mass of matter. [EU]

Molecule: A chemical made up of two or more atoms. The atoms in a molecule can be the same (an oxygen molecule has two oxygen atoms) or different (a water molecule has two hydrogen atoms and one oxygen atom). Biological molecules, such as proteins and DNA, can be made up of many thousands of atoms. [NIH]

Monitor: An apparatus which automatically records such physiological signs as respiration, pulse, and blood pressure in an anesthetized patient or one undergoing surgical or other procedures. [NIH]

Monoamine: Enzyme that breaks down dopamine in the astrocytes and microglia. [NIH]

Monoamine Oxidase: An enzyme that catalyzes the oxidative deamination of naturally occurring monoamines. It is a flavin-containing enzyme that is localized in mitochondrial membranes, whether in nerve terminals, the liver, or other organs. Monoamine oxidase is important in regulating the metabolic degradation of catecholamines and serotonin in neural or target tissues. Hepatic monoamine oxidase has a crucial defensive role in inactivating circulating monoamines or those, such as tyramine, that originate in the gut and are absorbed into the portal circulation. (From Goodman and Gilman's, The Pharmacological Basis of Therapeutics, 8th ed, p415) EC 1.4.3.4. [NIH]

Monoclonal: An antibody produced by culturing a single type of cell. It therefore consists of a single species of immunoglobulin molecules. [NIH]

Monocytes: Large, phagocytic mononuclear leukocytes produced in the vertebrate bone marrow and released into the blood; contain a large, oval or somewhat indented nucleus surrounded by voluminous cytoplasm and numerous organelles. [NIH]

Mononuclear: A cell with one nucleus. [NIH]

Monophosphate: So called second messenger for neurotransmitters and hormones. [NIH]

Morphine: The principal alkaloid in opium and the prototype opiate analgesic and narcotic. Morphine has widespread effects in the central nervous system and on smooth muscle. [NIH]

Morphogenesis: The development of the form of an organ, part of the body, or organism. [NIH]

Morphological: Relating to the configuration or the structure of live organs. [NIH]

Morphology: The science of the form and structure of organisms (plants, animals, and other forms of life). [NIH]

Motility: The ability to move spontaneously. [EU]

Motion Sickness: Sickness caused by motion, as sea sickness, train sickness, car sickness, and air sickness. [NIH]

Mucosa: A mucous membrane, or tunica mucosa. [EU]

Multiple sclerosis: A disorder of the central nervous system marked by weakness, numbness, a loss of muscle coordination, and problems with vision, speech, and bladder control. Multiple sclerosis is thought to be an autoimmune disease in which the body's immune system destroys myelin. Myelin is a substance that contains both protein and fat (lipid) and serves as a nerve insulator and helps in the transmission of nerve signals. [NIH]

Muscle Contraction: A process leading to shortening and/or development of tension in muscle tissue. Muscle contraction occurs by a sliding filament mechanism whereby actin filaments slide inward among the myosin filaments. [NIH]

Muscle Fibers: Large single cells, either cylindrical or prismatic in shape, that form the basic unit of muscle tissue. They consist of a soft contractile substance enclosed in a tubular sheath. [NIH]

Muscle Relaxation: That phase of a muscle twitch during which a muscle returns to a resting position. [NIH]

Mutagenesis: Process of generating genetic mutations. It may occur spontaneously or be induced by mutagens. [NIH]

Mutagens: Chemical agents that increase the rate of genetic mutation by interfering with the function of nucleic acids. A clastogen is a specific mutagen that causes breaks in chromosomes. [NIH]

Mydriatic: 1. Dilating the pupil. 2. Any drug that dilates the pupil. [EU]

Myelin: The fatty substance that covers and protects nerves. [NIH]

Myocardial infarction: Gross necrosis of the myocardium as a result of interruption of the blood supply to the area; it is almost always caused by atherosclerosis of the coronary arteries, upon which coronary thrombosis is usually superimposed. [NIH]

Myocardial Ischemia: A disorder of cardiac function caused by insufficient blood flow to the muscle tissue of the heart. The decreased blood flow may be due to narrowing of the coronary arteries (coronary arteriosclerosis), to obstruction by a thrombus (coronary thrombosis), or less commonly, to diffuse narrowing of arterioles and other small vessels within the heart. Severe interruption of the blood supply to the myocardial tissue may result in necrosis of cardiac muscle (myocardial infarction). [NIH]

Myocardium: The muscle tissue of the heart composed of striated, involuntary muscle known as cardiac muscle. [NIH]

Myosin: Chief protein in muscle and the main constituent of the thick filaments of muscle fibers. In conjunction with actin, it is responsible for the contraction and relaxation of muscles. [NIH]

Myotonia: Prolonged failure of muscle relaxation after contraction. This may occur after voluntary contractions, muscle percussion, or electrical stimulation of the muscle. Myotonia is a characteristic feature of myotonic disorders. [NIH]

Naloxone: A specific opiate antagonist that has no agonist activity. It is a competitive antagonist at mu, delta, and kappa opioid receptors. [NIH]

Naltrexone: Derivative of noroxymorphone that is the N-cyclopropylmethyl congener of naloxone. It is a narcotic antagonist that is effective orally, longer lasting and more potent than naloxone, and has been proposed for the treatment of heroin addiction. The FDA has approved naltrexone for the treatment of alcohol dependence. [NIH]

Narcotic: 1. Pertaining to or producing narcosis. 2. An agent that produces insensibility or stupor, applied especially to the opioids, i.e. to any natural or synthetic drug that has morphine-like actions. [EU]

Nasal Cavity: The proximal portion of the respiratory passages on either side of the nasal septum, lined with ciliated mucosa, extending from the nares to the pharynx. [NIH]

Nasal Septum: The partition separating the two nasal cavities in the midplane, composed of cartilaginous, membranous and bony parts. [NIH]

Nausea: An unpleasant sensation in the stomach usually accompanied by the urge to vomit. Common causes are early pregnancy, sea and motion sickness, emotional stress, intense pain, food poisoning, and various enteroviruses. [NIH]

NCI: National Cancer Institute. NCI, part of the National Institutes of Health of the United States Department of Health and Human Services, is the federal government's principal agency for cancer research. NCI conducts, coordinates, and funds cancer research, training, health information dissemination, and other programs with respect to the cause, diagnosis, prevention, and treatment of cancer. Access the NCI Web site at http://cancer.gov. [NIH]

Necrosis: A pathological process caused by the progressive degradative action of enzymes that is generally associated with severe cellular trauma. It is characterized by mitochondrial swelling, nuclear flocculation, uncontrolled cell lysis, and ultimately cell death. [NIH]

Need: A state of tension or dissatisfaction felt by an individual that impels him to action toward a goal he believes will satisfy the impulse. [NIH]

Neonatal: Pertaining to the first four weeks after birth. [EU]

Neoplasms: New abnormal growth of tissue. Malignant neoplasms show a greater degree of anaplasia and have the properties of invasion and metastasis, compared to benign neoplasms. [NIH]

Neoplastic: Pertaining to or like a neoplasm (= any new and abnormal growth); pertaining to neoplasia (= the formation of a neoplasm). [EU]

Nephritis: Inflammation of the kidney; a focal or diffuse proliferative or destructive process which may involve the glomerulus, tubule, or interstitial renal tissue. [EU]

Nephrologist: A doctor who treats patients with kidney problems or hypertension. [NIH]

Nephropathy: Disease of the kidneys. [EU]

Nerve: A cordlike structure of nervous tissue that connects parts of the nervous system with other tissues of the body and conveys nervous impulses to, or away from, these tissues. [NIH]

Nervous System: The entire nerve apparatus composed of the brain, spinal cord, nerves and ganglia. [NIH]

Networks: Pertaining to a nerve or to the nerves, a meshlike structure of interlocking fibers or strands. [NIH]

Neural: 1. Pertaining to a nerve or to the nerves. 2. Situated in the region of the spinal axis, as the neutral arch. [EU]

Neurogenic: Loss of bladder control caused by damage to the nerves controlling the bladder. [NIH]

Neurologic: Having to do with nerves or the nervous system. [NIH]

Neuromuscular: Pertaining to muscles and nerves. [EU]

Neuronal: Pertaining to a neuron or neurons (= conducting cells of the nervous system). [EU]

Neurons: The basic cellular units of nervous tissue. Each neuron consists of a body, an axon, and dendrites. Their purpose is to receive, conduct, and transmit impulses in the nervous system. [NIH]

Neuropathy: A problem in any part of the nervous system except the brain and spinal cord. Neuropathies can be caused by infection, toxic substances, or disease. [NIH]

Neuropeptide: A member of a class of protein-like molecules made in the brain. Neuropeptides consist of short chains of amino acids, with some functioning as neurotransmitters and some functioning as hormones. [NIH]

Neuropsychology: A branch of psychology which investigates the correlation between experience or behavior and the basic neurophysiological processes. The term neuropsychology stresses the dominant role of the nervous system. It is a more narrowly defined field than physiological psychology or psychophysiology. [NIH]

Neurosecretory Systems: A system of neurons that has the specialized function to produce and secrete hormones, and that constitutes, in whole or in part, an endocrine organ or system. [NIH]

Neurotransmitters: Endogenous signaling molecules that alter the behavior of neurons or effector cells. Neurotransmitter is used here in its most general sense, including not only messengers that act directly to regulate ion channels, but also those that act through second messenger systems, and those that act at a distance from their site of release. Included are neuromodulators, neuroregulators, neuromediators, and neurohumors, whether or not acting at synapses. [NIH]

Neutrons: Electrically neutral elementary particles found in all atomic nuclei except light hydrogen; the mass is equal to that of the proton and electron combined and they are unstable when isolated from the nucleus, undergoing beta decay. Slow, thermal, epithermal, and fast neutrons refer to the energy levels with which the neutrons are ejected from heavier nuclei during their decay. [NIH]

Neutrophil: A type of white blood cell. [NIH]

Nickel: A trace element with the atomic symbol Ni, atomic number 28, and atomic weight 58.69. It is a cofactor of the enzyme urease. [NIH]

Nitrates: Inorganic or organic salts and esters of nitric acid. These compounds contain the NO3- radical. [NIH]

Nitric acid: A toxic, corrosive, colorless liquid used to make fertilizers, dyes, explosives, and other chemicals. [NIH]

Nitric Oxide: A free radical gas produced endogenously by a variety of mammalian cells. It is synthesized from arginine by a complex reaction, catalyzed by nitric oxide synthase. Nitric oxide is endothelium-derived relaxing factor. It is released by the vascular endothelium and mediates the relaxation induced by some vasodilators such as acetylcholine and bradykinin. It also inhibits platelet aggregation, induces disaggregation of aggregated platelets, and inhibits platelet adhesion to the vascular endothelium. Nitric oxide activates cytosolic guanylate cyclase and thus elevates intracellular levels of cyclic GMP. [NIH]

Nitrogen: An element with the atomic symbol N, atomic number 7, and atomic weight 14. Nitrogen exists as a diatomic gas and makes up about 78% of the earth's atmosphere by volume. It is a constituent of proteins and nucleic acids and found in all living cells. [NIH]

Nitroglycerin: A highly volatile organic nitrate that acts as a dilator of arterial and venous smooth muscle and is used in the treatment of angina. It provides relief through improvement of the balance between myocardial oxygen supply and demand. Although total coronary blood flow is not increased, there is redistribution of blood flow in the heart when partial occlusion of coronary circulation is effected. [NIH]

Nitroprusside: (OC-6-22)-Pentakis(cyano-C)nitrosoferrate(2-). A powerful vasodilator used in emergencies to lower blood pressure or to improve cardiac function. It is also an indicator for free sulfhydryl groups in proteins. [NIH]

Nocturia: Excessive urination at night. [EU]

Non-small cell lung cancer: A group of lung cancers that includes squamous cell carcinoma, adenocarcinoma, and large cell carcinoma. [NIH]

Nonverbal Communication: Transmission of emotions, ideas, and attitudes between individuals in ways other than the spoken language. [NIH]

Norepinephrine: Precursor of epinephrine that is secreted by the adrenal medulla and is a widespread central and autonomic neurotransmitter. Norepinephrine is the principal transmitter of most postganglionic sympathetic fibers and of the diffuse projection system in the brain arising from the locus ceruleus. It is also found in plants and is used pharmacologically as a sympathomimetic. [NIH]

Nuclear: A test of the structure, blood flow, and function of the kidneys. The doctor injects a mildly radioactive solution into an arm vein and uses x-rays to monitor its progress through the kidneys. [NIH]

Nuclear Family: A family composed of spouses and their children. [NIH]

Nuclei: A body of specialized protoplasm found in nearly all cells and containing the chromosomes. [NIH]

Nucleic acid: Either of two types of macromolecule (DNA or RNA) formed by polymerization of nucleotides. Nucleic acids are found in all living cells and contain the information (genetic code) for the transfer of genetic information from one generation to the next. [NIH]

Nucleus: A body of specialized protoplasm found in nearly all cells and containing the chromosomes. [NIH]

Nursing Care: Care given to patients by nursing service personnel. [NIH]

Occult: Obscure; concealed from observation, difficult to understand. [EU]

Ocular: 1. Of, pertaining to, or affecting the eye. 2. Eyepiece. [EU]

Odds Ratio: The ratio of two odds. The exposure-odds ratio for case control data is the ratio of the odds in favor of exposure among cases to the odds in favor of exposure among noncases. The disease-odds ratio for a cohort or cross section is the ratio of the odds in favor of disease among the exposed to the odds in favor of disease among the unexposed. The prevalence-odds ratio refers to an odds ratio derived cross-sectionally from studies of prevalent cases. [NIH]

Odour: A volatile emanation that is perceived by the sense of smell. [EU]

Office Visits: Visits made by patients to health service providers' offices for diagnosis, treatment, and follow-up. [NIH]

Ointments: Semisolid preparations used topically for protective emollient effects or as a vehicle for local administration of medications. Ointment bases are various mixtures of fats, waxes, animal and plant oils and solid and liquid hydrocarbons. [NIH]

Oliguria: Clinical manifestation of the urinary system consisting of a decrease in the amount of urine secreted. [NIH]

Oncology: The study of cancer. [NIH]

On-line: A sexually-reproducing population derived from a common parentage. [NIH]

Opacity: Degree of density (area most dense taken for reading). [NIH]

Ophthalmologic: Pertaining to ophthalmology (= the branch of medicine dealing with the eye). [EU]

Opium: The air-dried exudate from the unripe seed capsule of the opium poppy, Papaver somniferum, or its variant, P. album. It contains a number of alkaloids, but only a few - morphine, codeine, and papaverine - have clinical significance. Opium has been used as an analgesic, antitussive, antidiarrheal, and antispasmodic. [NIH]

Opsin: A protein formed, together with retinene, by the chemical breakdown of meta-rhodopsin. [NIH]

Optic Chiasm: The X-shaped structure formed by the meeting of the two optic nerves. At the optic chiasm the fibers from the medial part of each retina cross to project to the other side of the brain while the lateral retinal fibers continue on the same side. As a result each half of the brain receives information about the contralateral visual field from both eyes. [NIH]

Optic Disk: The portion of the optic nerve seen in the fundus with the ophthalmoscope. It is formed by the meeting of all the retinal ganglion cell axons as they enter the optic nerve. [NIH]

Organelles: Specific particles of membrane-bound organized living substances present in eukaryotic cells, such as the mitochondria; the golgi apparatus; endoplasmic reticulum; lysomomes; plastids; and vacuoles. [NIH]

Orgasm: The crisis of sexual excitement in either humans or animals. [NIH]

Ornithine: An amino acid produced in the urea cycle by the splitting off of urea from arginine. [NIH]

Osmotic: Pertaining to or of the nature of osmosis (= the passage of pure solvent from a solution of lesser to one of greater solute concentration when the two solutions are separated by a membrane which selectively prevents the passage of solute molecules, but is permeable to the solvent). [EU]

Osteoarthritis: A progressive, degenerative joint disease, the most common form of arthritis, especially in older persons. The disease is thought to result not from the aging process but from biochemical changes and biomechanical stresses affecting articular cartilage. In the foreign literature it is often called osteoarthrosis deformans. [NIH]

Osteoporosis: Reduction of bone mass without alteration in the composition of bone, leading to fractures. Primary osteoporosis can be of two major types: postmenopausal osteoporosis and age-related (or senile) osteoporosis. [NIH]

Outpatient: A patient who is not an inmate of a hospital but receives diagnosis or treatment in a clinic or dispensary connected with the hospital. [NIH]

Ovaries: The pair of female reproductive glands in which the ova, or eggs, are formed. The ovaries are located in the pelvis, one on each side of the uterus. [NIH]

Ovary: Either of the paired glands in the female that produce the female germ cells and secrete some of the female sex hormones. [NIH]

Ovum: A female germ cell extruded from the ovary at ovulation. [NIH]

Oxalate: A chemical that combines with calcium in urine to form the most common type of kidney stone (calcium oxalate stone). [NIH]

Oxidation: The act of oxidizing or state of being oxidized. Chemically it consists in the increase of positive charges on an atom or the loss of negative charges. Most biological oxidations are accomplished by the removal of a pair of hydrogen atoms (dehydrogenation) from a molecule. Such oxidations must be accompanied by reduction of an acceptor molecule. Univalent o. indicates loss of one electron; divalent o., the loss of two electrons. [EU]

Oxidative Stress: A disturbance in the prooxidant-antioxidant balance in favor of the former, leading to potential damage. Indicators of oxidative stress include damaged DNA bases, protein oxidation products, and lipid peroxidation products (Sies, Oxidative Stress, 1991, pxv-xvi). [NIH]

Oxytocin: A nonapeptide posterior pituitary hormone that causes uterine contractions and stimulates lactation. [NIH]

Palliative: 1. Affording relief, but not cure. 2. An alleviating medicine. [EU]

Palpation: Application of fingers with light pressure to the surface of the body to determine consistence of parts beneath in physical diagnosis; includes palpation for determining the outlines of organs. [NIH]

Pancreas: A mixed exocrine and endocrine gland situated transversely across the posterior abdominal wall in the epigastric and hypochondriac regions. The endocrine portion is comprised of the Islets of Langerhans, while the exocrine portion is a compound acinar gland that secretes digestive enzymes. [NIH]

Pancreatic: Having to do with the pancreas. [NIH]

Panic: A state of extreme acute, intense anxiety and unreasoning fear accompanied by disorganization of personality function. [NIH]

Panic Disorder: A type of anxiety disorder characterized by unexpected panic attacks that last minutes or, rarely, hours. Panic attacks begin with intense apprehension, fear or terror and, often, a feeling of impending doom. Symptoms experienced during a panic attack include dyspnea or sensations of being smothered; dizziness, loss of balance or faintness; choking sensations; palpitations or accelerated heart rate; shakiness; sweating; nausea or other form of abdominal distress; depersonalization or derealization; paresthesias; hot flashes or chills; chest discomfort or pain; fear of dying and fear of not being in control of oneself or going crazy. Agoraphobia may also develop. Similar to other anxiety disorders, it may be inherited as an autosomal dominant trait. [NIH]

Papaverine: An alkaloid found in opium but not closely related to the other opium alkaloids in its structure or pharmacological actions. It is a direct-acting smooth muscle relaxant used in the treatment of impotence and as a vasodilator, especially for cerebral vasodilation. The mechanism of its pharmacological actions is not clear, but it apparently can inhibit phosphodiesterases and it may have direct actions on calcium channels. [NIH]

Parasympathetic Nervous System: The craniosacral division of the autonomic nervous system. The cell bodies of the parasympathetic preganglionic fibers are in brain stem nuclei and in the sacral spinal cord. They synapse in cranial autonomic ganglia or in terminal ganglia near target organs. The parasympathetic nervous system generally acts to conserve resources and restore homeostasis, often with effects reciprocal to the sympathetic nervous system. [NIH]

Parenteral: Not through the alimentary canal but rather by injection through some other route, as subcutaneous, intramuscular, intraorbital, intracapsular, intraspinal, intrasternal, intravenous, etc. [EU]

Paresthesias: Abnormal touch sensations, such as burning or prickling, that occur without an outside stimulus. [NIH]

Parkinsonism: A group of neurological disorders characterized by hypokinesia, tremor, and muscular rigidity. [EU]

Paroxysmal: Recurring in paroxysms (= spasms or seizures). [EU]

Particle: A tiny mass of material. [EU]

Parturition: The act or process of given birth to a child. [EU]

Patch: A piece of material used to cover or protect a wound, an injured part, etc.: a patch over the eye. [NIH]

Pathogenesis: The cellular events and reactions that occur in the development of disease. [NIH]

Pathologic: 1. Indicative of or caused by a morbid condition. 2. Pertaining to pathology (= branch of medicine that treats the essential nature of the disease, especially the structural and functional changes in tissues and organs of the body caused by the disease). [EU]

Pathologic Processes: The abnormal mechanisms and forms involved in the dysfunctions of tissues and organs. [NIH]

Pathologies: The study of abnormality, especially the study of diseases. [NIH]

Pathophysiology: Altered functions in an individual or an organ due to disease. [NIH]

Patient Care Management: Generating, planning, organizing, and administering medical and nursing care and services for patients. [NIH]

Patient Education: The teaching or training of patients concerning their own health needs. [NIH]

Patient Satisfaction: The degree to which the individual regards the health care service or product or the manner in which it is delivered by the provider as useful, effective, or beneficial. [NIH]

Patient Selection: Criteria and standards used for the determination of the appropriateness of the inclusion of patients with specific conditions in proposed treatment plans and the criteria used for the inclusion of subjects in various clinical trials and other research protocols. [NIH]

Pelvic: Pertaining to the pelvis. [EU]

Penile Erection: The state of the penis when the erectile tissue becomes filled with blood and causes the penis to become rigid and elevated. [NIH]

Penile Implantation: Surgical insertion of cylindric hydraulic devices for the treatment of organic impotence. [NIH]

Penile Prosthesis: Rigid, semi-rigid, or inflatable cylindric hydraulic devices, with either combined or separate reservoir and pumping systems, implanted for the surgical treatment of organic impotence. [NIH]

Penis: The external reproductive organ of males. It is composed of a mass of erectile tissue enclosed in three cylindrical fibrous compartments. Two of the three compartments, the corpus cavernosa, are placed side-by-side along the upper part of the organ. The third compartment below, the corpus spongiosum, houses the urethra . [NIH]

Pentoxifylline: A methylxanthine derivative that inhibits phosphodiesterase and affects blood rheology. It improves blood flow by increasing erythrocyte and leukocyte flexibility. It also inhibits platelet aggregation. Pentoxifylline modulates immunologic activity by stimulating cytokine production. [NIH]

Pepsin: An enzyme made in the stomach that breaks down proteins. [NIH]

Pepsin A: Formed from pig pepsinogen by cleavage of one peptide bond. The enzyme is a single polypeptide chain and is inhibited by methyl 2-diaazoacetamidohexanoate. It cleaves peptides preferentially at the carbonyl linkages of phenylalanine or leucine and acts as the principal digestive enzyme of gastric juice. [NIH]

Peptide: Any compound consisting of two or more amino acids, the building blocks of proteins. Peptides are combined to make proteins. [NIH]

Perception: The ability quickly and accurately to recognize similarities and differences among presented objects, whether these be pairs of words, pairs of number series, or multiple sets of these or other symbols such as geometric figures. [NIH]

Percutaneous: Performed through the skin, as injection of radiopacque material in radiological examination, or the removal of tissue for biopsy accomplished by a needle. [EU]

Perfusion: Bathing an organ or tissue with a fluid. In regional perfusion, a specific area of the body (usually an arm or a leg) receives high doses of anticancer drugs through a blood vessel. Such a procedure is performed to treat cancer that has not spread. [NIH]

Perineal: Pertaining to the perineum. [EU]

Perineum: The area between the anus and the sex organs. [NIH]

Peripheral blood: Blood circulating throughout the body. [NIH]

Peripheral Nervous System: The nervous system outside of the brain and spinal cord. The peripheral nervous system has autonomic and somatic divisions. The autonomic nervous system includes the enteric, parasympathetic, and sympathetic subdivisions. The somatic nervous system includes the cranial and spinal nerves and their ganglia and the peripheral sensory receptors. [NIH]

Peripheral Neuropathy: Nerve damage, usually affecting the feet and legs; causing pain, numbness, or a tingling feeling. Also called "somatic neuropathy" or "distal sensory polyneuropathy." [NIH]

Peripheral Vascular Disease: Disease in the large blood vessels of the arms, legs, and feet. People who have had diabetes for a long time may get this because major blood vessels in their arms, legs, and feet are blocked and these limbs do not receive enough blood. The signs of PVD are aching pains in the arms, legs, and feet (especially when walking) and foot sores that heal slowly. Although people with diabetes cannot always avoid PVD, doctors say they have a better chance of avoiding it if they take good care of their feet, do not smoke, and keep both their blood pressure and diabetes under good control. [NIH]

Peritoneal: Having to do with the peritoneum (the tissue that lines the abdominal wall and covers most of the organs in the abdomen). [NIH]

Peritoneal Cavity: The space enclosed by the peritoneum. It is divided into two portions, the greater sac and the lesser sac or omental bursa, which lies behind the stomach. The two sacs are connected by the foramen of Winslow, or epiploic foramen. [NIH]

Peritoneal Dialysis: Dialysis fluid being introduced into and removed from the peritoneal cavity as either a continuous or an intermittent procedure. [NIH]

Peritoneum: Endothelial lining of the abdominal cavity, the parietal peritoneum covering the inside of the abdominal wall and the visceral peritoneum covering the bowel, the mesentery, and certain of the organs. The portion that covers the bowel becomes the serosal layer of the bowel wall. [NIH]

Perivascular: Situated around a vessel. [EU]

Peroral: Performed through or administered through the mouth. [EU]

Personal Health Services: Health care provided to individuals. [NIH]

Personality Disorders: A major deviation from normal patterns of behavior. [NIH]

Phagocytosis: The engulfing of microorganisms, other cells, and foreign particles by phagocytic cells. [NIH]

Pharmaceutical Solutions: Homogeneous liquid preparations that contain one or more chemical substances dissolved, i.e., molecularly dispersed, in a suitable solvent or mixture of mutually miscible solvents. For reasons of their ingredients, method of preparation, or use, they do not fall into another group of products. [NIH]

Pharmacologic: Pertaining to pharmacology or to the properties and reactions of drugs. [EU]

Pharmacotherapy: A regimen of using appetite suppressant medications to manage obesity by decreasing appetite or increasing the feeling of satiety. These medications decrease appetite by increasing serotonin or catecholamine—two brain chemicals that affect mood and appetite. [NIH]

Pharynx: The hollow tube about 5 inches long that starts behind the nose and ends at the top of the trachea (windpipe) and esophagus (the tube that goes to the stomach). [NIH]

Phenotype: The outward appearance of the individual. It is the product of interactions between genes and between the genotype and the environment. This includes the killer phenotype, characteristic of yeasts. [NIH]

Phenoxybenzamine: An alpha-adrenergic anatagonist with long duration of action. It has been used to treat hypertension and as a peripheral vasodilator. [NIH]

Phentolamine: A nonselective alpha-adrenergic antagonist. It is used in the treatment of hypertension and hypertensive emergencies, pheochromocytoma, vasospasm of Raynaud's disease and frostbite, clonidine withdrawal syndrome, impotence, and peripheral vascular disease. [NIH]

Phenyl: Ingredient used in cold and flu remedies. [NIH]

Phenylalanine: An aromatic amino acid that is essential in the animal diet. It is a precursor of melanin, dopamine, noradrenalin, and thyroxine. [NIH]

Phimosis: The inability to retract the foreskin over the glans penis due to tightness of the prepuce. [NIH]

Phobias: An exaggerated and invariably pathological dread of some specific type of stimulus or situation. [NIH]

Phorbol: Class of chemicals that promotes the development of tumors. [NIH]

Phorbol Esters: Tumor-promoting compounds obtained from croton oil (Croton tiglium). Some of these are used in cell biological experiments as activators of protein kinase C. [NIH]

Phosphodiesterase: Effector enzyme that regulates the levels of a second messenger, the cyclic GMP. [NIH]

Phosphodiesterase Inhibitors: Compounds which inhibit or antagonize the biosynthesis or actions of phosphodiesterases. [NIH]

Phospholipases: A class of enzymes that catalyze the hydrolysis of phosphoglycerides or glycerophosphatidates. EC 3.1.-. [NIH]

Phospholipids: Lipids containing one or more phosphate groups, particularly those derived from either glycerol (phosphoglycerides; glycerophospholipids) or sphingosine (sphingolipids). They are polar lipids that are of great importance for the structure and function of cell membranes and are the most abundant of membrane lipids, although not stored in large amounts in the system. [NIH]

Phosphoprotein Phosphatase: A group of enzymes removing the serine- or threonine-bound phosphate groups from a wide range of phosphoproteins, including a number of enzymes which have been phosphorylated under the action of a kinase. (Enzyme Nomenclature, 1992) EC 3.1.3.16. [NIH]

Phosphorus: A non-metallic element that is found in the blood, muscles, nevers, bones, and teeth, and is a component of adenosine triphosphate (ATP; the primary energy source for the body's cells.) [NIH]

Phosphorylated: Attached to a phosphate group. [NIH]

Phosphorylation: The introduction of a phosphoryl group into a compound through the formation of an ester bond between the compound and a phosphorus moiety. [NIH]

Physical Examination: Systematic and thorough inspection of the patient for physical signs of disease or abnormality. [NIH]

Physician Assistants: Persons academically trained, licensed, or credentialed to provide medical care under the supervision of a physician. The concept does not include nurses, but does include orthopedic assistants, surgeon's assistants, and assistants to other specialists. [NIH]

Physiologic: Having to do with the functions of the body. When used in the phrase "physiologic age," it refers to an age assigned by general health, as opposed to calendar age. [NIH]

Physiology: The science that deals with the life processes and functions of organismus, their cells, tissues, and organs. [NIH]

Pigment: A substance that gives color to tissue. Pigments are responsible for the color of skin, eyes, and hair. [NIH]

Pilot Projects: Small-scale tests of methods and procedures to be used on a larger scale if the pilot study demonstrates that these methods and procedures can work. [NIH]

Pilot study: The initial study examining a new method or treatment. [NIH]

Pinocytosis: The engulfing of liquids by cells by a process of invagination and closure of the cell membrane to form fluid-filled vacuoles. [NIH]

Piperidines: A family of hexahydropyridines. Piperidine itself is found in the pepper plant as the alkaloid piperine. [NIH]

Pituitary Gland: A small, unpaired gland situated in the sella turcica tissue. It is connected to the hypothalamus by a short stalk. [NIH]

Placebos: Any dummy medication or treatment. Although placebos originally were medicinal preparations having no specific pharmacological activity against a targeted condition, the concept has been extended to include treatments or procedures, especially those administered to control groups in clinical trials in order to provide baseline measurements for the experimental protocol. [NIH]

Placenta: A highly vascular fetal organ through which the fetus absorbs oxygen and other nutrients and excretes carbon dioxide and other wastes. It begins to form about the eighth day of gestation when the blastocyst adheres to the decidua. [NIH]

Plague: An acute infectious disease caused by Yersinia pestis that affects humans, wild rodents, and their ectoparasites. This condition persists due to its firm entrenchment in sylvatic rodent-flea ecosystems throughout the world. Bubonic plague is the most common form. [NIH]

Plants: Multicellular, eukaryotic life forms of the kingdom Plantae. They are characterized by a mainly photosynthetic mode of nutrition; essentially unlimited growth at localized regions of cell divisions (meristems); cellulose within cells providing rigidity; the absence of organs of locomotion; absense of nervous and sensory systems; and an alteration of haploid and diploid generations. [NIH]

Plaque: A clear zone in a bacterial culture grown on an agar plate caused by localized destruction of bacterial cells by a bacteriophage. The concentration of infective virus in a fluid can be estimated by applying the fluid to a culture and counting the number of. [NIH]

Plasma: The clear, yellowish, fluid part of the blood that carries the blood cells. The proteins that form blood clots are in plasma. [NIH]

Plasma cells: A type of white blood cell that produces antibodies. [NIH]

Plasticity: In an individual or a population, the capacity for adaptation: a) through gene changes (genetic plasticity) or b) through internal physiological modifications in response to changes of environment (physiological plasticity). [NIH]

Platelet Activation: A series of progressive, overlapping events triggered by exposure of the platelets to subendothelial tissue. These events include shape change, adhesiveness, aggregation, and release reactions. When carried through to completion, these events lead to the formation of a stable hemostatic plug. [NIH]

Platelet Aggregation: The attachment of platelets to one another. This clumping together can be induced by a number of agents (e.g., thrombin, collagen) and is part of the mechanism leading to the formation of a thrombus. [NIH]

Platelet-Derived Growth Factor: Mitogenic peptide growth hormone carried in the alpha-granules of platelets. It is released when platelets adhere to traumatized tissues. Connective tissue cells near the traumatized region respond by initiating the process of replication. [NIH]

Platelets: A type of blood cell that helps prevent bleeding by causing blood clots to form. Also called thrombocytes. [NIH]

Platinum: Platinum. A heavy, soft, whitish metal, resembling tin, atomic number 78, atomic weight 195.09, symbol Pt. (From Dorland, 28th ed) It is used in manufacturing equipment for laboratory and industrial use. It occurs as a black powder (platinum black) and as a spongy substance (spongy platinum) and may have been known in Pliny's time as "alutiae". [NIH]

Poisoning: A condition or physical state produced by the ingestion, injection or inhalation of, or exposure to a deleterious agent. [NIH]

Policy Making: The decision process by which individuals, groups or institutions establish policies pertaining to plans, programs or procedures. [NIH]

Polycystic: An inherited disorder characterized by many grape-like clusters of fluid-filled cysts that make both kidneys larger over time. These cysts take over and destroy working kidney tissue. PKD may cause chronic renal failure and end-stage renal disease. [NIH]

Polypeptide: A peptide which on hydrolysis yields more than two amino acids; called tripeptides, tetrapeptides, etc. according to the number of amino acids contained. [EU]

Polysaccharide: A type of carbohydrate. It contains sugar molecules that are linked together chemically. [NIH]

Pons: The part of the central nervous system lying between the medulla oblongata and the mesencephalon, ventral to the cerebellum, and consisting of a pars dorsalis and a pars ventralis. [NIH]

Popliteal: Compression of the nerve at the neck of the fibula. [NIH]

Popliteal Vein: The vein formed by the union of the anterior and posterior tibial veins; it courses through the popliteal space and becomes the femoral vein. [NIH]

Posterior: Situated in back of, or in the back part of, or affecting the back or dorsal surface of the body. In lower animals, it refers to the caudal end of the body. [EU]

Postmenopausal: Refers to the time after menopause. Menopause is the time in a woman's life when menstrual periods stop permanently; also called "change of life." [NIH]

Postnatal: Occurring after birth, with reference to the newborn. [EU]

Postoperative: After surgery. [NIH]

Postsynaptic: Nerve potential generated by an inhibitory hyperpolarizing stimulation. [NIH]

Postural: Pertaining to posture or position. [EU]

Potassium: An element that is in the alkali group of metals. It has an atomic symbol K, atomic number 19, and atomic weight 39.10. It is the chief cation in the intracellular fluid of muscle and other cells. Potassium ion is a strong electrolyte and it plays a significant role in the regulation of fluid volume and maintenance of the water-electrolyte balance. [NIH]

Potentiation: An overall effect of two drugs taken together which is greater than the sum of the effects of each drug taken alone. [NIH]

Practicability: A non-standard characteristic of an analytical procedure. It is dependent on the scope of the method and is determined by requirements such as sample throughout and costs. [NIH]

Practice Guidelines: Directions or principles presenting current or future rules of policy for the health care practitioner to assist him in patient care decisions regarding diagnosis, therapy, or related clinical circumstances. The guidelines may be developed by government agencies at any level, institutions, professional societies, governing boards, or by the convening of expert panels. The guidelines form a basis for the evaluation of all aspects of health care and delivery. [NIH]

Prazosin: A selective adrenergic alpha-1 antagonist used in the treatment of heart failure, hypertension, pheochromocytoma, Raynaud's syndrome, prostatic hypertrophy, and urinary retention. [NIH]

Preclinical: Before a disease becomes clinically recognizable. [EU]

Precursor: Something that precedes. In biological processes, a substance from which another, usually more active or mature substance is formed. In clinical medicine, a sign or symptom that heralds another. [EU]

Pregnancy in Diabetics: Previously diagnosed diabetics that become pregnant. This does not include either symptomatic diabetes or impaired glucose tolerance induced by pregnancy but resolved at the end of pregnancy (diabetes, gestational). [NIH]

Prepuce: A covering fold of skin; often used alone to designate the preputium penis. [EU]

Prevalence: The total number of cases of a given disease in a specified population at a designated time. It is differentiated from incidence, which refers to the number of new cases in the population at a given time. [NIH]

Priapism: Persistent abnormal erection of the penis, usually without sexual desire, and accompanied by pain and tenderness. It is seen in diseases and injuries of the spinal cord, and may be caused by vesical calculus and certain injuries to the penis. [EU]

Procaine: A local anesthetic of the ester type that has a slow onset and a short duration of action. It is mainly used for infiltration anesthesia, peripheral nerve block, and spinal block. (From Martindale, The Extra Pharmacopoeia, 30th ed, p1016). [NIH]

Progeny: The offspring produced in any generation. [NIH]

Progesterone: Pregn-4-ene-3,20-dione. The principal progestational hormone of the body, secreted by the corpus luteum, adrenal cortex, and placenta. Its chief function is to prepare the uterus for the reception and development of the fertilized ovum. It acts as an antiovulatory agent when administered on days 5-25 of the menstrual cycle. [NIH]

Progression: Increase in the size of a tumor or spread of cancer in the body. [NIH]

Progressive: Advancing; going forward; going from bad to worse; increasing in scope or severity. [EU]

Projection: A defense mechanism, operating unconsciously, whereby that which is emotionally unacceptable in the self is rejected and attributed (projected) to others. [NIH]

Prolactin: Pituitary lactogenic hormone. A polypeptide hormone with a molecular weight of about 23,000. It is essential in the induction of lactation in mammals at parturition and is synergistic with estrogen. The hormone also brings about the release of progesterone from lutein cells, which renders the uterine mucosa suited for the embedding of the ovum should fertilization occur. [NIH]

Prolactinoma: A pituitary adenoma which secretes prolactin, leading to hyperprolactinemia. Clinical manifestations include amenorrhea; galactorrhea; impotence; headache; visual disturbances; and cerebrospinal fluid rhinorrhea. [NIH]

Proline: A non-essential amino acid that is synthesized from glutamic acid. It is an essential component of collagen and is important for proper functioning of joints and tendons. [NIH]

Promoter: A chemical substance that increases the activity of a carcinogenic process. [NIH]

Prophase: The first phase of cell division, in which the chromosomes become visible, the nucleus starts to lose its identity, the spindle appears, and the centrioles migrate toward opposite poles. [NIH]

Prophylaxis: An attempt to prevent disease. [NIH]

Prospective study: An epidemiologic study in which a group of individuals (a cohort), all free of a particular disease and varying in their exposure to a possible risk factor, is followed over a specific amount of time to determine the incidence rates of the disease in the exposed and unexposed groups. [NIH]

Prostaglandin: Any of a group of components derived from unsaturated 20-carbon fatty acids, primarily arachidonic acid, via the cyclooxygenase pathway that are extremely potent mediators of a diverse group of physiologic processes. The abbreviation for prostaglandin is PG; specific compounds are designated by adding one of the letters A through I to indicate the type of substituents found on the hydrocarbon skeleton and a subscript (1, 2 or 3) to indicate the number of double bonds in the hydrocarbon skeleton e.g., PGE2. The predominant naturally occurring prostaglandins all have two double bonds and are synthesized from arachidonic acid (5,8,11,14-eicosatetraenoic acid) by the pathway shown in the illustration. The 1 series and 3 series are produced by the same pathway with fatty acids having one fewer double bond (8,11,14-eicosatrienoic acid or one more double bond (5,8,11,14,17-eicosapentaenoic acid) than arachidonic acid. The subscript a or ß indicates the configuration at C-9 (a denotes a substituent below the plane of the ring, ß, above the plane). The naturally occurring PGF's have the a configuration, e.g., PGF2a. All of the prostaglandins act by binding to specific cell-surface receptors causing an increase in the level of the intracellular second messenger cyclic AMP (and in some cases cyclic GMP also). The effect produced by the cyclic AMP increase depends on the specific cell type. In some cases there is also a positive feedback effect. Increased cyclic AMP increases prostaglandin synthesis leading to further increases in cyclic AMP. [EU]

Prostaglandin Endoperoxides: Precursors in the biosynthesis of prostaglandins and thromboxanes from arachidonic acid. They are physiologically active compounds, having effect on vascular and airway smooth muscles, platelet aggregation, etc. [NIH]

Prostaglandins A: (13E,15S)-15-Hydroxy-9-oxoprosta-10,13-dien-1-oic acid (PGA(1)); (5Z,13E,15S)-15-hydroxy-9-oxoprosta-5,10,13-trien-1-oic acid (PGA(2)); (5Z,13E,15S,17Z)-15-hydroxy-9-oxoprosta-5,10,13,17-tetraen-1-oic acid (PGA(3)). A group of naturally occurring secondary prostaglandins derived from PGE. PGA(1) and PGA(2) as well as their 19-hydroxy derivatives are found in many organs and tissues. [NIH]

Prostaglandins H: A group of physiologically active prostaglandin endoperoxides. They are precursors in the biosynthesis of prostaglandins and thromboxanes. The most frequently encountered member of this group is the prostaglandin H2. [NIH]

Prostate: A gland in males that surrounds the neck of the bladder and the urethra. It secretes a substance that liquifies coagulated semen. It is situated in the pelvic cavity behind the lower part of the pubic symphysis, above the deep layer of the triangular ligament, and rests upon the rectum. [NIH]

Prostate gland: A gland in the male reproductive system just below the bladder. It surrounds part of the urethra, the canal that empties the bladder, and produces a fluid that forms part of semen. [NIH]

Prostatectomy: Complete or partial surgical removal of the prostate. Three primary approaches are commonly employed: suprapubic - removal through an incision above the pubis and through the urinary bladder; retropubic - as for suprapubic but without entering the urinary bladder; and transurethral (transurethral resection of prostate). [NIH]

Prostatic Hyperplasia: Enlargement or overgrowth of the prostate gland as a result of an increase in the number of its constituent cells. [NIH]

Prostatitis: Inflammation of the prostate. [EU]

Prosthesis: An artificial replacement of a part of the body. [NIH]

Protease: Proteinase (= any enzyme that catalyses the splitting of interior peptide bonds in a protein). [EU]

Protective Agents: Synthetic or natural substances which are given to prevent a disease or disorder or are used in the process of treating a disease or injury due to a poisonous agent. [NIH]

Protein C: A vitamin-K dependent zymogen present in the blood, which, upon activation by thrombin and thrombomodulin exerts anticoagulant properties by inactivating factors Va and VIIIa at the rate-limiting steps of thrombin formation. [NIH]

Protein Engineering: Procedures by which nonrandom single-site changes are introduced into structural genes (site-specific mutagenesis) in order to produce mutant genes which can be coupled to promoters that direct the synthesis of a specifically altered protein, which is then analyzed for structural and functional properties and then compared with the predicted and sought-after properties. The design of the protein may be assisted by computer graphic technology and other advanced molecular modeling techniques. [NIH]

Protein Isoforms: Different forms of a protein that may be produced from different genes, or from the same gene by alternative splicing. [NIH]

Protein Kinases: A family of enzymes that catalyze the conversion of ATP and a protein to ADP and a phosphoprotein. EC 2.7.1.37. [NIH]

Protein S: The vitamin K-dependent cofactor of activated protein C. Together with protein C, it inhibits the action of factors VIIIa and Va. A deficiency in protein S can lead to recurrent venous and arterial thrombosis. [NIH]

Proteins: Polymers of amino acids linked by peptide bonds. The specific sequence of amino acids determines the shape and function of the protein. [NIH]

Proteinuria: The presence of protein in the urine, indicating that the kidneys are not working properly. [NIH]

Proteolytic: 1. Pertaining to, characterized by, or promoting proteolysis. 2. An enzyme that promotes proteolysis (= the splitting of proteins by hydrolysis of the peptide bonds with formation of smaller polypeptides). [EU]

Protocol: The detailed plan for a clinical trial that states the trial's rationale, purpose, drug or vaccine dosages, length of study, routes of administration, who may participate, and other aspects of trial design. [NIH]

Protons: Stable elementary particles having the smallest known positive charge, found in the nuclei of all elements. The proton mass is less than that of a neutron. A proton is the nucleus of the light hydrogen atom, i.e., the hydrogen ion. [NIH]

Protozoa: A subkingdom consisting of unicellular organisms that are the simplest in the animal kingdom. Most are free living. They range in size from submicroscopic to macroscopic. Protozoa are divided into seven phyla: Sarcomastigophora, Labyrinthomorpha, Apicomplexa, Microspora, Ascetospora, Myxozoa, and Ciliophora. [NIH]

Proximal: Nearest; closer to any point of reference; opposed to distal. [EU]

Psychiatric: Pertaining to or within the purview of psychiatry. [EU]

Psychiatry: The medical science that deals with the origin, diagnosis, prevention, and treatment of mental disorders. [NIH]

Psychic: Pertaining to the psyche or to the mind; mental. [EU]

Psychogenic: Produced or caused by psychic or mental factors rather than organic factors. [EU]

Psychology: The science dealing with the study of mental processes and behavior in man and animals. [NIH]

Psychophysiology: The study of the physiological basis of human and animal behavior. [NIH]

Psychosexual: Pertaining to the mental aspects of sex. [NIH]

Psychotherapy: A generic term for the treatment of mental illness or emotional disturbances primarily by verbal or nonverbal communication. [NIH]

Puberty: The period during which the secondary sex characteristics begin to develop and the capability of sexual reproduction is attained. [EU]

Public Policy: A course or method of action selected, usually by a government, from among alternatives to guide and determine present and future decisions. [NIH]

Publishing: "The business or profession of the commercial production and issuance of literature" (Webster's 3d). It includes the publisher, publication processes, editing and editors. Production may be by conventional printing methods or by electronic publishing. [NIH]

Pulmonary: Relating to the lungs. [NIH]

Pulmonary Artery: The short wide vessel arising from the conus arteriosus of the right ventricle and conveying unaerated blood to the lungs. [NIH]

Pulmonary Circulation: The circulation of blood through the lungs. [NIH]

Pulmonary Edema: An accumulation of an excessive amount of watery fluid in the lungs, may be caused by acute exposure to dangerous concentrations of irritant gasses. [NIH]

Pulmonary Fibrosis: Chronic inflammation and progressive fibrosis of the pulmonary alveolar walls, with steadily progressive dyspnea, resulting finally in death from oxygen lack or right heart failure. [NIH]

Pulmonary hypertension: Abnormally high blood pressure in the arteries of the lungs. [NIH]

Pulse: The rhythmical expansion and contraction of an artery produced by waves of pressure caused by the ejection of blood from the left ventricle of the heart as it contracts. [NIH]

Pupil: The aperture in the iris through which light passes. [NIH]

Purines: A series of heterocyclic compounds that are variously substituted in nature and are known also as purine bases. They include adenine and guanine, constituents of nucleic acids, as well as many alkaloids such as caffeine and theophylline. Uric acid is the metabolic end product of purine metabolism. [NIH]

Putrefaction: The process of decomposition of animal and vegetable matter by living organisms. [NIH]

Quality of Life: A generic concept reflecting concern with the modification and enhancement of life attributes, e.g., physical, political, moral and social environment. [NIH]

Quinine: An alkaloid derived from the bark of the cinchona tree. It is used as an antimalarial drug, and is the active ingredient in extracts of the cinchona that have been used for that purpose since before 1633. Quinine is also a mild antipyretic and analgesic and has been used in common cold preparations for that purpose. It was used commonly and as a bitter and flavoring agent, and is still useful for the treatment of babesiosis. Quinine is also useful in some muscular disorders, especially nocturnal leg cramps and myotonia congenita, because of its direct effects on muscle membrane and sodium channels. The mechanisms of its antimalarial effects are not well understood. [NIH]

Quinolones: Quinolines which are substituted in any position by one or more oxo groups. These compounds can have any degree of hydrogenation, any substituents, and fused ring systems. [NIH]

Race: A population within a species which exhibits general similarities within itself, but is both discontinuous and distinct from other populations of that species, though not sufficiently so as to achieve the status of a taxon. [NIH]

Radiation: Emission or propagation of electromagnetic energy (waves/rays), or the waves/rays themselves; a stream of electromagnetic particles (electrons, neutrons, protons, alpha particles) or a mixture of these. The most common source is the sun. [NIH]

Radiation therapy: The use of high-energy radiation from x-rays, gamma rays, neutrons, and other sources to kill cancer cells and shrink tumors. Radiation may come from a machine outside the body (external-beam radiation therapy), or it may come from radioactive material placed in the body in the area near cancer cells (internal radiation therapy, implant radiation, or brachytherapy). Systemic radiation therapy uses a radioactive substance, such as a radiolabeled monoclonal antibody, that circulates throughout the body. Also called radiotherapy. [NIH]

Radical prostatectomy: Surgery to remove the entire prostate. The two types of radical prostatectomy are retropubic prostatectomy and perineal prostatectomy. [NIH]

Radioactive: Giving off radiation. [NIH]

Radioimmunotherapy: Radiotherapy where cytotoxic radionuclides are linked to antibodies in order to deliver toxins directly to tumor targets. Therapy with targeted radiation rather than antibody-targeted toxins (immunotoxins) has the advantage that adjacent tumor cells, which lack the appropriate antigenic determinants, can be destroyed by radiation cross-fire.

Radioimmunotherapy is sometimes called targeted radiotherapy, but this latter term can also refer to radionuclides linked to non-immune molecules (radiotherapy). [NIH]

Radiolabeled: Any compound that has been joined with a radioactive substance. [NIH]

Radiological: Pertaining to radiodiagnostic and radiotherapeutic procedures, and interventional radiology or other planning and guiding medical radiology. [NIH]

Radionuclide Imaging: Process whereby a radionuclide is injected or measured (through tissue) from an external source, and a display is obtained from any one of several rectilinear scanner or gamma camera systems. The image obtained from a moving detector is called a scan, while the image obtained from a stationary camera device is called a scintiphotograph. [NIH]

Radiotherapy: The use of ionizing radiation to treat malignant neoplasms and other benign conditions. The most common forms of ionizing radiation used as therapy are x-rays, gamma rays, and electrons. A special form of radiotherapy, targeted radiotherapy, links a cytotoxic radionuclide to a molecule that targets the tumor. When this molecule is an antibody or other immunologic molecule, the technique is called radioimmunotherapy. [NIH]

Rage: Fury; violent, intense anger. [NIH]

Randomized: Describes an experiment or clinical trial in which animal or human subjects are assigned by chance to separate groups that compare different treatments. [NIH]

Randomized clinical trial: A study in which the participants are assigned by chance to separate groups that compare different treatments; neither the researchers nor the participants can choose which group. Using chance to assign people to groups means that the groups will be similar and that the treatments they receive can be compared objectively. At the time of the trial, it is not known which treatment is best. It is the patient's choice to be in a randomized trial. [NIH]

Randomized Controlled Trials: Clinical trials that involve at least one test treatment and one control treatment, concurrent enrollment and follow-up of the test- and control-treated groups, and in which the treatments to be administered are selected by a random process, such as the use of a random-numbers table. Treatment allocations using coin flips, odd-even numbers, patient social security numbers, days of the week, medical record numbers, or other such pseudo- or quasi-random processes, are not truly randomized and trials employing any of these techniques for patient assignment are designated simply controlled clinical trials. [NIH]

Reagent: A substance employed to produce a chemical reaction so as to detect, measure, produce, etc., other substances. [EU]

Receptor: A molecule inside or on the surface of a cell that binds to a specific substance and causes a specific physiologic effect in the cell. [NIH]

Receptors, Serotonin: Cell-surface proteins hat bind serotonin and trigger intracellular changes which influence the behavior of cells. Several types of serotonin receptors have been recognized which differ in their pharmacology, molecular biology, and mode of action. [NIH]

Recombinant: A cell or an individual with a new combination of genes not found together in either parent; usually applied to linked genes. [EU]

Recombination: The formation of new combinations of genes as a result of segregation in crosses between genetically different parents; also the rearrangement of linked genes due to crossing-over. [NIH]

Rectal: By or having to do with the rectum. The rectum is the last 8 to 10 inches of the large intestine and ends at the anus. [NIH]

Rectum: The last 8 to 10 inches of the large intestine. [NIH]

Reductase: Enzyme converting testosterone to dihydrotestosterone. [NIH]

Refer: To send or direct for treatment, aid, information, de decision. [NIH]

Reflex: An involuntary movement or exercise of function in a part, excited in response to a stimulus applied to the periphery and transmitted to the brain or spinal cord. [NIH]

Reflux: The term used when liquid backs up into the esophagus from the stomach. [NIH]

Refractory: Not readily yielding to treatment. [EU]

Regeneration: The natural renewal of a structure, as of a lost tissue or part. [EU]

Regimen: A treatment plan that specifies the dosage, the schedule, and the duration of treatment. [NIH]

Regurgitation: A backward flowing, as the casting up of undigested food, or the backward flowing of blood into the heart, or between the chambers of the heart when a valve is incompetent. [EU]

Relapse: The return of signs and symptoms of cancer after a period of improvement. [NIH]

Relative risk: The ratio of the incidence rate of a disease among individuals exposed to a specific risk factor to the incidence rate among unexposed individuals; synonymous with risk ratio. Alternatively, the ratio of the cumulative incidence rate in the exposed to the cumulative incidence rate in the unexposed (cumulative incidence ratio). The term relative risk has also been used synonymously with odds ratio. This is because the odds ratio and relative risk approach each other if the disease is rare (5 percent of population) and the number of subjects is large. [NIH]

Relaxant: 1. Lessening or reducing tension. 2. An agent that lessens tension. [EU]

Reliability: Used technically, in a statistical sense, of consistency of a test with itself, i. e. the extent to which we can assume that it will yield the same result if repeated a second time. [NIH]

Renal Artery: A branch of the abdominal aorta which supplies the kidneys, adrenal glands and ureters. [NIH]

Renal failure: Progressive renal insufficiency and uremia, due to irreversible and progressive renal glomerular tubular or interstitial disease. [NIH]

Renal Replacement Therapy: Procedures which temporarily or permanently remedy insufficient cleansing of body fluids by the kidneys. [NIH]

Reproductive system: In women, this system includes the ovaries, the fallopian tubes, the uterus (womb), the cervix, and the vagina (birth canal). The reproductive system in men includes the prostate, the testes, and the penis. [NIH]

Respiration: The act of breathing with the lungs, consisting of inspiration, or the taking into the lungs of the ambient air, and of expiration, or the expelling of the modified air which contains more carbon dioxide than the air taken in (Blakiston's Gould Medical Dictionary, 4th ed.). This does not include tissue respiration (= oxygen consumption) or cell respiration (= cell respiration). [NIH]

Response rate: The percentage of patients whose cancer shrinks or disappears after treatment. [NIH]

Reticular: Coarse-fibered, netlike dermis layer. [NIH]

Retina: The ten-layered nervous tissue membrane of the eye. It is continuous with the optic nerve and receives images of external objects and transmits visual impulses to the brain. Its outer surface is in contact with the choroid and the inner surface with the vitreous body. The outer-most layer is pigmented, whereas the inner nine layers are transparent. [NIH]

Retinal: 1. Pertaining to the retina. 2. The aldehyde of retinol, derived by the oxidative enzymatic splitting of absorbed dietary carotene, and having vitamin A activity. In the retina, retinal combines with opsins to form visual pigments. One isomer, 11-cis retinal combines with opsin in the rods (scotopsin) to form rhodopsin, or visual purple. Another, all-trans retinal (trans-r.); visual yellow; xanthopsin) results from the bleaching of rhodopsin by light, in which the 11-cis form is converted to the all-trans form. Retinal also combines with opsins in the cones (photopsins) to form the three pigments responsible for colour vision. Called also retinal, and retinene1. [EU]

Retinol: Vitamin A. It is essential for proper vision and healthy skin and mucous membranes. Retinol is being studied for cancer prevention; it belongs to the family of drugs called retinoids. [NIH]

Retinopathy: 1. Retinitis (= inflammation of the retina). 2. Retinosis (= degenerative, noninflammatory condition of the retina). [EU]

Retropubic: A potential space between the urinary bladder and the symphisis and body of the pubis. [NIH]

Retropubic prostatectomy: Surgery to remove the prostate through an incision made in the abdominal wall. [NIH]

Retrospective: Looking back at events that have already taken place. [NIH]

Retrospective study: A study that looks backward in time, usually using medical records and interviews with patients who already have or had a disease. [NIH]

Rheology: The study of the deformation and flow of matter, usually liquids or fluids, and of the plastic flow of solids. The concept covers consistency, dilatancy, liquefaction, resistance to flow, shearing, thixotrophy, and viscosity. [NIH]

Rhinitis: Inflammation of the mucous membrane of the nose. [NIH]

Rhinorrhea: The free discharge of a thin nasal mucus. [EU]

Ribose: A pentose active in biological systems usually in its D-form. [NIH]

Ribosome: A granule of protein and RNA, synthesized in the nucleolus and found in the cytoplasm of cells. Ribosomes are the main sites of protein synthesis. Messenger RNA attaches to them and there receives molecules of transfer RNA bearing amino acids. [NIH]

Rigidity: Stiffness or inflexibility, chiefly that which is abnormal or morbid; rigor. [EU]

Risk factor: A habit, trait, condition, or genetic alteration that increases a person's chance of developing a disease. [NIH]

Rod: A reception for vision, located in the retina. [NIH]

Rolipram: A phosphodiesterase inhibitor with antidepressant properties. [NIH]

Salivary: The duct that convey saliva to the mouth. [NIH]

Salivary glands: Glands in the mouth that produce saliva. [NIH]

Salvage Therapy: A therapeutic approach, involving chemotherapy, radiation therapy, or surgery, after initial regimens have failed to lead to improvement in a patient's condition. Salvage therapy is most often used for neoplastic diseases. [NIH]

Samarium: An element of the rare earth family of metals. It has the atomic symbol Sm, atomic number 62, and atomic weight 150.36. The oxide is used in the control rods of some nuclear reactors. [NIH]

Saponins: Sapogenin glycosides. A type of glycoside widely distributed in plants. Each consists of a sapogenin as the aglycon moiety, and a sugar. The sapogenin may be a steroid or a triterpene and the sugar may be glucose, galactose, a pentose, or a methylpentose.

Sapogenins are poisonous towards the lower forms of life and are powerful hemolytics when injected into the blood stream able to dissolve red blood cells at even extreme dilutions. [NIH]

Schizoid: Having qualities resembling those found in greater degree in schizophrenics; a person of schizoid personality. [NIH]

Schizophrenia: A mental disorder characterized by a special type of disintegration of the personality. [NIH]

Schizotypal Personality Disorder: A personality disorder in which there are oddities of thought (magical thinking, paranoid ideation, suspiciousness), perception (illusions, depersonalization), speech (digressive, vague, overelaborate), and behavior (inappropriate affect in social interactions, frequently social isolation) that are not severe enough to characterize schizophrenia. [NIH]

Schwannoma: A tumor of the peripheral nervous system that begins in the nerve sheath (protective covering). It is almost always benign, but rare malignant schwannomas have been reported. [NIH]

Sclerosis: A pathological process consisting of hardening or fibrosis of an anatomical structure, often a vessel or a nerve. [NIH]

Screening: Checking for disease when there are no symptoms. [NIH]

Scrotum: In males, the external sac that contains the testicles. [NIH]

Sebaceous: Gland that secretes sebum. [NIH]

Sebaceous gland: Gland that secretes sebum. [NIH]

Sebum: The oily substance secreted by sebaceous glands. It is composed of keratin, fat, and cellular debris. [NIH]

Second Messenger Systems: Systems in which an intracellular signal is generated in response to an intercellular primary messenger such as a hormone or neurotransmitter. They are intermediate signals in cellular processes such as metabolism, secretion, contraction, phototransduction, and cell growth. Examples of second messenger systems are the adenyl cyclase-cyclic AMP system, the phosphatidylinositol diphosphate-inositol triphosphate system, and the cyclic GMP system. [NIH]

Secondary tumor: Cancer that has spread from the organ in which it first appeared to another organ. For example, breast cancer cells may spread (metastasize) to the lungs and cause the growth of a new tumor. When this happens, the disease is called metastatic breast cancer, and the tumor in the lungs is called a secondary tumor. Also called secondary cancer. [NIH]

Secretion: 1. The process of elaborating a specific product as a result of the activity of a gland; this activity may range from separating a specific substance of the blood to the elaboration of a new chemical substance. 2. Any substance produced by secretion. [EU]

Secretory: Secreting; relating to or influencing secretion or the secretions. [NIH]

Sediment: A precipitate, especially one that is formed spontaneously. [EU]

Segmental: Describing or pertaining to a structure which is repeated in similar form in successive segments of an organism, or which is undergoing segmentation. [NIH]

Semen: The thick, yellowish-white, viscid fluid secretion of male reproductive organs discharged upon ejaculation. In addition to reproductive organ secretions, it contains spermatozoa and their nutrient plasma. [NIH]

Seminal vesicles: Glands that help produce semen. [NIH]

Semisynthetic: Produced by chemical manipulation of naturally occurring substances. [EU]

Senile: Relating or belonging to old age; characteristic of old age; resulting from infirmity of old age. [NIH]

Sensitization: 1. Administration of antigen to induce a primary immune response; priming; immunization. 2. Exposure to allergen that results in the development of hypersensitivity. 3. The coating of erythrocytes with antibody so that they are subject to lysis by complement in the presence of homologous antigen, the first stage of a complement fixation test. [EU]

Sensor: A device designed to respond to physical stimuli such as temperature, light, magnetism or movement and transmit resulting impulses for interpretation, recording, movement, or operating control. [NIH]

Sequester: A portion of dead bone which has become detached from the healthy bone tissue, as occurs in necrosis. [NIH]

Serine: A non-essential amino acid occurring in natural form as the L-isomer. It is synthesized from glycine or threonine. It is involved in the biosynthesis of purines, pyrimidines, and other amino acids. [NIH]

Serotonin: A biochemical messenger and regulator, synthesized from the essential amino acid L-tryptophan. In humans it is found primarily in the central nervous system, gastrointestinal tract, and blood platelets. Serotonin mediates several important physiological functions including neurotransmission, gastrointestinal motility, hemostasis, and cardiovascular integrity. Multiple receptor families (receptors, serotonin) explain the broad physiological actions and distribution of this biochemical mediator. [NIH]

Serous: Having to do with serum, the clear liquid part of blood. [NIH]

Serum: The clear liquid part of the blood that remains after blood cells and clotting proteins have been removed. [NIH]

Sex Characteristics: Those characteristics that distinguish one sex from the other. The primary sex characteristics are the ovaries and testes and their related hormones. Secondary sex characteristics are those which are masculine or feminine but not directly related to reproduction. [NIH]

Sex Education: Education which increases the knowledge of the functional, structural, and behavioral aspects of human reproduction. [NIH]

Sexual Partners: Married or single individuals who share sexual relations. [NIH]

Shivering: Involuntary contraction or twitching of the muscles. It is a physiologic method of heat production in man and other mammals. [NIH]

Shock: The general bodily disturbance following a severe injury; an emotional or moral upset occasioned by some disturbing or unexpected experience; disruption of the circulation, which can upset all body functions: sometimes referred to as circulatory shock. [NIH]

Shunt: A surgically created diversion of fluid (e.g., blood or cerebrospinal fluid) from one area of the body to another area of the body. [NIH]

Sibutramine: A drug used for the management of obesity that helps reduce food intake and is indicated for weight loss and maintenance of weight loss when used in conjunction with a reduced-calorie diet. It works to suppress the appetite primarily by inhibiting the reuptake of the neurotransmitters norepinephrine and serotonin. Side effects include dry mouth, headache, constipation, insomnia, and a slight increase in average blood pressure. In some patients it causes a higher blood pressure increase. [NIH]

Side effect: A consequence other than the one(s) for which an agent or measure is used, as the adverse effects produced by a drug, especially on a tissue or organ system other than the one sought to be benefited by its administration. [EU]

Signal Transduction: The intercellular or intracellular transfer of information (biological activation/inhibition) through a signal pathway. In each signal transduction system, an activation/inhibition signal from a biologically active molecule (hormone, neurotransmitter) is mediated via the coupling of a receptor/enzyme to a second messenger system or to an ion channel. Signal transduction plays an important role in activating cellular functions, cell differentiation, and cell proliferation. Examples of signal transduction systems are the GABA-postsynaptic receptor-calcium ion channel system, the receptor-mediated T-cell activation pathway, and the receptor-mediated activation of phospholipases. Those coupled to membrane depolarization or intracellular release of calcium include the receptor-mediated activation of cytotoxic functions in granulocytes and the synaptic potentiation of protein kinase activation. Some signal transduction pathways may be part of larger signal transduction pathways; for example, protein kinase activation is part of the platelet activation signal pathway. [NIH]

Signs and Symptoms: Clinical manifestations that can be either objective when observed by a physician, or subjective when perceived by the patient. [NIH]

Silicon: A trace element that constitutes about 27.6% of the earth's crust in the form of silicon dioxide. It does not occur free in nature. Silicon has the atomic symbol Si, atomic number 14, and atomic weight 28.09. [NIH]

Silicon Dioxide: Silica. Transparent, tasteless crystals found in nature as agate, amethyst, chalcedony, cristobalite, flint, sand, quartz, and tridymite. The compound is insoluble in water or acids except hydrofluoric acid. [NIH]

Skeletal: Having to do with the skeleton (boney part of the body). [NIH]

Skeleton: The framework that supports the soft tissues of vertebrate animals and protects many of their internal organs. The skeletons of vertebrates are made of bone and/or cartilage. [NIH]

Skin Care: Maintenance of the hygienic state of the skin under optimal conditions of cleanliness and comfort. Effective in skin care are proper washing, bathing, cleansing, and the use of soaps, detergents, oils, etc. In various disease states, therapeutic and protective solutions and ointments are useful. The care of the skin is particularly important in various occupations, in exposure to sunlight, in neonates, and in decubitus ulcer. [NIH]

Skin graft: Skin that is moved from one part of the body to another. [NIH]

Skull: The skeleton of the head including the bones of the face and the bones enclosing the brain. [NIH]

Sleep apnea: A serious, potentially life-threatening breathing disorder characterized by repeated cessation of breathing due to either collapse of the upper airway during sleep or absence of respiratory effort. [NIH]

Small cell lung cancer: A type of lung cancer in which the cells appear small and round when viewed under the microscope. Also called oat cell lung cancer. [NIH]

Small intestine: The part of the digestive tract that is located between the stomach and the large intestine. [NIH]

Smooth muscle: Muscle that performs automatic tasks, such as constricting blood vessels. [NIH]

Soaps: Sodium or potassium salts of long chain fatty acids. These detergent substances are obtained by boiling natural oils or fats with caustic alkali. Sodium soaps are harder and are used as topical anti-infectives and vehicles in pills and liniments; potassium soaps are soft, used as vehicles for ointments and also as topical antimicrobials. [NIH]

Social Conditions: The state of society as it exists or influx. While it usually refers to society as a whole in a specified geographical or political region, it is applicable also to restricted strata of a society. [NIH]

Social Environment: The aggregate of social and cultural institutions, forms, patterns, and processes that influence the life of an individual or community. [NIH]

Social Isolation: The separation of individuals or groups resulting in the lack of or minimizing of social contact and/or communication. This separation may be accomplished by physical separation, by social barriers and by psychological mechanisms. In the latter, there may be interaction but no real communication. [NIH]

Social Support: Support systems that provide assistance and encouragement to individuals with physical or emotional disabilities in order that they may better cope. Informal social support is usually provided by friends, relatives, or peers, while formal assistance is provided by churches, groups, etc. [NIH]

Sodium: An element that is a member of the alkali group of metals. It has the atomic symbol Na, atomic number 11, and atomic weight 23. With a valence of 1, it has a strong affinity for oxygen and other nonmetallic elements. Sodium provides the chief cation of the extracellular body fluids. Its salts are the most widely used in medicine. (From Dorland, 27th ed) Physiologically the sodium ion plays a major role in blood pressure regulation, maintenance of fluid volume, and electrolyte balance. [NIH]

Soft tissue: Refers to muscle, fat, fibrous tissue, blood vessels, or other supporting tissue of the body. [NIH]

Solid tumor: Cancer of body tissues other than blood, bone marrow, or the lymphatic system. [NIH]

Solitary Nucleus: Gray matter located in the dorsomedial part of the medulla oblongata associated with the solitary tract. The solitary nucleus receives inputs from most organ systems including the terminations of the facial, glossopharyngeal, and vagus nerves. It is a major coordinator of autonomic nervous system regulation of cardiovascular, respiratory, gustatory, gastrointestinal, and chemoreceptive aspects of homeostasis. The solitary nucleus is also notable for the large number of neurotransmitters which are found therein. [NIH]

Solvent: 1. Dissolving; effecting a solution. 2. A liquid that dissolves or that is capable of dissolving; the component of a solution that is present in greater amount. [EU]

Soma: The body as distinct from the mind; all the body tissue except the germ cells; all the axial body. [NIH]

Somatic: 1. Pertaining to or characteristic of the soma or body. 2. Pertaining to the body wall in contrast to the viscera. [EU]

Spasm: An involuntary contraction of a muscle or group of muscles. Spasms may involve skeletal muscle or smooth muscle. [NIH]

Spasmolytic: Checking spasms; antispasmodic. [EU]

Spastic: 1. Of the nature of or characterized by spasms. 2. Hypertonic, so that the muscles are stiff and the movements awkward. 3. A person exhibiting spasticity, such as occurs in spastic paralysis or in cerebral palsy. [EU]

Spatial disorientation: Loss of orientation in space where person does not know which way is up. [NIH]

Specialist: In medicine, one who concentrates on 1 special branch of medical science. [NIH]

Species: A taxonomic category subordinate to a genus (or subgenus) and superior to a subspecies or variety, composed of individuals possessing common characters distinguishing them from other categories of individuals of the same taxonomic level. In taxonomic nomenclature, species are designated by the genus name followed by a Latin or Latinized adjective or noun. [EU]

Specificity: Degree of selectivity shown by an antibody with respect to the number and types of antigens with which the antibody combines, as well as with respect to the rates and the extents of these reactions. [NIH]

Spectrophotometry: The art or process of comparing photometrically the relative intensities of the light in different parts of the spectrum. [NIH]

Spectrum: A charted band of wavelengths of electromagnetic vibrations obtained by refraction and diffraction. By extension, a measurable range of activity, such as the range of bacteria affected by an antibiotic (antibacterial s.) or the complete range of manifestations of a disease. [EU]

Sperm: The fecundating fluid of the male. [NIH]

Sphincter: A ringlike band of muscle fibres that constricts a passage or closes a natural orifice; called also musculus sphincter. [EU]

Spina bifida: A defect in development of the vertebral column in which there is a central deficiency of the vertebral lamina. [NIH]

Spinal cord: The main trunk or bundle of nerves running down the spine through holes in the spinal bone (the vertebrae) from the brain to the level of the lower back. [NIH]

Spinal Cord Injuries: Penetrating and non-penetrating injuries to the spinal cord resulting from traumatic external forces (e.g., wounds, gunshot; whiplash injuries; etc.). [NIH]

Spinal Nerves: The 31 paired peripheral nerves formed by the union of the dorsal and ventral spinal roots from each spinal cord segment. The spinal nerve plexuses and the spinal roots are also included. [NIH]

Spirochete: Lyme disease. [NIH]

Spleen: An organ that is part of the lymphatic system. The spleen produces lymphocytes, filters the blood, stores blood cells, and destroys old blood cells. It is located on the left side of the abdomen near the stomach. [NIH]

Squamous: Scaly, or platelike. [EU]

Squamous cell carcinoma: Cancer that begins in squamous cells, which are thin, flat cells resembling fish scales. Squamous cells are found in the tissue that forms the surface of the skin, the lining of the hollow organs of the body, and the passages of the respiratory and digestive tracts. Also called epidermoid carcinoma. [NIH]

Squamous cell carcinoma: Cancer that begins in squamous cells, which are thin, flat cells resembling fish scales. Squamous cells are found in the tissue that forms the surface of the skin, the lining of the hollow organs of the body, and the passages of the respiratory and digestive tracts. Also called epidermoid carcinoma. [NIH]

Stabilization: The creation of a stable state. [EU]

Staging: Performing exams and tests to learn the extent of the cancer within the body, especially whether the disease has spread from the original site to other parts of the body. [NIH]

Steel: A tough, malleable, iron-based alloy containing up to, but no more than, two percent carbon and often other metals. It is used in medicine and dentistry in implants and instrumentation. [NIH]

Stem Cells: Relatively undifferentiated cells of the same lineage (family type) that retain the ability to divide and cycle throughout postnatal life to provide cells that can become specialized and take the place of those that die or are lost. [NIH]

Stents: Devices that provide support for tubular structures that are being anastomosed or for body cavities during skin grafting. [NIH]

Sterility: 1. The inability to produce offspring, i.e., the inability to conceive (female s.) or to induce conception (male s.). 2. The state of being aseptic, or free from microorganisms. [EU]

Steroid: A group name for lipids that contain a hydrogenated cyclopentanoperhydrophenanthrene ring system. Some of the substances included in this group are progesterone, adrenocortical hormones, the gonadal hormones, cardiac aglycones, bile acids, sterols (such as cholesterol), toad poisons, saponins, and some of the carcinogenic hydrocarbons. [EU]

Stimulant: 1. Producing stimulation; especially producing stimulation by causing tension on muscle fibre through the nervous tissue. 2. An agent or remedy that produces stimulation. [EU]

Stimulus: That which can elicit or evoke action (response) in a muscle, nerve, gland or other excitable issue, or cause an augmenting action upon any function or metabolic process. [NIH]

Stomach: An organ of digestion situated in the left upper quadrant of the abdomen between the termination of the esophagus and the beginning of the duodenum. [NIH]

Stool: The waste matter discharged in a bowel movement; feces. [NIH]

Stress: Forcibly exerted influence; pressure. Any condition or situation that causes strain or tension. Stress may be either physical or psychologic, or both. [NIH]

Stricture: The abnormal narrowing of a body opening. Also called stenosis. [NIH]

Stroke: Sudden loss of function of part of the brain because of loss of blood flow. Stroke may be caused by a clot (thrombosis) or rupture (hemorrhage) of a blood vessel to the brain. [NIH]

Structure-Activity Relationship: The relationship between the chemical structure of a compound and its biological or pharmacological activity. Compounds are often classed together because they have structural characteristics in common including shape, size, stereochemical arrangement, and distribution of functional groups. Other factors contributing to structure-activity relationship include chemical reactivity, electronic effects, resonance, and inductive effects. [NIH]

Struvite: A type of kidney stone caused by infection. [NIH]

Subacute: Somewhat acute; between acute and chronic. [EU]

Subarachnoid: Situated or occurring between the arachnoid and the pia mater. [EU]

Subclinical: Without clinical manifestations; said of the early stage(s) of an infection or other disease or abnormality before symptoms and signs become apparent or detectable by clinical examination or laboratory tests, or of a very mild form of an infection or other disease or abnormality. [EU]

Subcutaneous: Beneath the skin. [NIH]

Sublingual: Located beneath the tongue. [EU]

Subspecies: A category intermediate in rank between species and variety, based on a smaller number of correlated characters than are used to differentiate species and generally conditioned by geographical and/or ecological occurrence. [NIH]

Substance P: An eleven-amino acid neurotransmitter that appears in both the central and peripheral nervous systems. It is involved in transmission of pain, causes rapid contractions of the gastrointestinal smooth muscle, and modulates inflammatory and immune responses. [NIH]

Substrate: A substance upon which an enzyme acts. [EU]

Substrate Specificity: A characteristic feature of enzyme activity in relation to the kind of substrate on which the enzyme or catalytic molecule reacts. [NIH]

Suction: The removal of secretions, gas or fluid from hollow or tubular organs or cavities by means of a tube and a device that acts on negative pressure. [NIH]

Sulfotransferases: Enzymes which transfer sulfate groups to various acceptor molecules. They are involved in posttranslational sulfation of proteins and sulfate conjugation of exogenous chemicals and bile acids. EC 2.8.2. [NIH]

Superoxide: Derivative of molecular oxygen that can damage cells. [NIH]

Supplementation: Adding nutrients to the diet. [NIH]

Support group: A group of people with similar disease who meet to discuss how better to cope with their cancer and treatment. [NIH]

Suppositories: A small cone-shaped medicament having cocoa butter or gelatin at its basis and usually intended for the treatment of local conditions in the rectum. [NIH]

Suppression: A conscious exclusion of dsapproved desire contrary with repression, in which the process of exclusion is not conscious. [NIH]

Sympathetic Nervous System: The thoracolumbar division of the autonomic nervous system. Sympathetic preganglionic fibers originate in neurons of the intermediolateral column of the spinal cord and project to the paravertebral and prevertebral ganglia, which in turn project to target organs. The sympathetic nervous system mediates the body's response to stressful situations, i.e., the fight or flight reactions. It often acts reciprocally to the parasympathetic system. [NIH]

Sympathomimetic: 1. Mimicking the effects of impulses conveyed by adrenergic postganglionic fibres of the sympathetic nervous system. 2. An agent that produces effects similar to those of impulses conveyed by adrenergic postganglionic fibres of the sympathetic nervous system. Called also adrenergic. [EU]

Symphysis: A secondary cartilaginous joint. [NIH]

Symptomatic: Having to do with symptoms, which are signs of a condition or disease. [NIH]

Symptomatic treatment: Therapy that eases symptoms without addressing the cause of disease. [NIH]

Synapses: Specialized junctions at which a neuron communicates with a target cell. At classical synapses, a neuron's presynaptic terminal releases a chemical transmitter stored in synaptic vesicles which diffuses across a narrow synaptic cleft and activates receptors on the postsynaptic membrane of the target cell. The target may be a dendrite, cell body, or axon of another neuron, or a specialized region of a muscle or secretory cell. Neurons may also communicate through direct electrical connections which are sometimes called electrical synapses; these are not included here but rather in gap junctions. [NIH]

Synapsis: The pairing between homologous chromosomes of maternal and paternal origin during the prophase of meiosis, leading to the formation of gametes. [NIH]

Synaptic: Pertaining to or affecting a synapse (= site of functional apposition between neurons, at which an impulse is transmitted from one neuron to another by electrical or chemical means); pertaining to synapsis (= pairing off in point-for-point association of homologous chromosomes from the male and female pronuclei during the early prophase of meiosis). [EU]

Synergistic: Acting together; enhancing the effect of another force or agent. [EU]

Syphilis: A contagious venereal disease caused by the spirochete Treponema pallidum. [NIH]

Systemic: Affecting the entire body. [NIH]

Systemic disease: Disease that affects the whole body. [NIH]

Systemic lupus erythematosus: SLE. A chronic inflammatory connective tissue disease marked by skin rashes, joint pain and swelling, inflammation of the kidneys, inflammation of the fibrous tissue surrounding the heart (i.e., the pericardium), as well as other problems. Not all affected individuals display all of these problems. May be referred to as lupus. [NIH]

Systolic: Indicating the maximum arterial pressure during contraction of the left ventricle of the heart. [EU]

Tacrolimus: A macrolide isolated from the culture broth of a strain of Streptomyces tsukubaensis that has strong immunosuppressive activity in vivo and prevents the activation of T-lymphocytes in response to antigenic or mitogenic stimulation in vitro. [NIH]

Temporal: One of the two irregular bones forming part of the lateral surfaces and base of the skull, and containing the organs of hearing. [NIH]

Testicles: The two egg-shaped glands found inside the scrotum. They produce sperm and male hormones. Also called testes. [NIH]

Testicular: Pertaining to a testis. [EU]

Testis: Either of the paired male reproductive glands that produce the male germ cells and the male hormones. [NIH]

Testosterone: A hormone that promotes the development and maintenance of male sex characteristics. [NIH]

Therapeutics: The branch of medicine which is concerned with the treatment of diseases, palliative or curative. [NIH]

Thermal: Pertaining to or characterized by heat. [EU]

Thermogenesis: The generation of heat in order to maintain body temperature. The uncoupled oxidation of fatty acids contained within brown adipose tissue and shivering are examples of thermogenesis in mammals. [NIH]

Thermoregulation: Heat regulation. [EU]

Thigh: A leg; in anatomy, any elongated process or part of a structure more or less comparable to a leg. [NIH]

Third Ventricle: A narrow cleft inferior to the corpus callosum, within the diencephalon, between the paired thalami. Its floor is formed by the hypothalamus, its anterior wall by the lamina terminalis, and its roof by ependyma. It communicates with the fourth ventricle by the cerebral aqueduct, and with the lateral ventricles by the interventricular foramina. [NIH]

Thoracic: Having to do with the chest. [NIH]

Thorax: A part of the trunk between the neck and the abdomen; the chest. [NIH]

Threonine: An essential amino acid occurring naturally in the L-form, which is the active form. It is found in eggs, milk, gelatin, and other proteins. [NIH]

Threshold: For a specified sensory modality (e. g. light, sound, vibration), the lowest level (absolute threshold) or smallest difference (difference threshold, difference limen) or intensity of the stimulus discernible in prescribed conditions of stimulation. [NIH]

Thrombin: An enzyme formed from prothrombin that converts fibrinogen to fibrin. (Dorland, 27th ed) EC 3.4.21.5. [NIH]

Thrombocytes: Blood cells that help prevent bleeding by causing blood clots to form. Also called platelets. [NIH]

Thrombomodulin: A cell surface glycoprotein of endothelial cells that binds thrombin and serves as a cofactor in the activation of protein C and its regulation of blood coagulation.

[NIH]

Thrombophlebitis: Inflammation of a vein associated with thrombus formation. [NIH]

Thrombosis: The formation or presence of a blood clot inside a blood vessel. [NIH]

Thromboxanes: Physiologically active compounds found in many organs of the body. They are formed in vivo from the prostaglandin endoperoxides and cause platelet aggregation, contraction of arteries, and other biological effects. Thromboxanes are important mediators of the actions of polyunsaturated fatty acids transformed by cyclooxygenase. [NIH]

Thrombus: An aggregation of blood factors, primarily platelets and fibrin with entrapment of cellular elements, frequently causing vascular obstruction at the point of its formation. Some authorities thus differentiate thrombus formation from simple coagulation or clot formation. [EU]

Thymus: An organ that is part of the lymphatic system, in which T lymphocytes grow and multiply. The thymus is in the chest behind the breastbone. [NIH]

Thyroid: A gland located near the windpipe (trachea) that produces thyroid hormone, which helps regulate growth and metabolism. [NIH]

Thyrotropin: A peptide hormone secreted by the anterior pituitary. It promotes the growth of the thyroid gland and stimulates the synthesis of thyroid hormones and the release of thyroxine by the thyroid gland. [NIH]

Time Factors: Elements of limited time intervals, contributing to particular results or situations. [NIH]

Tin: A trace element that is required in bone formation. It has the atomic symbol Sn, atomic number 50, and atomic weight 118.71. [NIH]

Tinnitus: Sounds that are perceived in the absence of any external noise source which may take the form of buzzing, ringing, clicking, pulsations, and other noises. Objective tinnitus refers to noises generated from within the ear or adjacent structures that can be heard by other individuals. The term subjective tinnitus is used when the sound is audible only to the affected individual. Tinnitus may occur as a manifestation of cochlear diseases; vestibulocochlear nerve diseases; intracranial hypertension; craniocerebral trauma; and other conditions. [NIH]

Tissue: A group or layer of cells that are alike in type and work together to perform a specific function. [NIH]

Tolazamide: A sulphonylurea hypoglycemic agent with actions and uses similar to those of chlorpropamide. [NIH]

Tolerance: 1. The ability to endure unusually large doses of a drug or toxin. 2. Acquired drug tolerance; a decreasing response to repeated constant doses of a drug or the need for increasing doses to maintain a constant response. [EU]

Tomography: Imaging methods that result in sharp images of objects located on a chosen plane and blurred images located above or below the plane. [NIH]

Tonic: 1. Producing and restoring the normal tone. 2. Characterized by continuous tension. 3. A term formerly used for a class of medicinal preparations believed to have the power of restoring normal tone to tissue. [EU]

Tonicity: The normal state of muscular tension. [NIH]

Tooth Loss: The failure to retain teeth as a result of disease or injury. [NIH]

Topical: On the surface of the body. [NIH]

Toxic: Having to do with poison or something harmful to the body. Toxic substances usually cause unwanted side effects. [NIH]

Toxicity: The quality of being poisonous, especially the degree of virulence of a toxic microbe or of a poison. [EU]

Toxicology: The science concerned with the detection, chemical composition, and pharmacologic action of toxic substances or poisons and the treatment and prevention of toxic manifestations. [NIH]

Toxins: Specific, characterizable, poisonous chemicals, often proteins, with specific biological properties, including immunogenicity, produced by microbes, higher plants, or animals. [NIH]

Trace element: Substance or element essential to plant or animal life, but present in extremely small amounts. [NIH]

Trachea: The cartilaginous and membranous tube descending from the larynx and branching into the right and left main bronchi. [NIH]

Traction: The act of pulling. [NIH]

Transdermal: Entering through the dermis, or skin, as in administration of a drug applied to the skin in ointment or patch form. [EU]

Transduction: The transfer of genes from one cell to another by means of a viral (in the case of bacteria, a bacteriophage) vector or a vector which is similar to a virus particle (pseudovirion). [NIH]

Transfection: The uptake of naked or purified DNA into cells, usually eukaryotic. It is analogous to bacterial transformation. [NIH]

Transferases: Transferases are enzymes transferring a group, for example, the methyl group or a glycosyl group, from one compound (generally regarded as donor) to another compound (generally regarded as acceptor). The classification is based on the scheme "donor:acceptor group transferase". (Enzyme Nomenclature, 1992) EC 2. [NIH]

Translation: The process whereby the genetic information present in the linear sequence of ribonucleotides in mRNA is converted into a corresponding sequence of amino acids in a protein. It occurs on the ribosome and is unidirectional. [NIH]

Translocation: The movement of material in solution inside the body of the plant. [NIH]

Transmitter: A chemical substance which effects the passage of nerve impulses from one cell to the other at the synapse. [NIH]

Transplantation: Transference of a tissue or organ, alive or dead, within an individual, between individuals of the same species, or between individuals of different species. [NIH]

Transurethral: Performed through the urethra. [EU]

Transurethral Resection of Prostate: Resection of the prostate using a cystoscope passed through the urethra. [NIH]

Trauma: Any injury, wound, or shock, must frequently physical or structural shock, producing a disturbance. [NIH]

Treatment Outcome: Evaluation undertaken to assess the results or consequences of management and procedures used in combating disease in order to determine the efficacy, effectiveness, safety, practicability, etc., of these interventions in individual cases or series. [NIH]

Triglyceride: A lipid carried through the blood stream to tissues. Most of the body's fat tissue is in the form of triglycerides, stored for use as energy. Triglycerides are obtained primarily from fat in foods. [NIH]

Tryptophan: An essential amino acid that is necessary for normal growth in infants and for nitrogen balance in adults. It is a precursor serotonin and niacin. [NIH]

Tuberculosis: Any of the infectious diseases of man and other animals caused by species of Mycobacterium. [NIH]

Type 2 diabetes: Usually characterized by a gradual onset with minimal or no symptoms of metabolic disturbance and no requirement for exogenous insulin. The peak age of onset is 50 to 60 years. Obesity and possibly a genetic factor are usually present. [NIH]

Tyramine: An indirect sympathomimetic. Tyramine does not directly activate adrenergic receptors, but it can serve as a substrate for adrenergic uptake systems and monoamine oxidase so it prolongs the actions of adrenergic transmitters. It also provokes transmitter release from adrenergic terminals. Tyramine may be a neurotransmitter in some invertebrate nervous systems. [NIH]

Tyrosine: A non-essential amino acid. In animals it is synthesized from phenylalanine. It is also the precursor of epinephrine, thyroid hormones, and melanin. [NIH]

Ultrasonography: The visualization of deep structures of the body by recording the reflections of echoes of pulses of ultrasonic waves directed into the tissues. Use of ultrasound for imaging or diagnostic purposes employs frequencies ranging from 1.6 to 10 megahertz. [NIH]

Unconscious: Experience which was once conscious, but was subsequently rejected, as the "personal unconscious". [NIH]

Urea: A compound (CO(NH2)2), formed in the liver from ammonia produced by the deamination of amino acids. It is the principal end product of protein catabolism and constitutes about one half of the total urinary solids. [NIH]

Uremia: The illness associated with the buildup of urea in the blood because the kidneys are not working effectively. Symptoms include nausea, vomiting, loss of appetite, weakness, and mental confusion. [NIH]

Ureter: One of a pair of thick-walled tubes that transports urine from the kidney pelvis to the bladder. [NIH]

Urethra: The tube through which urine leaves the body. It empties urine from the bladder. [NIH]

Urethritis: Inflammation of the urethra. [EU]

Urinalysis: Examination of urine by chemical, physical, or microscopic means. Routine urinalysis usually includes performing chemical screening tests, determining specific gravity, observing any unusual color or odor, screening for bacteriuria, and examining the sediment microscopically. [NIH]

Urinary: Having to do with urine or the organs of the body that produce and get rid of urine. [NIH]

Urinary Calculi: Calculi in any part of the urinary tract. According to their composition or pattern of chemical composition distribution, urinary calculi types may include alternating or combination, cystine, decubitus, encysted, fibrin, hemp seed, matrix, mulberry, oxalate, struvite, urostealith, and xanthic calculi. [NIH]

Urinary Retention: Inability to urinate. The etiology of this disorder includes obstructive, neurogenic, pharmacologic, and psychogenic causes. [NIH]

Urinary tract: The organs of the body that produce and discharge urine. These include the kidneys, ureters, bladder, and urethra. [NIH]

Urinary tract infection: An illness caused by harmful bacteria growing in the urinary tract. [NIH]

Urine: Fluid containing water and waste products. Urine is made by the kidneys, stored in the bladder, and leaves the body through the urethra. [NIH]

Urine Testing: Checking urine to see if it contains glucose (sugar) and ketones. Special strips of paper or tablets (called reagents) are put into a small amount of urine or urine plus water. Changes in the color of the strip show the amount of glucose or ketones in the urine. Urine testing is the only way to check for the presence of ketones, a sign of serious illness. However, urine testing is less desirable then blood testing for monitoring the level of glucose in the body. [NIH]

Urodynamic: Measures of the bladder's ability to hold and release urine. [NIH]

Urogenital: Pertaining to the urinary and genital apparatus; genitourinary. [EU]

Urogenital System: All the organs involved in reproduction and the formation and release of urine. It includes the kidneys, ureters, bladder, urethra, and the organs of reproduction - ovaries, uterus, fallopian tubes, vagina, and clitoris in women and the testes, seminal vesicles, prostate, seminal ducts, and penis in men. [NIH]

Urologist: A doctor who specializes in diseases of the urinary organs in females and the urinary and sex organs in males. [NIH]

Urology: A surgical specialty concerned with the study, diagnosis, and treatment of diseases of the urinary tract in both sexes and the genital tract in the male. It includes the specialty of andrology which addresses both male genital diseases and male infertility. [NIH]

Uterine Contraction: Contraction of the uterine muscle. [NIH]

Uterus: The small, hollow, pear-shaped organ in a woman's pelvis. This is the organ in which a fetus develops. Also called the womb. [NIH]

Vaccine: A substance or group of substances meant to cause the immune system to respond to a tumor or to microorganisms, such as bacteria or viruses. [NIH]

Vacuoles: Any spaces or cavities within a cell. They may function in digestion, storage, secretion, or excretion. [NIH]

Vagina: The muscular canal extending from the uterus to the exterior of the body. Also called the birth canal. [NIH]

Vaginal: Of or having to do with the vagina, the birth canal. [NIH]

Vascular: Pertaining to blood vessels or indicative of a copious blood supply. [EU]

Vascular endothelial growth factor: VEGF. A substance made by cells that stimulates new blood vessel formation. [NIH]

Vasculitis: Inflammation of a blood vessel. [NIH]

Vasectomy: An operation to cut or tie off the two tubes that carry sperm out of the testicles. [NIH]

Vasoactive: Exerting an effect upon the calibre of blood vessels. [EU]

Vasoconstriction: Narrowing of the blood vessels without anatomic change, for which constriction, pathologic is used. [NIH]

Vasodilatation: A state of increased calibre of the blood vessels. [EU]

Vasodilation: Physiological dilation of the blood vessels without anatomic change. For dilation with anatomic change, dilatation, pathologic or aneurysm (or specific aneurysm) is used. [NIH]

Vasodilator: An agent that widens blood vessels. [NIH]

VE: The total volume of gas either inspired or expired in one minute. [NIH]

Vector: Plasmid or other self-replicating DNA molecule that transfers DNA between cells in nature or in recombinant DNA technology. [NIH]

Vein: Vessel-carrying blood from various parts of the body to the heart. [NIH]

Venereal: Pertaining or related to or transmitted by sexual contact. [EU]

Venous: Of or pertaining to the veins. [EU]

Venous blood: Blood that has given up its oxygen to the tissues and carries carbon dioxide back for gas exchange. [NIH]

Venous Thrombosis: The formation or presence of a thrombus within a vein. [NIH]

Ventricle: One of the two pumping chambers of the heart. The right ventricle receives oxygen-poor blood from the right atrium and pumps it to the lungs through the pulmonary artery. The left ventricle receives oxygen-rich blood from the left atrium and pumps it to the body through the aorta. [NIH]

Ventricular: Pertaining to a ventricle. [EU]

Venules: The minute vessels that collect blood from the capillary plexuses and join together to form veins. [NIH]

Vertebrae: A bony unit of the segmented spinal column. [NIH]

Vertebral: Of or pertaining to a vertebra. [EU]

Vesicoureteral: An abnormal condition in which urine backs up into the ureters, and occasionally into the kidneys, raising the risk of infection. [NIH]

Vesicular: 1. Composed of or relating to small, saclike bodies. 2. Pertaining to or made up of vesicles on the skin. [EU]

Vestibulocochlear Nerve: The 8th cranial nerve. The vestibulocochlear nerve has a cochlear part (cochlear nerve) which is concerned with hearing and a vestibular part (vestibular nerve) which mediates the sense of balance and head position. The fibers of the cochlear nerve originate from neurons of the spiral ganglion and project to the cochlear nuclei (cochlear nucleus). The fibers of the vestibular nerve arise from neurons of Scarpa's ganglion and project to the vestibular nuclei. [NIH]

Vestibulocochlear Nerve Diseases: Diseases of the vestibular and/or cochlear (acoustic) nerves, which join to form the vestibulocochlear nerve. Vestibular neuritis, cochlear neuritis, and acoustic neuromas are relatively common conditions that affect these nerves. Clinical manifestations vary with which nerve is primarily affected, and include hearing loss, vertigo, and tinnitus. [NIH]

Veterinary Medicine: The medical science concerned with the prevention, diagnosis, and treatment of diseases in animals. [NIH]

Viral: Pertaining to, caused by, or of the nature of virus. [EU]

Virilism: Development of masculine traits in the female. [NIH]

Virulence: The degree of pathogenicity within a group or species of microorganisms or viruses as indicated by case fatality rates and/or the ability of the organism to invade the tissues of the host. [NIH]

Virus: Submicroscopic organism that causes infectious disease. In cancer therapy, some viruses may be made into vaccines that help the body build an immune response to, and kill, tumor cells. [NIH]

Viscera: Any of the large interior organs in any one of the three great cavities of the body, especially in the abdomen. [NIH]

Visceral: , from viscus a viscus) pertaining to a viscus. [EU]

Visceral Afferents: The sensory fibers innervating the viscera. [NIH]

Vitreous Hemorrhage: Hemorrhage into the vitreous body. [NIH]

Vitro: Descriptive of an event or enzyme reaction under experimental investigation occurring outside a living organism. Parts of an organism or microorganism are used together with artificial substrates and/or conditions. [NIH]

Vivo: Outside of or removed from the body of a living organism. [NIH]

Volition: Voluntary activity without external compulsion. [NIH]

Weight Gain: Increase in body weight over existing weight. [NIH]

White blood cell: A type of cell in the immune system that helps the body fight infection and disease. White blood cells include lymphocytes, granulocytes, macrophages, and others. [NIH]

Windpipe: A rigid tube, 10 cm long, extending from the cricoid cartilage to the upper border of the fifth thoracic vertebra. [NIH]

Withdrawal: 1. A pathological retreat from interpersonal contact and social involvement, as may occur in schizophrenia, depression, or schizoid avoidant and schizotypal personality disorders. 2. (DSM III-R) A substance-specific organic brain syndrome that follows the cessation of use or reduction in intake of a psychoactive substance that had been regularly used to induce a state of intoxication. [EU]

Wound Healing: Restoration of integrity to traumatized tissue. [NIH]

Wounds, Gunshot: Disruption of structural continuity of the body as a result of the discharge of firearms. [NIH]

Xanthine: An urinary calculus. [NIH]

Xanthine Oxidase: An iron-molybdenum flavoprotein containing FAD that oxidizes hypoxanthine, some other purines and pterins, and aldehydes. Deficiency of the enzyme, an autosomal recessive trait, causes xanthinuria. EC 1.1.3.22. [NIH]

Xenobiotics: Chemical substances that are foreign to the biological system. They include naturally occurring compounds, drugs, environmental agents, carcinogens, insecticides, etc. [NIH]

Xenograft: The cells of one species transplanted to another species. [NIH]

X-ray: High-energy radiation used in low doses to diagnose diseases and in high doses to treat cancer. [NIH]

Yeasts: A general term for single-celled rounded fungi that reproduce by budding. Brewers' and bakers' yeasts are Saccharomyces cerevisiae; therapeutic dried yeast is dried yeast. [NIH]

Yohimbine: A plant alkaloid with alpha-2-adrenergic blocking activity. Yohimbine has been used as a mydriatic and in the treatment of impotence. It is also alleged to be an aphrodisiac. [NIH]

Zoster: A virus infection of the Gasserian ganglion and its nerve branches, characterized by discrete areas of vesiculation of the epithelium of the forehead, the nose, the eyelids, and the cornea together with subepithelial infiltration. [NIH]

Zygote: The fertilized ovum. [NIH]

Zymogen: Inactive form of an enzyme which can then be converted to the active form, usually by excision of a polypeptide, e. g. trypsinogen is the zymogen of trypsin. [NIH]

INDEX

Printed in the United Kingdom
by Lightning Source UK Ltd.
102710UKS00001B/28